Economic Stress, Human Capital, and Families in Asia

Quality of Life in Asia

Volume 4

This series, the first of its kind, will examine both the objective and subjective dimensions of life quality in Asia, especially East Asia. It will unravel and compare the contours, dynamics and patterns of building nations, offering innovative works that discuss basic and applied research, emphasizing interand multi-disciplinary approaches to the various domains of life quality. Thus, the series will appeal to a variety of fields in humanities, social sciences and other professional disciplines. Asia is the largest, most populous continent on Earth, and it is home to the world's most dynamic region, East Asia. In the past three decades, East Asia has been the most successful region in the world in expanding its economies and integrating them into the global economy, offering lessons on how poor countries, even with limited natural resources, can achieve rapid economic development. Yet while scholars and policymakers have focused on why East Asia has prospered, little has been written on how its economic expansion has affected the quality of life of its citizens. The series will publish several volumes a year, either single or multiple-authored monographs or collections of essays.

For further volumes:
http://www.springer.com/series/8416

Wei-Jun Jean Yeung • Mui Teng Yap
Editors

Economic Stress, Human Capital, and Families in Asia

Research and Policy Challenges

Springer

Editors
Wei-Jun Jean Yeung
Department of Sociology & Asia Research
National University of Singapore
Singapore

Mui Teng Yap
Lee Kuan Yew School of Public Policy
Institute of Policy Studies
National University of Singapore
Singapore

ISSN 2211-0550 ISSN 2211-0569 (electronic)
ISBN 978-94-007-7385-1 ISBN 978-94-007-7386-8 (eBook)
DOI 10.1007/978-94-007-7386-8
Springer Dordrecht Heidelberg New York London

Library of Congress Control Number: 2013954521

Printed on acid-free paper

Springer is part of Springer Science+Business Media (www.springer.com)

Foreword

It has long been understood by social scientists that changing economic conditions at both the macro and micro levels shape and alter family forms and processes in predictable ways. The grand theorists of modern social science – Karl Marx, Max Weber, Adam Smith and Emile Durkheim – all posited in one way or another the proposition that economic systems are a primary determinant of how families are organized and how they operate in everyday life. These seminal writers have spawned long traditions of research exploring links between economic change and family adaptations in the contemporary disciplines of anthropology, sociology, psychology, and, of course, economics.

Despite this history spanning more than a century, many central questions remain unexplored. This excellent volume examining the consequences of recent economic events on families and individuals in Asia provides an abundance of fresh evidence and insights for both researchers and policy makers. The chapters provide a starting point for broader and deeper investigations into how global economic events set off a succession of changing conditions that challenge the workings of families and the wellbeing of individuals.

Translating theories and ideas conceived in the West to Asia is no simple matter because culture and institutional forms across regions of the world and specific countries moderate the nexus between economic events and responses by families and individuals. The spread of free market capitalism from the West is a powerful impetus for change everywhere, but the nature of the change at the family and individual levels may differ depending on local conditions. Or, put differently, we might say that individuals experience and define changing economic circumstances differently because they view it through particular cultural and institutional lenses. This collection demonstrates just how complicated the task of creating broad generalization about the link between economic change and individual behavior is when adaptations to change are refracted by conditions on the ground.

Jean Yeung's preface to this volume provides a brief history of the conference in 2010 that brought together scholars and policy makers from both the West and a large number of Asian countries to begin to think about how the Great Recession may be affecting cohorts of children and the elderly. She sets the ambitious goal of providing "a systematic understanding of the experiences of families in Asia when under economic stress." In one way or another, all the chapters share a common concern about how changing (typically declining) levels of resources ramify through family systems, affecting the welfare of both the next generation and older generations who rely on economic and social assistance from family members.

In fact, when the conference occurred, the Great Recession had already ended in a strictly technical sense. As we now know, the timing and severity of The Great Recession varied in countries in North America, Europe, and Asia complicating many of the analyses that attempt to examine cross-national impacts. Indeed, the lingering effects of the recession continue for families in the United States and Europe even 5 years after it ended. A cohort of young adults in a large number of countries in the West and the developing world continues to struggle to find secure working conditions. The most immediate impacts are high rates of unemployment, growing levels of poverty, and delayed home leaving. Accompanying these changes, we are beginning to notice that young adults are further delaying marriage and childbearing. The long-term effects of postponement of family formation have yet to be calculated, but they will surely aggravate secular declines in marriage and fertility.

These changes in turn may erode the already tenuous support that is being provided to the elderly in many Asian nations that lack the social security systems that are widespread in the West. In China, the crisis of the elderly, already acute, may become even worse in the next generation as the number of productive family members dwindles as a result of the one-child policy. The already heavy demands on adults at mid-life are likely to grow as they try to spread their limited resources between their parents and their children.

The growing body of evidence reported in the chapter by Duncan and Magnuson that an absence of resources in early childhood creates a form of cognitive stunting helps to explain the widening social class differences that are becoming more pronounced in the West, particularly in countries with inadequate family supports. While poverty broadly figures in this volume, the widening of social class differences is barely touched upon. However, it is clear that the ideal of meritocracy is seriously undermined when children begin life in such varying circumstances. Among the affluent both in the West and in Asia, children start out with enormous advantages that only widen as they enter the educational system. Poor children and even those from middle-income families, unless they are provided with considerable assistance, are likely to flounder in school.

The policy challenges of addressing a better system of managing the shocks of economic recession, not to mention economic crises brought on by natural disasters, are immense. Currently, the tools at the hands of policy makers are crude and insufficient. Clearly, the family cannot be left to shoulder the responsibilities of caring for the young and the elderly without more governmental assistance. However, it is challenging to put social insurance systems in place in nations that have traditionally relied on the family to care for its members. The family is not likely to be up to the task unless it receives greater help in the childbearing and childrearing years. Indeed, in this sense, low fertility may be a predictable adaptation, as it appears to be in many of the more economically developed Asian nations such as Japan, Korea, and Taiwan.

As traditional Confucian values come into conflict with modern educational systems and job markets designed to maximize human capital, how can traditional gender roles be maintained or modified? Issues of gender lie at the heart of the crisis of the Asian family as it attempts to navigate new economic demands. Thus far, it is proving to be difficult in Asia to adopt the patterns of gender change followed in the West. Can Asian societies invent new ways of how men and women perform family roles that are distinctively different from Western models? It is simply too soon to tell.

One bright note in the rather gloomy picture that emerges from this volume about the current capacities of families to manage uncertain economic conditions is that we are developing far better ways of monitoring what is happening to families and individuals through data collection. Data does not necessarily solve problems, but it surely exposes them. I foresee a time when policy makers are equipped with much better data systems that permit researchers to examine how children and the elderly are faring in real time to current economic circumstances. There is an urgent need for systems of data that permit better country-level comparisons than are currently possible with episodic surveys and penetrating qualitative case studies. Common data systems across the region will heighten the ability of policy makers to compare the impact of particular interventions much as has been done with the growth of contingent cash family supplements in Latin America. Parallel panel studies in Asia will provide necessary information to help understand how families respond to economic vicissitudes and to craft policies that do a better job of assisting children and the elderly.

Some day in the not-too-distant future we will look back at this volume as a pioneering attempt to bring better alignment between the economic systems of Asia nations and the needs of their populations.

The Zellerbach Family Professor of Sociology Frank F. Furstenberg, Ph.D.
University of Pennsylvania
Philadelphia, PA, USA
July 2013

Preface

Two months after I relocated to Singapore in 2008, the global financial crisis struck. As in other parts of the world, in Asia the crisis led to a reduction in economic growth and pushed millions more people below the poverty line. This financial crisis compounded the economic distress wrought upon families across Asia by the slew of natural disasters that had struck over the past decade. Together, these calamities exposed the extent to which Asian families bear the weight of economic stress, how vulnerable families in Asia can be to that stress, and how inadequate social safety nets are in the region. One may be quick to attribute the prevalence of and vulnerability to economic stress to seemingly chance disasters such as these, but in truth the perils exist even during economic good times.

The brunt of the financial crisis should awaken us to the fact that, at all times, a large proportion of the Asian population suffers from economic deprivation as a result of job instability, a rising cost of living, illness, death or absence of adult family members, marital dissolution, low-wage jobs, or natural disasters. The family unit is under duress. To ignore this is to ignore that when family falters, individuals' well-being and human capital erode and society is threatened. We must confront the danger by first taking the time to understand the experiences of these families.

Having spent much of my career studying the effect of poverty on family and individuals' life chances, I felt a pressing need to investigate the impact of economic deprivation on families in Asia. My prior research focused on families in the USA, which are considerably distinct from the family contexts in Asia. In general, compared to their American counterparts, the more prevalent extended families and religious practices here may provide Asian families buffers during economic hard times less available in the Western societies. However, Asian families are shrinking at a faster pace, have lower income, face weaker public safety nets, affected to a greater extent by migration, and live in societies that are ageing more rapidly. Moreover, I quickly learned after arriving in Singapore that there is no universal Asian family context; Asia consists of many incredibly diverse cultural and political systems and families across Asia are being challenged in vastly different ways. This distinct context demands a careful study of the unique experiences of families in various Asian countries.

My colleagues, Professor Gavin Jones, Associate Professor Angelique Chan, Dr. Mui Teng Yap and I raised funds to convene a conference, the *International Conference on Economic Stress, Human Capital, and Families in Asia: Research and Policy Challenges*, on 3 and 4 June, 2010, in the National University of Singapore, to explore how economic stress impacts human lives in this part of the world. About 200 eminent policy-makers, practitioners, researchers, academics, and non-governmental organisations from 18 countries, including Thailand, Korea, China, Indonesia, India, Vietnam, Australia, Singapore, the UK, USA, Sweden, Pakistan and the Netherlands, gathered to address challenges that Asian families face today under the changing family institution, financial crises, natural disasters and the revamping of social safety nets in the past few decades.

We express our gratitude to Singapore's Ministry of Community Development, Youth, and Sports (MCYS) and the Family Research Network, NUS Changing Family in Asia Cluster, Asia Research Institute, the Faculty of Arts and Social Sciences, Institute of Policy Studies (IPS), Lee Kuan Yew School of Public Policy, and Department of Epidemiology and Public Health (EPH), Yong Loo Lin School of Medicine for their generous funding of this two-day conference. My heartfelt appreciation goes to the guest-of-honour then-Minister of Community Development, Youth and Sports, Singapore, Dr. Vivian Balakrishnan, NUS President Professor Tan Chorh Chuan, Provost Professor Tan Eng Chye, and the keynote speakers, Dr. Noeleen Heyzer, Professors Greg J. Duncan, Sheila B. Kamerman and Elizabeth Frankenberg, for their unwavering support of this conference.

At that time, there had not yet been much new data on the recent crises, but what was presented was an important start. The authors of the chapters explore an assortment of vital issues: Who is most vulnerable to economic stress? How does economic stress affect parenting behaviour and children's well-being? What is the aftermath of tsunamis and earthquakes in Indonesia and China? How has the birth rate been affected in Korea or other countries that are also struggling with an ultra-low fertility? How effective are the Singapore Work Support programmes for families under stress? How will China care for the financially distressed elderly given her plunged age structure and skewed sex ratio as a result of the one-child policy? Does financial stress trigger domestic violence in the family? To what extent do private and public social support networks buffer a family's economic stress? These chapters comprise the majority of this volume which is divided into five parts: an overview of how the recent financial crisis has affected families and children in the region and the lessons we have learned about the long-term effects of poverty; women, children and economic stress; economic stress and health; social support during economic hardships; and economic stress and public policy.

I am deeply indebted to Professor Gavin Jones, Associate Professor Angelique Chan, and Dr. Mui Teng Yap for collaborating with me and supporting me to organise the conference and to compile this volume. The contributions from all authors and participants of the conference cannot be overstated. I am most grateful to Ms. Saharah Abubakar who has provided expert and tireless assistance in editing and coordinating among authors and the publisher.

The primary goal of this collection is to provide a systematic understanding of the experiences of families in Asia when under economic stress. I hope the analysis will provide students and scholars in Asia and in other parts of the world, particularly those of family, poverty, education, health, and public policy, with a richer understanding of Asian contexts as they develop further research. Ultimately, the objective is to arm policymakers with a nuanced and deep insight that will guide them in supporting families through economic distress.

Professor, National University of Singapore
Department of Sociology & Asia Research Institute
Singapore, Singapore
June 2013

Wei-Jun Jean Yeung

Contents

Contributors

Janet M. Arnado Research Institute for Gender and Women, Inc., Malaybalay City, Philippines

Adam K.L. Cheung Asia Research Institute, National University of Singapore, Singapore

Susanne Y.P. Choi Department of Sociology, The Chinese University of Hong Kong, Hong Kong

Greg J. Duncan University of California, Irvine, CA, USA

Shirley Gatenio Gabel Graduate School of Social Service, Fordham University, NY, USA

Noeleen Heyzer United Nations ESCAP, Bangkok, Thailand

Kong Weng Ho Department of Economics, National University of Singapore, Singapore

Sheila B. Kamerman School of Social Work, Columbia University, NY, USA

Doo-Sub Kim Department of Sociology, Hanyang University, Seoul, South Korea

Katherine Magnuson University of Wisconsin, Madison, WI, USA

Irene Y.H. Ng Department of Social Work, National University of Singapore, Singapore

Mahesh S. Patel UNICEF East Asia and Pacific Regional Office, Bangkok, Thailand

Phua Kai Hong Lee Kuan Yew School of Public Policy, National University of Singapore, Singapore

Phua Kai Lit Jeffrey Cheah School of Medicine and Health Sciences, Monash University, Selangor, Malaysia

Kattika Thanakwang Institute of Nursing, Suranaree University of Technology, Nakhon Ratchasima, Thailand

Samman J. Thapa UNICEF Regional Office for the Middle East and North Africa, Amman, Jordan

Sam Wong School of Environmental Sciences, University of Liverpool, Merseyside, UK

Zhenhua Xu Department of Sociology, University of North Carolina at Chapel Hill, NC, USA

Mui Teng Yap Institute of Policy Studies, Lee Kuan Yew School of Public Policy, National University of Singapore, Singapore

Wei-Jun Jean Yeung Department of Sociology & Asia Research, National University of Singapore, Singapore

Zhao Yandong Institute of Science, Technology and Society, Chinese Academy of Science and Technology for Development, Beijing, China

Chapter 1
Economic Stress, Human Capital, and Families in Asia: Research and Policy Challenges

Wei-Jun Jean Yeung

Background

The changing demographic landscape, globalization, natural disasters, financial crises, and the revamping of social safety nets in many Asian countries in the past few decades have subjected countless people to economic stress (Cameron 2002; Fallon and Lucas 2002; Kim and Park 2006; Nobles and Buttenheim 2006; Thomas and Frankenberg 2007; United Nations 2009). Job and income loss, volatile gasoline and food prices, and growing residential insecurity top the list of sources of family economic stress in recent years (Lokshine and Yemtsov 2004; Madhavan and DeRose 2008). Research has shown that economic stress is linked to poor human capital development, emotional distress, health problems, unstable marriages, curtailed family consumption, modified employment behavior of family members, changing union formation and fertility patterns, more frequent geographic movement, and harsher parenting behavior (Catalano et al. 2005; Conger and Conger 2008; Friedman and Thomas 2009; Frankenberg et al. 2005; Ruhm 2000; Stuckler et al. 2009). Falling incomes and rising poverty may also erode a family's social support networks, leaving them isolated and unable to engage in social exchange.

Previous research in western societies shows that changes in opportunity structure do not affect all households in the same manner. Family wealth, human capital, and support networks help buffer families from sudden economic shocks (Yeung and Hofferth 1998). Community resources, public assistance, and local labor market conditions also affect families' ability to cope with adversity. Certain groups, such as unskilled workers, the working poor, single-parent families, or

W.-J.J. Yeung (✉)
Department of Sociology & Asia Research Institute, National University of Singapore, Block AS1, 11 Arts Link, 117570 Singapore, Singapore
e-mail: socywj@nus.edu.sg; ariywj@nus.edu.sg

W.J.J. Yeung and M.T. Yap (eds.), *Economic Stress, Human Capital, and Families in Asia: Research and Policy Challenges*, Quality of Life in Asia 4,
DOI 10.1007/978-94-007-7386-8_1, © Springer Science+Business Media Dordrecht 2013

ethnic minorities, are at greater risk of economic hardship. Families with multiple barriers are especially vulnerable to economic stress. However, research in the USA reveals that middle-class families or highly skilled workers are not immune to these economic uncertainties either (Duncan et al. 1996). Research also shows that family members carry unequal burdens, with more adverse impact typically on women, children, and the elderly. The ability of families and governments to adapt to changes in the economy has long-lasting implications for human capital development, intergenerational mobility, and future economic growth of a society.

Research from western countries may not be applicable to Asia where many countries still have a relatively lower income, public safety nets are more tenuous than in many American or European countries, family ties are shrinking with low marriage and fertility rates, and populations aging more rapidly than in many Western countries. There is a pressing need to understand how Asian families are faring under economic stress in recent years.

This book presents findings about the consequences and policy implications of economic stress for human capital development and family well-being in Asia. These papers were originally presented in an international conference "Economic Stress, Human Capital and Families in Asia: Research and Policy Challenges" held in the National University of Singapore on 3rd and 4th of June 2010, convened by W. Jean Yeung, Gavin Jones, Angelique Chan, and Mui Teng Yap. The objective of the conference was to discuss the consequences of economic stress, adaptation behavior, and the policy implications for human capital development and family well-being specific to Asia Pacific countries. More than 50 professionals and academics from 18 countries presented a total of 37 papers featuring experiences of countries in the Asia Pacific region. A subset of these papers is included in this volume.

The scope of these articles goes beyond the impact of the recent financial crisis to include the effects of economic deprivation families in Asia experience as a result of job loss, marital dissolution, low-wage employment, and catastrophic natural calamities. It is important to note that economic stress affects a significant segment of the population not only during financial crisis but also during economic good times, although it does not usually receive due attention unless we are hit by a financial crisis. The papers address a wide spectrum of themes in different panels, including social safety nets; physical and mental health; vulnerability and resiliency; social support networks; children and youth well-being; parenting, gender, and family relations; natural disasters; and migration. Using both quantitative and qualitative methods, the papers bring perspectives from multiple disciplines such as sociology, economics, social work, demography, public health, anthropology, and public policy. The authors seek answers to questions such as what is the aftermath of the earthquake in China, how has the birthrate been affected in Korea or other countries that are also struggling with an ultra-low fertility rate, how has economic stress affected migrant women and their children's well-being in Hong Kong, and how will China care for the elderly given her sharply altered age structure and a highly skewed sex ratio as a result of the one-child policy? It should come as no surprise that these questions defy simple answers. What we learn from previous experience is that economic stress exacts many social and psychological costs on the quality of individual and family life, and if we ignore the potential consequences of economic stress, the cost is high. We hope findings from this collection of papers could inform future family and developmental policies and stimulate future research.

Main Questions Addressed

Economic stress is defined in this book to include substantial loss in work hours, income, or assets, the experience of material hardships such as food insecurity and inadequate housing or health care, or failure to make ends meet. Main questions addressed in these chapters include:

(a) The nature of economic stress

- To what extent have Asian families experienced economic stress in the last few decades?
- What types of economic stress have Asian families experienced?
- Who are most vulnerable to economic stress?

(b) Coping behavior

- What adaptation strategies do families use when they are under economic stress?
- To what extent have families' economic activities changed in terms of family member's employment behavior and how families manage their economic resources (income and assets such as savings and financial investment) or time?
- To what extent is economic stress related to family expenditures on children's development?
- How does economic stress affect health-care utilization? How might economic stress (food related or otherwise) contribute to health-care utilization or physical and mental health of family members?
- To what extent do private and public social support networks buffer family's economic stress, e.g., the availability and impact of assistance from family and friends or government assistance programs?

(c) Potential consequences of economic stress

- To what extent is economic stress related to the individual's physical and mental health status?
- To what extent is economic stress related to the individual's expectation and behavior in marriage and fertility?
- To what extent is economic stress related to family dynamics, for example, intergenerational relations and transfers?

Conceptual Framework

An overarching framework, depicted below, is used to summarize how authors in this collection conceptualize the nature and impact of economic stress. This framework integrates two theoretical traditions to examine the household response to economic setbacks: (1) the family stress theory that takes sociopsychological factors into account and (2) microeconomic theories that see family members pooling resources together and smoothing life course consumptions over time.

The crisis model originally developed by Hill (1949) forms the central concept of the family stress theory. The model begins with certain stressor events such as job loss which precipitate changes in patterns of one or more of the following: family interaction, family goals, roles of family members, and values. Such changes potentially may destabilize the balance in the family necessary for effective family functioning. The objective economic stress, measured by indicators such as major income or assets loss, often triggers a certain level of subjective economic strain/pressure among family members. The degree to which a family adjusts depends upon the family's social-psychological and financial resources to meet the changes and the family's subjective perception of the stressor events. Stress theory also considers the social context of the family and community resources. This basic framework was later extended by McCubbin et al. (1982) in a longitudinal study of family stress and crisis and elaborated upon by other researchers (George 1993; Zimmerman 1988). Empirical research in the USA shows that economic problems may alter the socioemotional balance in the family which may result in marital discord and conflict and, perhaps, lead to divorce (Conger et al. 1990; Elder et al. 1984; Elder 1999; Liem and Liem 1988). Conger and his colleagues further developed the family stress model to show the adverse effect of financial difficulties on parents' emotions, behaviors, and relationship, which, in turn, affects their parenting behavior and children's developmental outcomes (Conger and Conger 2002, 2008; Conger and Elder 1994).

In microeconomic theory, a family is viewed as an economic unit in which family members pool resources and make joint decisions about consumption to achieve their optimum well-being or utility. Economic theory emphasizes the concept of permanent income (Blau and Ferber 1992), which states that a family's level of consumption is based upon the potential flow of income through time. The concept of permanent income also states that a family's level of consumption typically is indicated by the educational level of the head of the family or by the family's income averaged over a number of years rather than by the family's income at any point in time. Thus, families save in good times and borrow in times of need. Families also manage by modifying the labor supply of family members. Wives and older children historically have been a source of additional income when needed by the family economy, which is the added worker hypothesis (Sassier 1995).

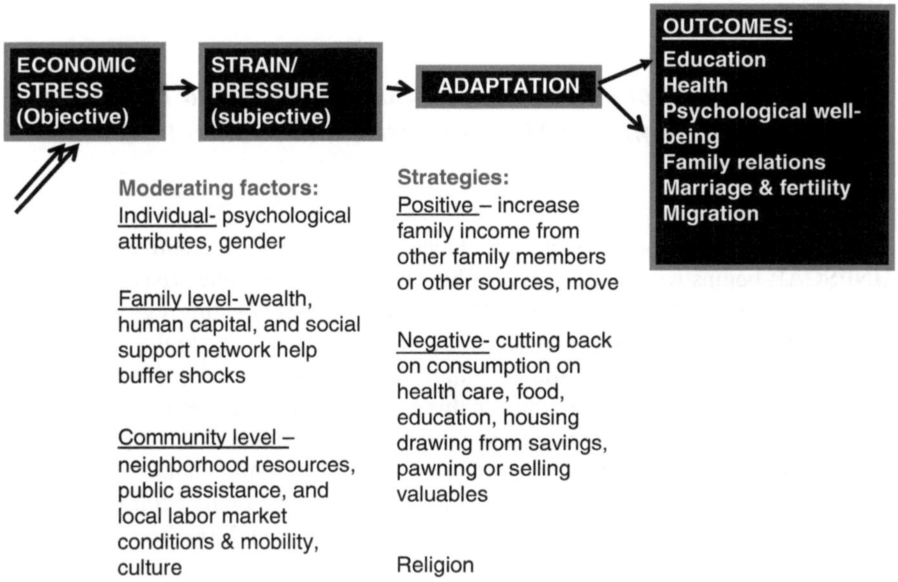

Fig. 1.1 Conceptual framework

When a family experiences economic stress, family members tend to adapt to the change with various strategies, such as cutting back on consumption on health care, food, education, or housing, going on public assistance, drawing from savings, borrowing money, obtaining a loan, or selling assets (Yeung and Hofferth 1998). They may also seek alternative sources of income, move to a different location, send other family members to the labor market, or seek spiritual support. Throughout this process, family members' life satisfaction and outlook to the future may change.

Figure 1.1 depicts a set of moderators at individual, family, and community levels that may shape how economic stress affects a family. These moderators include the psychological attributes of the individual and family members, stock of family wealth (savings and assets) and human capital, and social support networks that may buffer the economic stress, as well as community resources such as public assistance or local labor market conditions.

Many of the chapters in this volume examine the factors that influence a family's adaption strategies and how these changes in resources and adaptation behavior relate to family members' physical and mental health, education, family relations, marriage and fertility behavior, and patterns of geographic moves. In the remainder of this chapter, we summarize the main findings from these chapters and discuss their policy implications.

Part I: Overview

Addressing the Economic Crisis on Communities and Families in Asia Pacific: Toward a More Inclusive and Resilient Development

Noeleen Heyzer, Under Secretary General, UN and Executive Secretary, UNESCAP, begins with an overview of how the recent economic crisis has affected the communities and families in Asia Pacific and suggests how this region can move toward attaining a more inclusive and resilient development. She highlights how the global financial crisis had, by the third quarter of 2008, affected Asian economies, leading to rising unemployment rates in this region. Exports dropped sharply at rates that were almost twice as large as and more widespread than those experienced in past crises. Heyzer shows that since the first global economic contraction hit Asia and the Pacific late in 2008, economic growth among developing economies of the region decelerated sharply from 9.1 % in 2007 to 4.0 % in 2009. The growth rate remained positive as a result of the continuing rapid growth in China (8.7 %) and India (7.2 %). She points out that if these two powerhouses are excluded, growth of developing economies in the rest of the region actually contracted to 0.6 %, not unlike the rest of the world.

The decline in growth rates was followed by massive job losses in many of the key export manufacturing industries in the region. According to UN estimates, by 2009 the number of unemployed in the Asia Pacific region had increased by ten million relative to 2007, thus increasing the unemployment rate to 5.0 %. These trends, combined with the weakening family and community support structure in the context of increasing urbanization, migration, and aging populations, could result in adverse social consequences that will take many years to reverse.

Heyzer cautions that while the region is experiencing a healthy recovery, this recovery has several downside risks, including premature withdrawal of the fiscal stimulus, protectionism, return of inflation, and financial and exchange rate instability. She notes that the recent global financial crisis has revealed the limits of this region's export-oriented, low-cost, labor-intensive growth model. She argues that the region has to address its own macroeconomic, social, ecological, and development imbalances and development gaps and that this could be done by empowering the poor and generating growth which is more inclusive of the poor and which is more ecologically sustainable. She also makes the following suggestions:

- First, strengthening social protection should be a high priority. If poor households can rely on social protection systems that will automatically trigger social safety nets at times of adversity, they will be able to maintain food intake and continue to use education and health services.
- Second, as the majority of the poor live in rural areas and derive most of their income from agriculture, they are likely to benefit from agricultural growth.

Thus, a more knowledge-intensive green revolution that combines advances in science and agricultural engineering with the region's unique traditional knowledge and makes agriculture more environmentally resilient is needed.

- Third, the Asia Pacific economies should develop new and greener industries and businesses based on innovations that will save energy and materials. This will provide more affordable products for the poor while maintaining growth and promoting environmental sustainability.
- Fourth, the financial system has to be more inclusive so that millions of the unbanked can gain access to modern financial services and small and medium enterprises can be assisted to contribute to development.

In addition, a more resilient and inclusive social protection system is needed and the state and the private sector need to rethink how it could invest in new human capacity development. A change is needed in the way social protection strategies are formulated and implemented, and the goal and structure of social protection programs and interventions must be transformed from a welfare strategy to an investment one.

The Impact of the Economic Crisis on Children in East Asia and the Pacific: A UNICEF Perspective (2009–2010)

Samman J. Thapa and Mahesh S. Patel present a UNICEF perspective on the swift and severe impact of the financial crisis since 2008 on children in East Asia and the Pacific (EAP), threatening to reverse progress toward the Millennium Development Goals. They note that children face more severe risks than adults during economic crises and caution about the adverse impact on children's health and education and the increase in child labor. In particular, they call for special attention to countries that have low income, are most affected by the financial crisis, and have minimal fiscal cushions to cope with shock.

They note that the different countries in EAP were affected at various levels by the crises and the recoveries have been similarly varied. This has important implications for the abilities of different nations to maintain social commitments for the poor and vulnerable, especially children.

They highlight the crucial role of China in the recovery of Asia. For instance, its US$ 600 billion stimulus program and monetary easing that led banks to dole out US$ 1.2 trillion in 2009 have been effective in ensuring the growth it experienced in 2009 (*The Financial Times* 2009). Emerging Asia too grew by over 5 %, while Advanced Economies contracted by 3.2 % (IMF 2010). The growth gap between these two groups has never been wider (*The Economist* 2009). The report also shows that EAP economies overall have made a "V" shaped comeback, largely due to China's strong performance.

Despite the overall bright long-term growth prospects in East Asia and the Pacific (EAP), the authors point out that countries such as Cambodia, Mongolia, Papua New

Guinea, and the Pacific Islands that are hard hit but have minimal fiscal ability to recover are facing severe challenges. The situation is particularly dire for children in these countries.

Thapa and Patel also illustrate how economic crisis can potentially turn into a crisis for children with Mendoza's framework (2009) that captures how the world economic crisis can transmit through different channels to children. When exogenous shock in the form of financial crisis hits the world economy, the goods and services trade, private investments, foreign aid, and other linkages in the national economy are adversely affected. At the microlevel, the household economy is in turn affected when it is deprived of access to public services, employment, financial services and basic goods, and remittances. The increased deprivations caused by these transmission channels of exogenous shocks in turn have the potential to exacerbate child poverty in the region.

For the poorest and most vulnerable, the twin shocks of higher food prices and falling or lost incomes could result in adverse coping strategies such as withdrawal of children from school, delay in school payments, or reduction in health-care expenditure, further worsening life conditions of vulnerable children. In terms of health outcomes, they quote another study done by UNICEF Cambodia which revealed that wasting among poor urban children in the country increased from 6 % in 2005 to 15.9 % (above the 15 % threshold of a "humanitarian emergency") in 2008, primarily due to rising food prices (Cambodia Anthropometrics Survey 2008).

They explain how wasting, stunting, and underweight levels among children in EAP are very high once the regional aggregates for these indicators are decomposed. Stunting rates of 40 % or above in countries such as Indonesia, Cambodia, and Lao PDR are comparable to levels observed in countries in South Asia and sub-Saharan Africa. Poor households in the region spend up to 75–80 % (ADB 2008) of their income on food, and lowered purchasing power due to higher food prices, reduced incomes, and higher fuel/commodity prices could lead families to adopt adverse coping strategies such as cutting down on their food intake that may permanently jeopardize the healthy development of their children.

The authors also use data collected from real-time monitoring initiatives from countries such as Indonesia, Lao PDR, Vietnam, and Mongolia to highlight notable government responses that can potentially avert or mitigate the impact of financial crisis on children. UNICEF has played a key role in supporting these initiatives. They note that the EAP region has borne significant social costs for children during the 1997 Asian crisis and argue that it is critical to invest in social protection of children, which not only is morally desirable but makes economic and political sense, during the recent global economic recession.

The Long Reach of Early Childhood Poverty

Greg J. Duncan and Katherine Magnuson bring the lessons learned about the long-term impact of poverty on adult outcomes based on experiences primarily from western societies. They note that international comparison shows that the USA has one of the highest poverty rates among industrialized countries. Drawing the poverty line at 50 % of median disposable income (about US$29,000 for a family of three in today's dollars) classifies 16 % of the US population as poor. Poverty rate is lower in the UK and continental Europe and lowest in Scandinavian countries. The authors note that the two Asian countries that participate in the Luxembourg Income Study program – Taiwan and South Korea – have poverty rates that are in between those of the USA and most other Western countries.

More striking, the child poverty rates in the USA are particularly high, with nearly one-quarter of US children classified as poor, using the 50 % of median standard. In particular, deep poverty for US children is considerably more pervasive than among children in most Western industrialized countries.

Duncan and Magnuson investigate the question of whether childhood poverty compromises one's life chances and how it does so. They examine the relationships between early childhood income and later adult outcomes based on data from a longitudinal study in the USA – the Panel Study of Income Dynamics – on children born between 1968 and 1975. Adult outcomes were collected between ages 30 and 37.

Compared with children whose families had incomes of at least twice the poverty line during their early childhood, the authors note that poor children completed two fewer years of schooling, earned less than half as much, worked 451 fewer hours per year, received US$826 per year more in food stamps as adults, and were nearly three times as likely to report poor overall health. Poor males were more than twice as likely to be arrested. For females, poverty was associated with a more than fivefold increase in the likelihood of bearing a child out of wedlock prior to age 21. Their analysis shows that for families with an average early childhood income below $25,000, a $3,000 annual boost to family income was associated with a 17 % increase in adult earning.

A $3,000 annual increase in the prenatal to age-five income of low-income families was associated with 135 additional work hours per year after age 25. In contrast, increments to early childhood income for children in high-income families were not significantly associated with higher adult earnings or work hours.

They also find long-term impact of early childhood income on adult attainment measures. Income increases in early childhood were generally favorable in terms of earnings, work hours, the absence of receipt of welfare income, and "on-time" completed schooling in adulthood. In contrast, most adult behavior and health measures were more likely to be responsive to income increases later in childhood as well, although the patterns were not nearly as consistent as those found for the attainment measures.

With regard to policies, Duncan and Magnuson conclude that we should ensure that sanctions and other regulations do not deny benefits to families with very young children. Providing income support to working poor parents through wage supplements has been shown to improve children's achievement, according to data from experimental welfare reform evaluation studies undertaken during the

1990s. Thus income may play a causal role in younger children's achievement, and beneficial welfare reform programs should increase both income and parental employment.

Part II: Impact of Economic Stress on Women and Children

How economic stress affects parenting behavior and children's well-being is the theme of several papers at the conference. Among them, Doo-Sub Kim explores the effects of the 1997 Asian economic crisis on the levels of achieved and desired fertility of Korean couples. Janet Arnado describes another strategy to cope with economic stress employed frequently by Filipino women – going abroad as migrant workers. She argues that such coping strategy is strongly intertwined with gender relations at home. Adam K. L. Cheung and Susanne Y. P. Choi examine how financial stress could trigger domestic violence in the family.

The Recent Economic Crisis, Changes in the Pattern of Achieved Fertility and Ideal Number of Children in Korea

Based on data from the 2006 Korean National Fertility Survey, Doo-Sub Kim's research examines the extent to which the 1997 Asian economic crisis has affected the level of desired and achieved fertility for couples of different socioeconomic status. He finds that the economic crisis has had a significant negative impact on the number of children ever born (CEB) to Korean couples even though it has not reduced Korean women's ideal number of children (INC).

He compares fertility between women married before 1997 and those first married in 1997 or thereafter. The gap between INC and CEB became wider after the 1997 Asian economic crisis. For those who were married before 1997, the gap between INC and CEB was not found to be meaningful and did not appear dependent on the socioeconomic status of the couple (measured by wife's level of education). However, for those who were married for the first time in 1997 or thereafter, the gap between desired and achieved fertility turned out to be widest among those with the lowest socioeconomic status and the narrowest among those with middle or upper-middle status.

Kim notes that the economic crisis appeared to have altered the causal mechanisms of Korean fertility. The post-crisis fertility shows a different pattern from before, according to the socioeconomic status of the couple. In the ultralow fertility context after the economic crisis, level of recent fertility was highest among those with upper-middle socioeconomic status, followed by those with the highest socioeconomic status, and finally those with the lowest socioeconomic status.

These results suggest that the economic crisis has likely created the greatest economic stress for the segment of the population that has low social capital and income to the extent that they are unable to have as many children as they desire to. Kim notes that the current level of lowest-low fertility in Korea is mainly due to a strong sense of job insecurity among young couples in an uncertain economic environment. To encourage young people to marry earlier and have children, the author contends, overall improvements in the security of the labor market is needed. In addition, Kim argues that policy makers should focus pro-natal programs on least educated couples to effectively boost fertility and priority should be given to selected groups that show a wider gap between achieved and desired fertility.

Economic Stress, Gender Relations, and Migration of Filipinas to Singapore

In the Philippines, economic stress takes yet another form. The Philippine President admitted in 2001 that the local job market was tough and that the national economy relied on remittances from overseas workers as the country had not been able to recover from its recession since the seventies. Arnado cites Faist's study in 2000 that shows that the Philippines has a disproportionately high emigration level, with roughly 10 % of its total population (about eight million) working overseas as compared with the 2 % total world migrant population.

Arnado illustrates with ethnographic data that many Filipino families cope with economic stress by sending family members abroad to work and strive for survival through the remittances from their labor and the global structural opportunities. She argues that such coping strategy is strongly intertwined with gender relations at home. For example, past researchers have found an association between economic stress and domestic violence, such as marital violence and engagement in vices such as drugs and alcohol. And economic stress and domestic violence affect marital relations and parent-child relationships. Thus, the need to cope with family economic stress and strained gender relations motivates Filipino women to migrate to Singapore, even when they have very little information about the country. Having been abandoned or husband abandonment is often a hidden reason behind the migration for work among these women. This strategy provides economic relief and space for emotional recovery for them.

In view of the country's high unemployment rate, Arnado speculates that labor will continue to dominate the Philippines' export commodity in the future. Many family members will continue to live apart and rely on technological devices to communicate. Abused women may find solace in other countries or they may be victimized by their employers. Women who have never been married are very likely to have a harder time finding a marital partner given the sexual, time, and space restrictions in their workplaces in Singapore.

Financial Stress and Domestic Violence in Hong Kong

Adam Cheung and Susanne Choi examine how financial stress can affect family dynamics in the context of Hong Kong. Although in general the Hong Kong economy is gradually recovering from the economic recession since the 1997 financial crisis and the outbreak of SARS, income inequality and growing poverty are becoming more acute in Hong Kong. In the context where husbands are expected to be the primary breadwinner of the family and, violence in the family is widely considered as a private matter, men's economic insecurity can affect the power dynamic in the household and subsequently increase the risk of domestic violence.

Past theoretical literature suggests that husbands may use violence as an instrument to maintain their authority in the household in times of economic hardship. Using the household survey data collected in 2007, Cheung and Choi empirically examine the impact of men's economic insecurity on the risk of husband-to-wife violence in Hong Kong, with a special focus on the mediating role of husband's power motive. According to the household survey data, about 10 % of the sampled couples reported at least one episode of husband-to-wife physical assault during one preceding year. The survey reveals that both subjective and objective indicators of husband's economic insecurity are positively related to the risk of husband-to-wife violence. Financially stressed husbands are more likely to act violently against the wives. Cheung and Choi also note that power dynamics in the relationship play a crucial role in mediating the relationship between some of the indicators of economic insecurity and domestic violence. The data show that a husband is more likely to feel the need to have more decision-making power when he is financially stressed, earning less than his wife, and is not employed full-time. The need for power in the relationship then provides a motivation for the husband to use violence.

While some recent studies show that men's economic role and dominance in the family are still the central elements in the construction of male identity in Hong Kong, some recent economic changes, such as the shrinkage of the manufacturing sectors, have particularly affected men's economic security. Ignoring the potential impacts of these economic changes on family relations may have a high cost on the society. In order to have a better understanding of the impact of economic changes on the risk of domestic violence, the authors note that longitudinal data are needed in future work.

Part III: Economic Stress and Health

Kattika Thanakwang examines the effects of economic strain on mental health among Thai elders. Jean Yeung and Zhenhua Xu investigate how economic stress affects health of China's oldest-olds.

Economic Strain and Psychological Well-Being Among Thai Elderly

Thanakwang first describes the aging population in Thailand as a result of declining fertility and prolonged life expectancy over the past several decades. She then notes that more than one-fourth of Thai elders have an annual income below the poverty line and are financially dependent on their children. Based on survey data collected in 2002, Thanakwang finds that only 24.3 % of the farmers aged 50–64 years were financially prepared for their old age and 31.3 % did not have savings or any financial assets.

Previous research shows that in Thailand, family members or children in particular are a main resource and assistance provider to their parents. The financial dependency on children is even higher for older persons aged 70 years old or above and for female elderly, whereas income from work decreases with age.

In line with previous research, Thanakwang finds a negative relationship between economic constraint and psychological health. Thai elders who needed financial support were 3.6 times more likely to suffer from financial strain than those who did not need financial assistance.

Given the increasing dependency ratio, the elderly will be supported by a shrinking class of working-age population, and the burden on family members caring for their elderly parents will increase significantly in the foreseeable future. With the low fertility rate in Thailand, Thanakwang estimates that some families may have no offspring to provide instrumental, emotional, and financial support. Thanakwang argues, therefore, that the financial security and well-being of the elderly will become a big challenge to Thai society. She concludes that future work needs to further examine the moderating or mediating mechanisms through which economic stress affects one's psychological well-being. Longitudinal study is needed to examine the effects of poverty and financial strain on both physical and psychological well-being of the elderly.

Economic Stress and Mortality Hazard for China's Oldest-Olds

Yeung and Xu examine the impact of economic stress on the mortality hazard of the elderly in rural China. Due to the one-child policy initiated in 1979, China is experiencing an even sharper increase in the dependency ratio than Thailand. The working-age population will begin to decline in about 15 years as a result of fewer children born (the proportion of population aged 0–14 halved from 40.7 to 22.9 % between 1964 and 2000). The proportion aged 60 and above has risen from 6 % in the 1960s to about 12 % today. In particular, the proportion of oldest-olds (those 80 and above) is estimated to be climbing most rapidly, from 14 % of the total elderly population in 2000 to 34.4 % in 2050, amounting to 114 million.

Yeung and Xu note that the social safety nets for the elderly in China have weakened since the economic reform in 1978, as a result of the privatization of health-care provision and the consequent increase in out-of-pocket medical cost and a large uninsured population. As a result, many Chinese elderly live in poverty. They cite a study conducted in 2000 which shows that 11.3 % of those aged 60–64 were poor. Among the oldest-olds, poverty was even more prevalent, with the proportion having increased dramatically to 22.6 % for those aged 75–79, 27.7 % for those aged 80–84, and 30.3 % for those aged 85–89.

Based on the data from the Chinese Longitudinal Healthy Longevity Survey, the authors show that 16 % of the rural oldest-olds in China were under economic stress in 2000. About two-thirds of the oldest-old mainly relied on their children as main source of income. This group was less likely to be under economic stress. Those who relied on other types of governmental assistance, own work, or grandchildren were more likely to be under economic stress. The majority of the oldest-old relied on family and children to pay for their medical costs and as their main caretakers during illness. Those who were responsible for their own medical costs were more likely to be under economic stress. The authors find that living under economic stress in 2000 increased mortality of the oldest-olds over the subsequent 5 years. By the end of the fifth year, 42 % of those who were under economic stress vs. 48 % who were not had survived. This negative effect on longevity was partly due to the detrimental impact of economic stress on the mental health of the elderly and the quality of health care.

Yeung and Xu point out that the upcoming generation of elderly, those who were born after the 1950s, has fewer children than their predecessors (and many have no son) to rely on in their old age due to the one-child policy. In addition, the skewed sex ratio means there are fewer daughters and daughters-in-law to perform the caregiving tasks which have traditionally been females' responsibility. These demographic changes will weaken family support for the elderly. They further caution that rural-urban migration has accelerated the aging process in the rural areas. Although pension reform is under way, a majority of the rural elderly population still do not have access to these government resources. Alleviating economic hardships of the elderly will become a major challenge for the Chinese government.

Part IV: Social Support During Economic Hardships

Social support is often viewed as critical resources that help buffer hardships in economic hard times. Investigating the role of social networks in times of disaster, Zhao Yandong illustrates the key role social networks play in the disaster relief and reconstruction process in areas affected by the Wenchuan earthquake in China. Sam Wong describes how social support for children is reduced for mainland migrant children in Hong Kong during the Asian financial crisis.

Social Networks and Reduction of Risk in Disasters: An Example of the Wenchuan Earthquake

Rescue efforts had been underway in China's Sichuan province after the devastating Wenchuan earthquake measuring 7.9 on the Richter scale struck in 2008. According to Xinhua news agency, nearly 15,000 people died in the disaster, with as many as 24,000 people trapped under rubble from collapsed buildings and another 14,000 declared missing. Based on data from a two-wave survey with about 4,000 households conducted in 2008 and 2009, Zhao Yandong finds that after the earthquake, around 95 % of survivors were rescued by relatives, neighbors, and other persons nearby. Only a very small proportion of trapped victims were rescued by external rescue personnel, such as PLA soldiers, professional rescue teams, or volunteers. Social networks played an indispensable role in facilitating information flow in the disaster area. After the earthquake, around 16 % of the residents in the earthquake area acquired information regarding the government's disaster-relief policies through relatives, friends, and other social ties.

Zhao finds that those with more heterogeneous networks found it easier to obtain new information. Some victims also received various types of support from social networks during recovery. Though the government was the main support provider, social networks provided important informal support. Larger networks also brought greater social support. More than 30 % of respondents considered social networks to be their most important source of support.

Zhao finds that social networks helped to provide emotional support, hence reducing the traumatic impact of disasters and maintaining good mental health for survivors. In addition members in the affected communities helped each other more actively and participated more in collective activities after the earthquake than before. Through this process, Zhao argues, new types of social capital were formed since the study finds that there was a higher level of trust among community members and a majority of members believed their communities had become stronger than before. Zhao thus stresses the critical role of social networks in facilitating the recovery and reconstruction process after a disaster and urges the government to tap on the existing social capital and invest in fostering strong new social networks.

Human and Social Capital Dynamics in Economic Crises: The Impact on Poor Chinese Migrant Children in Hong Kong During the Far East Economic Crisis

Sam Wong draws on empirical research on the experiences of poor mainland Chinese migrants in Hong Kong during the Far East economic crisis. He shows that the rising unemployment and reduced family salary have led to a decrease in family spending on social activities and involvement, thus adversely affecting children's social support network and investment in children's human capital. Wang cites the Hong Kong government's initiative in 2002 to set up a HK$300 million Community Investment and Inclusion Fund as an example of government policy designed to help migrant families during the difficult times.

Part V: Economic Stress and Public Policy

Several papers evaluate specific policies implemented in a number of Asian countries that aim at reducing poverty, alleviating deprivation, or increasing access to health care and children's access to schools. Shirley Gatenio Gabel and Sheila Kamerman discuss the Conditional Cash Transfer as a policy strategy to reduce child poverty in Asia. As noted by Phua Kai Hong and Phua Kai Lit, timely assessment of the health impact of the economic crisis is crucial in formulating evidenced-based policies to mitigate the impact of the financial crisis. Despite several previous studies, how economic stress has affected health in the Asia Pacific region has remained largely unexplored. Phua and Phua review past evidence of health impact of economic crises and draws lessons from experiences in Asia. Irene Y. H. Ng and Kong Weng Ho discuss how the Singapore government has responded to the needs of families that are experiencing multiple stressors after the recent global economic recession.

Conditional Cash Transfers (CCTs): A Child Policy Strategy in Asia

Gatenio Gabel and Kamerman review the effectiveness of Conditional Cash Transfers (CCTs), cash benefits that impose behavioral conditions on recipients, which is an increasingly popular tool for alleviating childhood poverty and for investing in children's future in less developed Asian countries such as India, Pakistan, Cambodia, Indonesia, Mongolia, and the Philippines. The education component of CCTs is usually a cash grant targeted at school-aged children which covers school-related fees and costs. The health and nutrition component covers the cost of food or offsets the opportunity costs of travel and waiting time for parents attending health-care centers, on condition that the children attend health clinics and women obtain prenatal care.

While early evidence shows that CCTs have been highly effective in reducing poverty in both developed and developing countries, recent evidence is mixed with regard to the value of conditionality. In addition, cash benefits alone are not adequate to achieve health and education goals. Gatenio Gabel and Kamerman focus on whether CCTs in these countries have achieved their goals of reducing child poverty, increasing school enrolment, and improving health and nutrition, especially in Asia, and discuss the conditions under which CCTs can be effective. They raise questions regarding the effectiveness and cost of CCTs relative to unconditional cash benefits, whether CCT is a viable option for all countries or only for those with an adequate level of resources, whether CCTs are more effective for girls than for boys, and how conditional and unconditional benefits can promote social inclusion and minimize risks of exclusion.

Gatenio Gabel and Kamerman conclude that the challenge for both unconditional and conditional cash transfers in developing countries is to ensure that in the longer term, these interventions develop into sustainable social policies for children that can be supported by national social protection systems.

The Health Impact of Economic Crises: Policy Implications and Lessons from Asia

The review of past evidence by Phua and Phua reveals that the Asian financial crisis in the late 1990s had had significant impact on the health risks, utilization of health services, and mental health of Asian population. Health risks associated with the financial crisis include an increase in mortality and incidence of infectious diseases, mental health and other related problems, malnutrition, decline in immunization level, and loss of health insurance. Quoting a 2009 UNICEF report, Phua and Phua note that child mortality rate increased during the East Asian financial crisis from 68.3 in 1995–1996 to 79.7 during 1997–1998 in countries that were most severely affected.

Partly due to a rise in the cost of imported drugs and supplies and the loss of job-linked health insurance after the financial crisis, there was a reduction in access to health services and a shift in demand for cheaper care from the private sector to the public sector and NGOs. Research shows that there was a tendency for individuals to delay care-seeking, to self-treat, or even forgo care-seeking from health-care providers.

Past research also suggests that financial crisis is related to an increase in substance abuse, depression, mental disorder, and related problems. For instance, research shows that in Japan, Korea, and Hong Kong, the suicide rates were higher in 1998 compared with 1997 (10,400 more) and this increase was associated with the economic crisis and with the rise in unemployment. Past experience reveals that vulnerable groups such as ethnic minorities, the poor, single mothers with children, the elderly, and the disabled often bear the brunt of cutbacks in public spending on health and social services. Foreign workers, dependent families, the elderly, and lower-skilled employees become the most immediate victims of retrenchment.

Phua and Phua warn that time lags in detection and treatment of health problems during crisis years would become worse considering the long-term effect on physical and mental health in later life. They argue that the 1997 financial crisis had revealed the weaknesses in social safety nets and the health-care financing system.

The 2009 UNICEF report underscores the role of government in providing social protection for vulnerable groups especially in view of the competing demands on government and the needs to strengthen social safety nets.

Phua and Phua suggest that the government should diversify social and health-care financing, reexamine priorities, and provide access to affordable essential health care. Urgent priority should be given to strengthening mental health services in anticipation of increased demand during economic crisis. In short, evidence-based health sector reforms which expand public health budgets and avoid long-term social and economic costs should be implemented. Phua and Phua conclude that investing in prevention, early detection, and treatment of illness is good public policy in times of economic crisis.

Policy Responses for Multi-stressed Low-Earning Families in Singapore

The paper by Irene Ng and Kong Weng Ho describes how the Singapore government had responded to the 2008 global recession, doling out a range of policies in aid of all levels of wage earners. This chapter argues that the measures were probably effective in helping many families tide through the recession, but not through longer-term hardships and also not for some families who faced multiple challenges. Based on a model of multi-stressed low-earning families and data from a small pilot study, the chapter demonstrates that low-income families in Singapore face multiple socioeconomic challenges that temporary financial assistance has limited ability to address.

The multi-stressed low-earning families model describes the interacting effects of low earnings with low education, irrelevant skills, physical and mental health, family relationships, children issues, and criminal record. In an unstable globalized economy, the income gap is widening and bottom wages are stagnating. Within such a context, multi-stressed low-income earners are disadvantaged in multiple ways.

Data from a pilot study of 50 low-income families demonstrate the high prevalence of the challenges found in the model. Two case studies illustrate how these challenges play out in respondents' lives. The 50 respondents in the study were recipients of the Work Support Program (WSP), a government assistance program. Administrative data show the temporary nature of WSP and the unchanged economic situations of WSP recipients who completed WSP in 2009.

Based on the above findings and policy direction, the article observes that the expanding social welfare programs in Singapore will continue to grow. It suggests that low-earning multi-stressed families need help beyond recession measures and economic assistance. It discusses implementation and eligibility issues that need to be looked into if assistance is to more holistically address both economic and social factors.

Summary

These chapters underscore how macro-level economic stress can filter down through households to affect individuals' economic and sociopsychological well-being. Collectively, the papers reveal a wide spectrum of economic stresses experienced by families in various Asian Pacific countries due to financial crises, natural calamity, reform of the social welfare system, or depressed economy. Countries have been affected to varying degrees and are coping at different rates. The bright prospect of regional economic growth led largely by China and India should not mask the considerable stress felt by many families and individuals, particularly among vulnerable groups such as children, women, the elderly, and the working poor. The economic shocks in the past several decades have exposed the vulnerability of the family institution and the weaknesses in this region's social protection system that can lead to detrimental long-term effects on human capital development.

Family and community responses to economic deprivation and uncertainties often weaken family ties or compromise individuals' life chances. As shown in these papers, such responses can include cutting back on social services, curtailing expenditures on children's food, education and health, taking youth out of school prematurely to engage in often dangerous trades, migrating away from family members, compromising health care, having more frequent family conflicts, and postponing or even foregoing having children.

As seen in Korea, the current lowest-low fertility rates are attributed, to a great extent, to the population's anxiety of the economic uncertainties. In areas struck by natural disasters, a large number of children have become orphans. Children in developing Asian countries, such as Indonesia, Cambodia, and Lao PDR, are experiencing stunting rates at levels comparable to those in South Asia and sub-Saharan Africa. Findings from longitudinal studies in the USA that illuminate the long-term adverse effects of childhood economic deprivation on individuals' achievements should alert us to pay special attention to such early deprivations.

Women are dealt multiple blows when families sacrifice female education, unemployment rise when labor-intensive industries shut down, public policies are ambivalent about providing assistance for single mothers, or when economic hardships lead girls to resort to early marriage or to become sex workers, as seen in the cases of Chinese and Filipino migrant women, single mothers in Malaysia, and girls in Indonesia, India, and Bangladesh, among others. In Hong Kong, women experience a higher incidence of domestic violence when their husbands are under financial stress.

With limited resources to buffer economic stress, the working poor and elderly often delay seeking health care or self-treat when medical cost is high and they have no access to health insurance, as we see in many countries. The studies on China and Thailand show that economic stress among the elderly is associated with greater emotional distress, greater incidence of chronic diseases, and higher mortality. Today's elderly in Asia depend heavily on their children for care. However, recent demographic trends suggest that the next generation of elderly cannot expect to rely on children to care for them in the same way.

Given the demographic changes in this region, family networks have become significantly smaller and the working-age population will start to decline soon in many countries. As the family institution undergoes rapid transition, the economies in Asia Pacific need to transform themselves to be more productive than before. Enhancing human capital, therefore, is critical for sustaining development in this region. As noted by Heyzer, however, the Asia Pacific has the lowest level of public expenditure on social protection. Expanding such effort for the most vulnerable groups should be a policy priority.

These chapters reveal that in times of intense economic stress, social support networks are crucial and their potential as resource provider could be tapped more vigorously. However, for the vulnerable population, such networks are fragile and sometimes reinforce existing social inequality as those in the networks of the deprived are often poor themselves and have limited sociopsychological resources. Public policies can be more poverty-sensitive and gender-sensitive to help strengthen family and community ties to help families and individuals tide over economic hard times.

References

Asian Development Bank. (2008). *Key indicators for Asia and the Pacific 2008*. Manila: The Asian Development Bank.

Blau, F. D., & Ferber, M. A. (Eds.). (1992). *The economics of women, men and work*. Englewood Cliffs: Prentice Hall.

Cameron, L. A. (2002). *The impact of the Indonesian financial crisis on children: Data from 100 villages survey* (World Bank Policy Research Working Paper No. 2799). Parkville: University of Melbourne, Department of Economics.

Catalano, R., Bruckner, T., Anderson, B., & Gould, J. (2005). Fetal death sex ratios: A test of the economic stress hypothesis. *International Journal of Epidemiology, 34*, 944–948.

Conger, R. D., & Conger, K. J. (2002). Resilience in Midwestern families: Selected findings from the first decade of a prospective, longitudinal study. *Journal of Marriage and the Family, 64*, 361–373.

Conger, R. D., & Conger, K. J. (2008). Understanding the processes through which economic hardship influences families and children. In D. R. Crane & T. B. Heaton (Eds.), *Handbook of families and poverty* (pp. 64–81). Thousand Oaks: Sage Publications.

Conger, R. D., & Elder, G. H., Jr. (1994). *Families in troubled times: Adapting to change in rural America*. New York: Aldine De Gruyter.

Conger, R. D., Elder, G. H., Jr., Lorenz, F. O., Conger, K. J., Simons, R. L., Whitbeck, L. B., Huck, S., & Melby, J. N. (1990). Linking economic hardship to marital quality and instability. *Journal of Marriage and the Family, 52*, 643–656.

Duncan, G. J., Boisjoly, J., & Smeeding, T. (1996). Economic mobility of young workers in the 1970s and 1980s. *Demography, 33*(4), 497–509.

Elder, G. H., Jr. (1999). *Children of the great depression: Social change in life experience* (25th anniversary ed.). Boulder: Westview Press.

Elder, G. H., Jr., Liker, J. K., & Cross, C. E. (1984). Parent–child behavior in the great depression: Life course and intergenerational influences. In P. B. Bates & O. G. Brim Jr. (Eds.), *Life-span development and behavior* (Vol. 6, pp. 109–158). New York: Academic.

Fallon, P., & Lucas, R. E. B. (2002). The impact of financial crises on labor markets, household income and poverty: A review of evidence. *World Bank Research Observer, 17*(1), 21–45.

Frankenberg, E., McKee, D., & Thomas, D. (2005). Health consequences of forest fires in Indonesia. *Demography, 42*(1), 109–129.

Friedman, J., & Duncan, T. (2009). Psychological health before, during, and after an economic crisis: Results from Indonesia, 1993–2000. *The World Bank Development Economic Review, 23*(1), 57–76.

George, L. K. (1993). Sociological perspectives on life transitions. *Annual Review of Sociology, 19*, 353–373.

Hill, R. (1949). *Families under stress: Adjustment to the crises of war separation and reunion.* New York: Harper & Brothers.

International Monetary Fund. (2010). *World economic outlook April 2010.* Washington, DC: International Monetary Fund.

Kim, A. E., & Park, I. (2006). Changing trends of work in South Korea: The rapid growth of unemployment and job insecurity. *Asian Survey, 46*(3), 437–456.

Liem, R., & Liem, J. H. (1988). The psychological effects of unemployment on workers and their families. *Journal of Social Issues, 44*, 87–105.

Lokshine, M., & Yemtsov, R. (2004). Household strategies of coping with shocks in post-crisis Russia. *Review of Development Economics, 8*(1), 15–32.

Madhavan, S., & DeRose, L. F. (2008, August 31). *Families and crisis in the developing world: Implications for responding to children affected by HIV/AIDS.* Joint Learning Initiative on Children and HIV/AIDS JILC. http://www.ovcsupport.net/s/library.php?ld=926

McCubbin, H. I., Cauble, A. E., & Patterson, J. M. (1982). *Family stress, coping and social support.* Springfield: C. C. Thomas.

Mendoza, R. (2009). Aggregate shocks, poor households and children: Transmission channels and policy responses. *Global Social Policy, 9*(Special Issue), 55–78.

Nobles, J., & Butterheim, A. (2008) Marriage and Socioeconomic Change in Contemporary Indonesia. *Journal of Marriage and Family, 70*(4), 904–918.

Ruhm, C. J. (2000). Are recession good for your health? *Quarterly Journal of Economics, 115*(2), 617–650.

Sassier, S. (1995). Trade-offs in the family: Sibling effects on daughters' activities in 1910. *Demography, 32*(4), 557–575.

Stuckler, D., King, L., & McKee, M. (2009). Mass privatisation and the post-communist mortality crisis. *Lancet, 373*, 399–407.

The Economist. (2009). From slump to jump. *The Economist.*http://www.economist.com/node/14133744?story_id=14133744. Accessed 5 Aug 2009.

The Financial Times. (2009, September 10). Asia economic weather map. *The Financial Times.*

Thomas, D., & Frankenberg, E. (2007). Household responses to the financial crisis in Indonesia: Longitudinal evidence on poverty, resources, and well-being. In A. E. Harrison (Ed.), *Globalization and poverty* (pp. 517–560). Chicago: University of Chicago Press.

UNICEF Cambodia. (2008). *Cambodia anthropometrics survey.* Phnom Penh.

United Nations. (2009). *The global economic and financial crisis: Regional impacts, responses and solutions.* New York: United Nations.

Yeung, W. J., & Hofferth, S. (1998). Family adaptations to income and job loss in the U.S. *Journal of Family and Economic Issues, 19*, 255–283.

Zimmerman, S. L. (1988). *Understanding family policy: Theoretical approaches.* Newbury Park: Sage Publications.

Part I
Overview

Chapter 2
Global Financial Crisis and Economic and Social Challenges for Asia and the Pacific

Noeleen Heyzer

Introduction: A Situationer

In recent years, the global financial crisis, volatile food and energy prices, and climate-related disasters have increased risks, vulnerabilities, and stress on families, and on people, beyond the existing pressures of living.

These interconnected crises have severely tested capacities – human and institutional – putting additional burden on the states and institutions, on family structures, and on the human capital required to manage complex responses to address the multiple threats to development and to turn them into opportunities for shared prosperity, social progress, and ecological sustainability.

A Synchronized Crisis

As the first global economic contraction in modern times hit Asia and the Pacific in late 2008, economic growth among developing economies of the region decelerated sharply from a pre-crisis level of 9.1 % in 2007 to 4.0 % in 2009. That the growth rate remained positive was due to continuous rapid growth in China (8.7 %) and India (7.2 %). If those two powerhouses were excluded, growth of developing economies in the rest of the region would have contracted to 0.6 %, not unlike in the rest of the world. The synchronized impact of the crisis is shown in Fig. 2.1.

N. Heyzer (✉)
Under-Secretary-General of the United Nations and Executive Secretary of the Economic and Social Commission for Asia and the Pacific, United Nations ESCAP, UN Building, Bangkok, Thailand
e-mail: heyzer@un.org

W.J.J. Yeung and M.T. Yap (eds.), *Economic Stress, Human Capital, and Families in Asia: Research and Policy Challenges*, Quality of Life in Asia 4,
DOI 10.1007/978-94-007-7386-8_2,

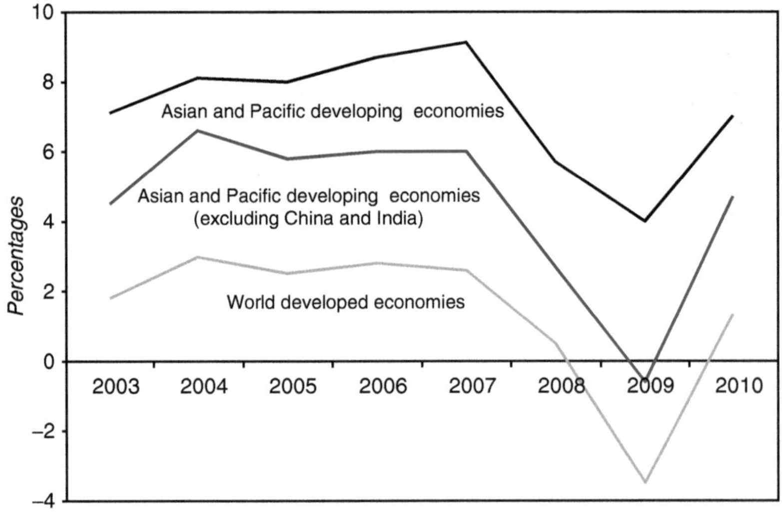

Fig. 2.1 Real GDP growth of Asian and Pacific developing and world developed economies, 2003–2010 (*Source*: ESCAP 2010a, figure 30)

Some countries were able to absorb the shock of the crisis through large fiscal stimulus. The countries best able to mount rapid and large public spending programs were those that entered the crisis with strong macroeconomic fundamentals. The massive additional fiscal spending helped reduce the impact of lowered exports and the falling demand for services such as tourism, as well as reduced growth of migrant remittances. Even more important, the stimulus also afforded some protection to the vulnerable workers who had lost their jobs.

Contraction of Exports

Among the channels of transmission of the recession in the West to the region, the sharp contraction of exports in 2008/2009 was the most immediate. The decline in exports, which started in mid 2008, was actually much sharper than the declines recorded during the Asian crisis of 1997 and the dotcom bust in 2001 (Fig. 2.2).

The contracting exports also led to a severe impact on the well-being of the poorest in our region. ESCAP's estimates suggest that the crisis has led to an additional 21 million people being pushed into poverty.

The impact of the crisis on employment is far from over. While GDP may be recovering across the region, we know from experience following the 1997 Asian Financial Crisis that it may be years before the poorest people are able to recover from the global crisis of the past 2 years.

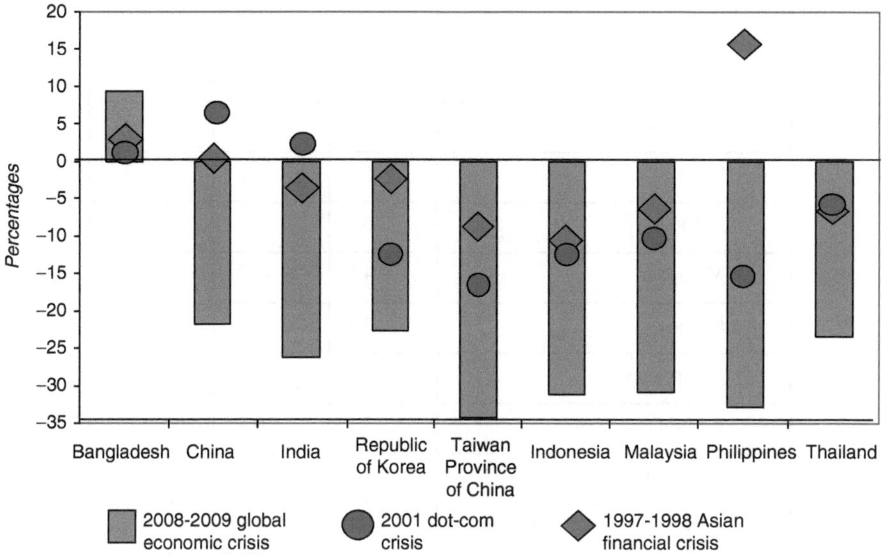

Fig. 2.2 Comparative growth performance of goods exports of major developing economies during three crises, 1997–2009 (*Source*: ESCAP 2010a, figure 6)

2010 Outlook for Key Countries

After bottoming out in the first quarter of 2009, growth has since been on the upswing across the region. The outlook for 2010 suggests a healthy recovery with developing ESCAP economies expected to grow at 7 % in 2010 compared to just 4 % in 2009 (Fig. 2.3).

China is expected to continue to be the best performer, expanding by 9.5 % in 2010, with investment in infrastructure helping to remove supply-side constraints and spur even faster growth beyond 2010. The expanding domestic consumption and investment will see India growing at a rate of around 8.3 %.

Among other major economies of the region, Indonesia is expected to grow at 5.5 %, and the Republic of Korea at 5.2 %. Other major export-led economies are expected to experience substantial growth recovery in 2010, such as Singapore (7.0 %), Malaysia (5.0 %), Thailand (4.0 %), and Philippines (3.5 %).

Downside Risks

The recovery, while expected to be strong, is subject to a number of critical downside risks.

The first is the risk that fiscal stimulus will be withdrawn prematurely, therefore stopping the growth momentum in its tracks and leading to a double-dip recession.

	2008	2009	2010
China	9.0	8.7	9.5
Hong Kong, China	2.4	−1.9	4.5
India	6.7	7.2	8.3
Indonesia	6.1	4.5	5.5
Malaysia	4.6	−1.7	5.0
Pakistan	4.1	2.0	3.2
Philippines	3.8	0.9	3.5
Republic of Korea	2.2	0.2	5.2
Singapore	1.1	−2.0	7.0
Taiwan Province of China	0.7	−1.9	4.5
Thailand	2.5	−2.3	4.0
Developing ESCAP economies	5.7	4.0	7.0

Fig. 2.3 Rates of economic growth of selected developing ESCAP economies (*Source*: ESCAP calculations adapted from the ESCAP 2010a, Table 7)

Therefore, the exit strategies for fiscal stimulus packages need to be carefully planned and have to be gradual, especially in the context of the European debt crisis.

There is also a serious threat of protectionist tendencies creeping up despite the call by G-20 leaders at their Summits. This would endanger the ongoing export recovery witnessed across the region.

Downside Risks and Policy Challenges

Another downside risk is the return of inflation. With recovery, inflationary pressures have been revived in several Asia-Pacific countries especially in South Asia, where food prices are rising sharply. Reminiscent of the food-fuel crisis of 2007, oil prices are also rising (Fig. 2.4).

With recovery taking hold, inflationary pressures are expected to rise in most countries in 2010. Therefore, controlling inflation is a major challenge for the region. As inflation adversely affects the poor disproportionately, it is a serious problem for many countries in the region with high incidence of poverty.

This situation implies a tough balancing act on the part of policy makers. While monetary tightening may be necessary to restrain inflationary pressures, as

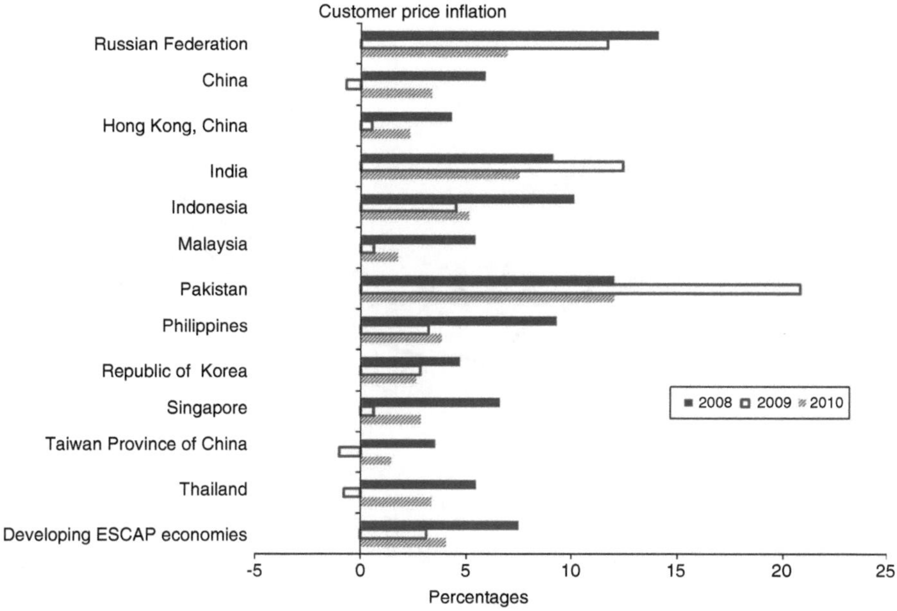

Fig. 2.4 Inflationary pressures (*Source*: ESCAP calculations adapted from the ESCAP 2010a, Table 10)

a number of central banks have begun doing, policy makers may be cautious about withdrawing fiscal stimulus policies lest the fledgling recovery process is disrupted.

The other key policy challenge that the policy makers are facing at the moment pertains to financial and exchange rate stability (Fig. 2.5).

Other than demand-side pressures, inflation has been caused by the return of large foreign portfolio inflows. There was a massive expansion of liquidity in the advanced countries in the wake of the crisis. Now that liquidity is finding its way to the emerging markets in the region leading to booming asset prices, stock prices have reached the pre-crisis peaks across the region. The inflows have also resulted in pressures on exchange rates which can threaten export recovery.

Here we support use of capital controls, where necessary, to moderate short-term capital flows in the emerging markets.

Infrastructure and Other Development Gaps

The Asia-Pacific region has close to one billion people living in poverty,[1] which, combined with other wide development gaps such as in the levels of infrastructure development (Fig. 2.6), provide it considerable headroom for augmenting

[1]ESCAP/ADB/UNDP (2010/2011, p. 8).

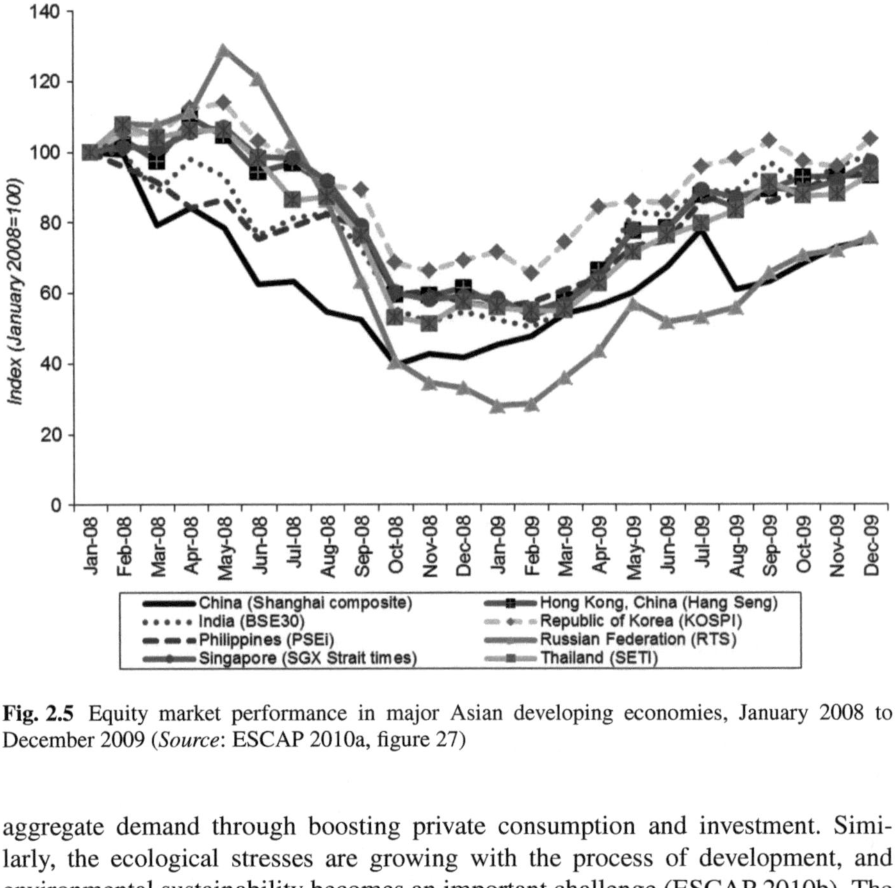

Fig. 2.5 Equity market performance in major Asian developing economies, January 2008 to December 2009 (*Source*: ESCAP 2010a, figure 27)

aggregate demand through boosting private consumption and investment. Similarly, the ecological stresses are growing with the process of development, and environmental sustainability becomes an important challenge (ESCAP 2010b). The forests, mangroves, coral reefs, aquifers, minerals, and other forms of natural capital that comprise the ecosystems are vital to the poor and non-poor alike for their livelihoods, particularly in developing countries. Natural capital constitutes only 5 % of national wealth in rich countries, while it constitutes an average of 40 % in low-income countries (ESCAP 2010a, b). Natural capital contributes over 40 % of household income in many rural areas (World Bank 2008). Unbridled exploitation of natural resources has eroded this capital and given rise to significant economic stresses. Soil fertility is declining and air and water pollution is increasing as unsustainable agricultural practices have taken hold. Excessive use of fossil fuel-based fertilizers and pesticides together with inefficient water management systems has added to the economic difficulties rural communities – where most of the poor live and work – have come to face. Urban pollution, congestion, and increasing waste have led to increased costs in maintaining urban services which are ultimately borne by the whole community through increased taxes, higher services fees, or lack of services or poorly maintained services.

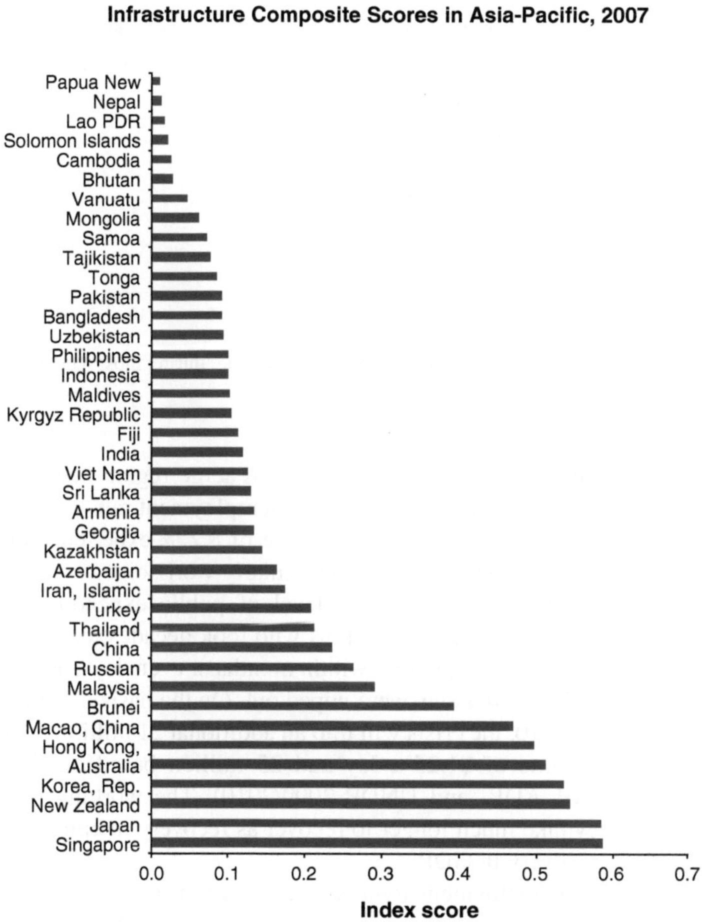

Fig. 2.6 Infrastructure composite scores in Asia and the Pacific, 2007 (*Source*: ESCAP 2010a, figure 61)

Part I: The Nature and Impact of the Economic Crisis

By the third quarter of 2008, what started as a housing crisis in the USA had turned into a global financial crisis affecting the real economy everywhere. This crisis presented Asia with its most difficult economic challenge in recent times. With its major trading partners in deep economic trouble, there is no way for Asia to "export" out of this crisis, unlike during the 1997 crisis.

The crisis revealed the limits of the region's export-oriented, low-cost, labor-intensive growth model. Exports dropped sharply at rates that were almost twice as large as and more widespread than those experienced in past crises. This was followed by massive job losses in many of the key export manufacturing industries in the region, including textiles, garments, electronics, and autos. We estimated that

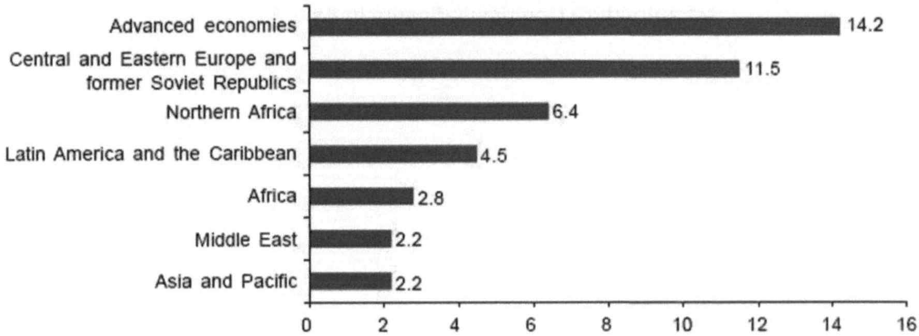

Fig. 2.7 Social expenditure as a percentage of GDP, worldwide, during most recent year available (*Source*: ILO 2009b)

by 2009, the number of unemployed in the Asia-Pacific region had increased by ten million compared to 2007, bringing up the unemployment rate to 5.0 %.[2] While some might argue that this rate is still below that of 8.2 % experienced by OECD countries, there are other features that are particularly worrisome.

First, as a region that has the lowest level of public expenditure on social protection, as illustrated in Fig. 2.7, millions who took decades to work their way out of poverty slipped back into poverty within months or even days, as any personal savings quickly dried up and assets were wiped out. On the basis of current growth estimates over 2009–2010, the crisis will trap an additional 21 million people below the extreme poverty line of $1.25-a-day and 25 million based on the $2-a-day poverty line (ESCAP, ADB, and UNDP 2009/2010). The working poor are the hardest hit, and they take much longer to recover as recovery in employment takes much longer than recovery in GDP.

Second, official unemployment figures, even in countries where they are collected at regular intervals, mask the depth of the problem. In the absence of social protection systems, unemployment is untenable for many workers who have lost their jobs or whose income is reduced. To survive and support families, people try to cope by switching jobs often from formal to informal and casual jobs, many of them falling prey to exploitative conditions and giving up rights at work (ESCAP 2010a, b). Such increases in informality are difficult to reverse; real wages take time to recover as does labor productivity. Previous economic crisis points towards a recovery lag in the labor market that can trail behind economic recovery by as long as 4–5 years (ESCAP 2010a, b). Unemployment figures in Asia are therefore a crude measurement that grossly underestimates the fallout from the crisis.

Third, severe economic recessions often lead to irreversible changes in the labor market and permanent job losses. Since the Asian financial crisis in 1997, unemployment rates in some of the Asian economies that were most affected by

[2]For more data, see ILO and Economic and Labour Market Analysis Department (2009).

that crisis, namely, Thailand, Indonesia, the Republic of Korea, Hong Kong, and China, have never fully recovered to their pre-crisis levels (ESCAP 2010a, b).

Poorer people are affected more because they have fewer buffers and because the range and effectiveness of their buffers are inadequate. Families may react to the declining income of primary wage earners and overall decline in a family's purchasing power by taking measures that continue to keep them poor. This includes reducing the number and quality of meals, reducing health and education expenditure, and pushing more family members out to work in difficult and often dangerous situations. Typically this involves more vulnerable family members, particularly young women, children, and sometimes the elderly. Children who cease schooling may never return. Girls who are trafficked to help their families survive may never recover from the social fallout. Women who are required to work longer hours are further relied on to provide care for the sick, elderly, and extended family, increasing their burden and their "crisis of time." Unemployed or underemployed youth quickly turn to petty crime resulting in increased criminality often linked to violence against women.

A recent study conducted by ESCAP, ADB, and UNDP analyzes the impact or vulnerability of women and children to the economic crisis (ESCAP, ADB and UNDP 2009/2010). For instance, the proportion of under-five children underweight who are most at risk to the economic crisis are from Armenia, Lao PDR, Cambodia, Nepal, and Pakistan. These countries already have very high levels of child malnutrition, to begin with, further exacerbated by the crisis. Similarly, women are particularly vulnerable in situations of economic shock. In Asia and the Pacific region, the majority of low-skilled, low-salaried, and temporary workers are women, and many of them have lost their jobs in the garment, textile, and electronics industries. In Thailand alone, the number of unemployed women increased by 47 % between May 2008 and May 2009 compared to 15 % for men. In Sri Lanka, the unemployment rate for women increased from 7.9 to 9.2 % between the first quarter and second quarters of 2009 (ILO 2009a).

Fourth, remittances have become an increasingly important source of external development finance, far larger than FDI flows, in many countries, thus not only providing balance of payments support but also providing income relief to the poorest households. However, during the crisis, total remittances fell by 1.5 % in East Asia and 1.8 % in South Asia in 2009.[3] While these falls are much smaller than the volatility experienced by other capital flows to developing countries, looking forward, there is a danger in over-reliance on such flows. With double digit unemployment levels and labor market conditions that are expected to remain depressed in most destination countries, sociopolitical pressures against migration are building and a number of countries have already introduced policies to restrict migrant workers' access to labor markets. The export of labor services may therefore also have reached the limits of its success, not unlike the export boom of manufactures. Similarly, with the economic crisis in the richer countries, high-end tourism has also been badly affected.

---

[3]For detailed information, see Ratha et al. (2009).

Part II: Sustaining Growth by Addressing Multiple Imbalances

If Asia cannot "trade" itself out of the crisis, Asia has "spent" itself out of the crisis. The good news is that Asia is experiencing a V-shaped recovery supported by massive fiscal stimulus packages. ESCAP's latest *Economic and Social Survey* projects a 7.0 % growth in 2010 of the Asia-Pacific developing economies, led by China growing at 9.5 % and India, at 8.3 %. However, the recovery is fragile besides further uncertainties created by the European debt crisis. Furthermore, rising inflation in a number of countries especially in food prices, growing asset bubbles, and appreciating exchange rates in a weak growth environment require a tough balancing act on fiscal and monetary policies and will make 2010 a year of complex policy making.

Beyond these short-term challenges, a serious consideration has to be given to the prospects of sustaining the recovery beyond the fiscal stimulus packages. It is not possible to return to "growth as usual" and "trade as usual" scenarios given global macroeconomic imbalances and the unwinding of debt-fuelled consumption. This clearly means that Asia has to develop new sources of demand that would make up for the shortfall in the advanced economies like the USA.

The key long-term challenge for the region is locating new drivers of growth to supplement the previous engine of demand in developed countries. The solution for the region lies in sustaining growth by addressing its own macroeconomic, social, ecological, and development imbalances and development gaps. This can be done by empowering the poor and making growth "greener." The result will be greater demand from within the region, as well as growth which is more inclusive of the poor and which is more ecologically sustainable.

The region has to address development gaps to drive growth. With 950 million people in poverty, Asia has large headroom for expanding aggregate demand and thus reducing dependence on external consumption. Asia is also lagging in terms of achieving many other Millennium Development Goals (MDG) targets. Wide infrastructure gaps in the region also provide an additional potential of generating demand in this region. Similarly, the ecological stresses are growing with the process of development and environmental sustainability becoming an important challenge.

ESCAP has come up with a four-pronged policy agenda for expanding domestic consumption and inclusive and sustainable growth:

- Firstly, we need to attach a high importance to strengthening social protection. If poor households can rely on systems of social protection that will automatically trigger social safety nets at times of adversity, they will be able to maintain food intake and continue to use education and health services. Just as important, in non-crisis times they will have less need to maintain precautionary savings and can use more of their income to meet their consumption needs.
- Second, as the majority of poor people live in the rural areas and derive most of their income from agriculture, they are likely to benefit from agricultural growth. We need a second, more knowledge-intensive green revolution that combines advances in science and agricultural engineering with the region's unique traditional knowledge to make agriculture more environmentally resilient.

- Third, the Asia-Pacific economies have the opportunity to develop new and greener industries and businesses based on innovations that are eco-efficient and will save energy, water, and value earth's resources. This way they can provide more affordable green products and services while maintaining growth and promoting environmental sustainability.
- And fourth, we need to make our financial system more inclusive so that millions of the unbanked can access modern financial services and small and medium enterprises can be assisted to contribute to development.

All this means investing in human capital so that Asia is able to shape a more knowledge-intensive and innovative economy of the future – one that is low in carbon but high in poverty reduction.

My fifth policy agenda is to exploit the potential of regional economic cooperation to complement the national policy actions to rebalance economic growth.

A number of initiatives have been taken over the past decade in the direction of regional cooperation in Asia at subregional, bilateral, and regional levels. These include a number of FTAs and comprehensive economic partnership arrangements. These arrangements need to be deepened and broadened to create a larger unified market. It is my belief that with some of the world's largest and fastest-growing economies, Asia can become an even greater economic powerhouse if it develops a more integrated regional market. In that direction the initiative taken by the East Asia Summit involving 16 countries at their Summit in Hua Hin to pursue a comprehensive economic partnership of East Asia (CEPEA) is an important one.[4]

Regional cooperation should also involve developing regional transportation networks and improving trade facilitation. Strengthening regional ICT connectivity is another important aspect. ESCAP has been assisting the region in developing regional transport networks, trade facilitation, and ICT connectivity as summarized in ESCAP's *Economic and Social Survey of Asia and the Pacific 2010*.

I must say that the discussions on reforming the international financial architecture at the G-20 and other forums need to find their counterpart within the region. The regional financial architecture in Asia is in its infancy and should be improved in line with the region's greater trade integration. Particular areas include designing a regional crisis management fund, boosting exchange rate coordination, and establishing a regional investment fund to direct regional reserves to regional needs. The multilateralization of the Chiang-Mai Initiative is an important step but with combined reserves of nearly $5 trillion, the possibilities are immense. The region now has the ability to develop a more ambitious regional cooperative architecture for serving its needs and in investing in itself.

We know from the 1997 Asian financial crisis that social recovery takes longer than economic recovery and cannot be taken for granted. We therefore need an agenda for social equity to ensure that governments invest in their people and build the foundation for inclusive and sustainable development.

---

[4]See Chairman's Statement, East Asia Summit, Hua Hin October 2009.

Part III: An Agenda for Social Protection

We can no longer expect families to be the shock absorbers of risks and vulnerabilities that we face. Risks and vulnerabilities are no longer sporadic. We now have to build new resilience in a constant climate of shocks from weather-related disasters to volatility in commodity prices, to global economic crises, to sudden illnesses or disabilities. Family structures have been stretched to breaking point. They are already changing due to factors such as delayed age of marriage, declining fertility, disruption of marriages, a rapidly aging population, international migration, rise in female-headed households, family members being dispersed and living apart due to global employment patterns, and displacement due to conflict and political unrest. With urbanization and urban housing patterns, there is also a shift from the extended family to the nuclear family.

Given these macro and micro changes, the state and the private sector need to rethink how it can invest in new human capacity development, resilient institutions, and state-corporation-citizen accountability interfaces as part of our twenty-first century reality of globalization and interdependence.

The region's most important asset is its peoples, and human capital is embodied in the quality of our future development. At the same time, the crisis exposed the need to create a new paradigm for inclusive economic growth within the Asia region – a paradigm that accelerates economic growth and sustains recovery by investing in people. It is built on the premise that there can be no further economic transformation without social transformation.

Let me outline some elements of this social transformation process:

Rising economic stresses and large-scale and persistent poverty in the region call for more resilient and inclusive social protection systems. This agenda must include four equally important policy goals:

(a) Reduce entrenched poverty and protect the population at large from the risk of falling into poverty as a result of not only economic crisis but also life-changing exogenous shocks such as disasters, illness, and disability
(b) Social inclusion for inclusive growth and political stability
(c) Human security as a basic right
(d) Achievement of MDGs

These goals can be addressed through social protection as a key component of broader economic and social development policies aimed at supporting household consumption and providing meaningful access to education, health, and other services that will pave the way to MDG achievement, promoting better chances of individual development, family well-being, and social cohesion.

At the same time, we must change the way we formulate and implement social protection strategies. I believe two major changes are required.

First, the goal and structure of social protection programs and interventions must be transformed from a solely welfare strategy to an investment strategy. In addition to targeting risks and vulnerabilities associated with crises and upheavals, the enhancement of social protection must be mindful of the structural elements that place social groups in a situation of exclusion and vulnerability in the first place. What are some examples?

- Spatial such as remote locations, isolated rural areas, and slums. These need to be connected to development services.
- Economic and financial, such as disparities in the distribution of incomes and productive assets as well as limited access to employment opportunities.
- Sociocultural, such as identity-based forms of exclusion – ethnicity, religion, gender, age, and physical ability.
- Legal, such as complicated registration systems for birth certificate and home registration, leading to statelessness or "people without papers."

Existing social protection frameworks rarely include social exclusion as a source of vulnerability.

These challenges need to be addressed by appropriate social protection investments if we are to have inclusive societies.

It is also important to acknowledge that risks and vulnerabilities are not static but dynamic processes. At the level of the individual, they are the result of changes over the life course of a person.

Conditions are dynamic also at the level of communities and nations, namely, demographic and economic shifts. Some of the changes that social protection strategies need to address are (1) urbanization and migration, (2) aging populations, and (3) the breakdown of informal support structures based on the extended family.

This leads to my final point, namely, that we need an approach that builds on the synergies between various social protection schemes and between social protection and other social and economic policies. To give you an example, conditional cash transfers for children to go to school will not be effective if schools are not properly staffed or the quality of teaching is poor. Furthermore, securing the intended effect of social protection strategies requires careful attention to potential impacts on the economy. For example, in countries where the population has started to age rapidly – or will be doing so in the near future – we will see an increased emphasis on how social protection is to be sustainably financed. Social protection must not simply be seen as a handout. It is an investment in inclusive growth. It is an investment in human capabilities to get people out of exclusion and poverty and to build resilience to risks and vulnerabilities.

The opportunity is now for Asia to emerge as a leader: in the global economy, in the realm of social progress, and in safeguarding our global environment. Asia's development relies on our ability to achieve three balances on our shared development journey:

First, balance between our economic growth, our social needs, and the limits of the earth: the three interconnected pillars of development.

Second, balance between the individual and the collective: how to transform the initiative of each into the common good for all.

Third, balance between the power of the market and the power of the state: the global financial crisis of the past 2 years underscores the limits of relying solely on the market to correct itself and the dangers of overregulation by the state.

In conclusion, alongside rapid growth and wealth generation, income inequalities, chronic poverty, and sociopolitical exclusion are all part of the Asian experience. Economic stresses bring to the fore complex policy challenges and opportunities. It is in those countries that maintain an explicit and unrelenting recognition that human development rests on the integration of economic and social policies that will build resilience to future crises. Working together, Asia can shape the forces of the economic recovery by investing in its people, its human capital, and its social foundations. As a region, we must build upon our collective strengths if we are not only to recover from the present crisis but make social progress that will see the region's peoples live longer, wealthier, healthier, and in solidarity with each other.

References

ESCAP. (2010a). *Economic and social survey of Asia and the Pacific 2010* (United Nations Publication, Sales No. E.10.II.F.2, figure 6). Retrieved from http://www.unescap.org/pdd/publications/survey2010/download/index.asp

ESCAP. (2010b). *Financing an inclusive and green growth: A supportive financial system and green growth for achieving the Millennium Development Goals in Asia and the Pacific 2010.* New York: United Nations Publication, chapter 4, page 63.

ESCAP, ADB, & UNDP. (2009/2010). *Achieving the millennium development goals in an era of global uncertainty, Asia-Pacific Regional Report 2009/10* (United Nations Publication, Sales No. E.10.II.F.10, p. 31). Retrieved from www.mdgasiapacific.org/regional-report-2009-10

ESCAP, ADB, & UNDP. (2010/2011). *Paths to 2015- MDG priorities in Asia and the Pacific: Asia-Pacific MDG Report 2010/11* (United Nations Publication, Sales No. E.10.II.F.20). Bangkok: ESCAP.

ILO. (2009a). *Key indicators of labour market* (6th ed.). Geneva: ILO.

ILO. (2009b). *The financial and economic crisis: A decent work response*. Geneva: ILO.

ILO, & Economic and Labour Market Analysis Department. (2009, October). *Trends econometric models*. www.ilo.org/empelm/what/projects/lang--en/WCMS_114246/index.htm. Accessed Oct 2009.

Ratha, D., Mohapatra, S., & Silwal, A. (2009). *Migration and remittance trends 2009: A better-than-expected outcome so far, but significant risks ahead* (Migration and Development Brief 11, p. 14). Washington, DC: World Bank.

World Bank. (2008). *Global monitoring report 2008: MDGs and the environment – Agenda for inclusive and sustainable development*. Washington, DC: World Bank.

Chapter 3
The Impact of the Economic Crisis on Children in East Asia and the Pacific: A UNICEF Perspective (2009–2010)

Samman J. Thapa and Mahesh S. Patel

Impacts of Economic and Other Crises in EAP Countries

The global economic crisis hit EAPR with remarkable speed and ferocity in mid-2008. Any expectations that "decoupled" East Asian economies, supposedly not tied to the fortunes of western economies anymore, would emerge unscathed from this downturn did not materialize. The latest estimates for 2009 suggest that East Asia excluding China experienced a mere 1.2 % growth in 2009 (World Bank 2010a). Even growth in China eased to 8.7 % from a phenomenal 13 % recorded in 2007 (ADB 2010). And while it took a little longer, low-income countries (LICs) in the region also felt the pinch. Cambodia's was the starkest case. An expansion of 10.2 % in 2007 turned into a contraction of 2.0 %, the largest difference over a 2-year period for any country in the region (World Bank 2010a, b). All of this compounded the adverse impacts of the food price rises and commodity price fluctuations. Countries that are not highly integrated into the global economy – such as Mongolia, Myanmar, Lao PDR, Papua New Guinea (PNG), and the Pacific Island countries – bore the brunt of the multiple shocks given their lack of fiscal space to react and dependence on few commodity exports.

Against this backdrop, how is the region faring a little over a year after the full onset of the crisis? Is the "worst recession since the great depression" (World Bank 2008) leaving a trail of economic disaster in its wake in EAPR as dire prognoses had proclaimed earlier?

Not really. Although the economic crisis has noticeably dented economies in EAPR, it has not been anywhere as bad as predictions from a year ago. Many analyses now state that Asia (particularly EAP) has been the first region to pull

S.J. Thapa (✉) • M.S. Patel
UNICEF Regional Office for the Middle East and North Africa,
P.O. Box 1551, Amman 11821, Jordan
e-mail: sthapa@unicef.org; mpatel@unicef.org

W.J.J. Yeung and M.T. Yap (eds.), *Economic Stress, Human Capital, and Families in Asia: Research and Policy Challenges*, Quality of Life in Asia 4,
DOI 10.1007/978-94-007-7386-8_3, © Springer Science+Business Media Dordrecht 2013

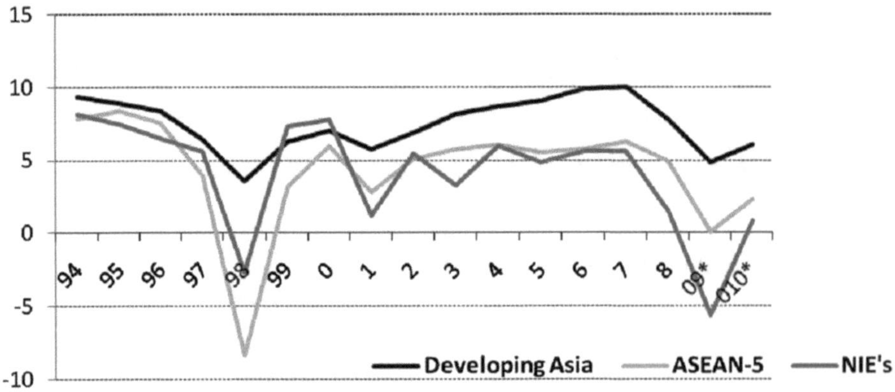

Fig. 3.1 Average annual growth rates (GDP, constant prices) (*Source*: IMF 2010)

out of the economic slump, even leading the global recovery. China's role in this is particularly crucial. Its US$ 600 billion stimulus program and monetary easing that led banks to dole out US$ 1.2 trillion in 2009 have been effective in ensuring the growth it experienced in 2009 (*The Financial Times* 2009a). Emerging Asia too grew by over 5 %, while advanced economies contracted by 3.2 % (IMF 2010). The growth gap between these two groups has never been wider (*Economist* 2009). EAP economies overall have made a "V"-shaped comeback (IMF 2010) as seen in Fig. 3.1, thanks largely to China's strong performance.

These developments need to be considered alongside the speed of economic development achieved by many countries in East Asia since the 1960s (World Bank 1993). This progress has been so spectacular that there has been much speculation as to when China and the other large economies (China plus Brazil, Russia, India, Indonesia, Mexico, and Turkey) will overtake the USA and the G-7 in terms of total output (PPP). A recent report expects the world's seven largest emerging economies (the "E-7"), mentioned above, to overtake the G-7 by 2020 (PWC 2010). As the graph below demonstrates, the gap in GDP growth between emerging economies, led by China, has never been wider. While per capita income equality is still relatively distant, this increase in total output and the outstanding performance of the "tigers" laid to rest the notion that developing countries were doomed forever to be economically inferior and their people doomed to eternal poverty (Patel 2000b) (Fig. 3.2).

Within this overall picture, however, it is important to note that different countries in EAP were affected differently by the crises and the recoveries have been similarly varied. This has important implications for the abilities of different nations to maintain social commitments for the poor and vulnerable, especially children. Since there are significant existing inter- and intracountry disparities within the region, this may complicate efforts to achieve the Millennium Development Goals (MDGs) with equity. Analyzing how the economic crisis has transmitted across countries provides a starting point in effectively addressing social concerns that the crisis has spawned

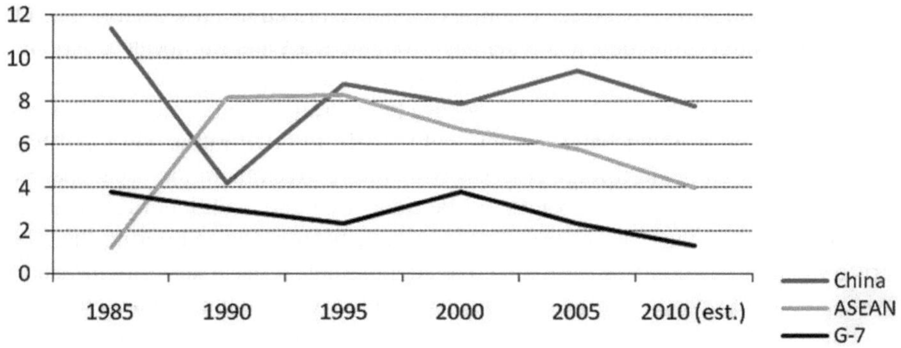

Fig. 3.2 Percentage change in real GDP (*Source*: EIU database 2009)

Fig. 3.3 Exports of goods and services as % of GDP and GDP growth (Q1, 2009) (*Source*: EIU database 2009)

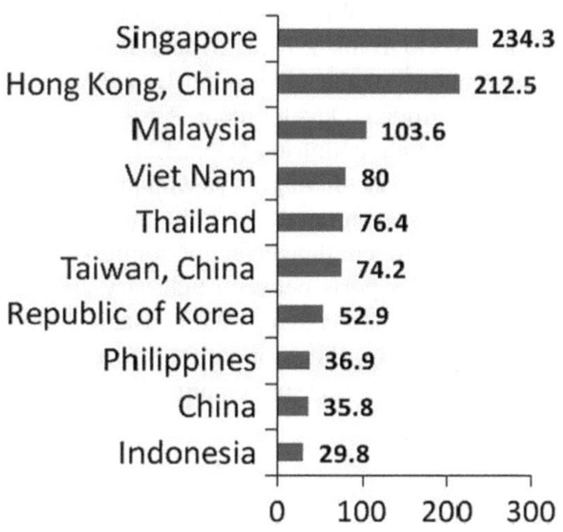

or ones that it may have exacerbated. Openness to international trade among countries, as the crisis struck in early 2009, is especially noteworthy in this regard.

The countries that were least hit have been ones which were not as interconnected to the Western economies and they have also recovered fastest. China and Indonesia are the most prominent countries in this category, with India being an example from South Asia. As Fig. 3.3 shows, China and Indonesia had some of the lowest exports (35.8 and 29.8 %, respectively) to GDP ratio and have indeed performed better than most economies in the region. The global nature of this crisis, unlike the homegrown one in 1997/1998, has meant that low trade exposure, strong domestic demand, and the diversified nature of these economies shielded them from the worst of the crisis.

More open economies such as Thailand, Malaysia, and Singapore bore the brunt of the crisis. Their financial interlinkages with western economies weakened post-1997 but their trade dependence to these economies increased in the same period.

Also, as most exports from these countries are concentrated in a few sectors (such as high-tech goods) which depend on demand from the USA and European economies, the sharp downturn in the latter economies affected them quickly. But chastened by their experience of the 1997 crisis, they have built strong macroeconomic positions (healthy current account balances, low public debt to GDP ratios, etc.) and have accumulated significant foreign reserves which have given them the fiscal space to react strongly. The stimuli packages in Malaysia, Thailand, and South Korea are all examples of this. Such a scenario could not have been envisaged during the 1997 crisis when these countries were forced to adopt stringent fiscal austerity measures, which required severe slashing of public expenditure even in the social sectors.

Finally, it is important to monitor how low-income countries (LICs) and/or commodity exporters such as Cambodia, Mongolia, Papua New Guinea, and the Pacific Island countries are faring as we transition from crisis to recovery since their fiscal positions are not as strong as those of the countries from the previous two categories. With global remittances having dropped by 6 % compared to 2008 (World Bank 2010a, b) and foreign aid too expected to suffer due to the global nature of the crisis – an UNCTAD study says there is a 30 % cumulative drop in Official Development Assistance (ODA) by the 5th year of a banking crisis in donor countries (UNCTAD 2009) – these countries will face the most challenges in achieving a sustainable recovery. Mongolia – heavily dependent on revenues generated by gold and copper exports – is a case in point for illustrating the challenge facing commodity-exporting countries. The sharp fall in the value of exports between February 2008 and February 2009 was equivalent to over 10 % of GDP there (World Bank 2009a). With relatively limited scope for deficit financing, the economic crisis may erode recent gains in education sector spending and put pressure on already depressed levels of health expenditure in these countries.

Implications for Children and Child Poverty

The social impacts of the economic downturn and the food price crisis too have transmitted differently across countries but their severity is undoubted. The full extent of this impact remains to be seen as past crises have demonstrated how the social impacts of a crisis take longer to transmit and be apparent (World Bank 2009a, b, c; Patel 2009a). A famous example is the time it took Indonesia after 1997/1998 to lower its income poverty rate to pre-crisis levels after that crisis.

But some effects have already been observed. Slower growth due to reduced global demand has induced massive job losses in export-dependent sectors. An estimated 25 million migrant workers in China lost their jobs in 2009, whereas 50,000 garment workers in Cambodia – 17 % of the total – are reported to have lost jobs since September 2008. This will have a severe impact in slowing poverty reduction in EAPR. The World Bank estimates that 14 million people in the region who would have escaped income poverty under normal circumstances will not be able to do so due to the crises (World Bank 2010a, b). Cambodia, Malaysia, Thailand, and Timor-Leste are expected to experience absolute rises in poverty (World Bank 2009a, b, c).

For the poorest and vulnerable, the twin shocks of higher food prices and falling or lost incomes could result in coping strategies like taking children out of school, delaying school payments or cutting down on healthcare expenditure, further worsening the condition of vulnerable children. There is already evidence of such incidences. A survey done by UNICEF among migrant communities most vulnerable to the crisis in Vietnam has revealed that many families of migrant workers are taking children out of school and/or delaying school payments or contemplating these as coping strategies. There is similar news coming from the Pacific Island countries (UNICEF 2009).

In terms of health outcomes, a study done by UNICEF Cambodia revealed that wasting among poor urban children in that country increased from 6 % in 2005 to 15.9 % (above the 15 % threshold of a "humanitarian emergency") in 2008, primarily due to rising food prices (Cambodia Anthropometrics Survey 2008). Modelling done by Bhutta et al. (2009) on the potential impact of this crisis on maternal and child health also shows that if unaddressed, the current crisis could increase rates of maternal anemia, prevalence of low birth weight, childhood stunting, wasting, and under five child mortality in EAPR. A special issue of the academic journal *Global Social Policy* dedicated to UNICEF studies released in September 2009 (available online at http://gsp.sagepub.com/content/vol9/1_suppl/) chronicles in further detail the specific implications of the crisis on children vis-à-vis different channels such as education, health, reduced family incomes, and child labor.

This economic crisis has also exacerbated the vulnerability of particular groups like women (heavily employed in export-oriented sectors), the urban poor, and migrants. In Cambodia, a UNIAP report pointed out that the economic crisis has led women to leave poorly paid work in the garment sector to take up employment in the sex sector.

Given these socioeconomic outcomes and their implications – including an unfortunate slowdown or even reversal of hard won gains in the achievement of MDGs – most governments across the region have been relatively quick to act, no doubt influenced by their experiences of the 1997 economic crisis' social dimension. Because of this and EAPR's rapid socioeconomic development over the past few decades, the particular focus on children may seem unclear.

It Is Anything but Out of Focus. The sense of optimism when considering EAP's progress is sometimes misplaced when it comes to delivering results for children. The graphs below show how wasting, stunting, and underweight levels among children in EAP are very high once the regional aggregates for these indicators are decomposed. As with general poverty figures, it is China's performance in improving these figures that has contributed to EAP's positive aggregate. Otherwise the levels of stunting in EAP countries even today – almost or above 40 % in countries such as Indonesia, Cambodia, and Lao PDR – are comparable to levels observed in countries in South Asia and sub-Saharan Africa. Stunting is perhaps

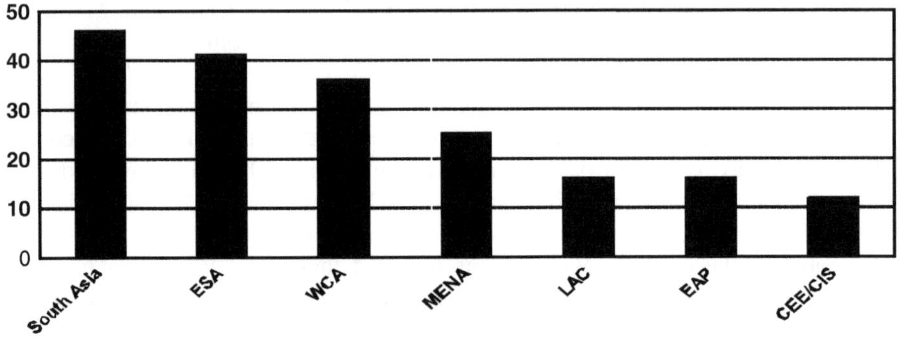

Fig. 3.4 Stunting by region (*Source*: UNICEF 2007)

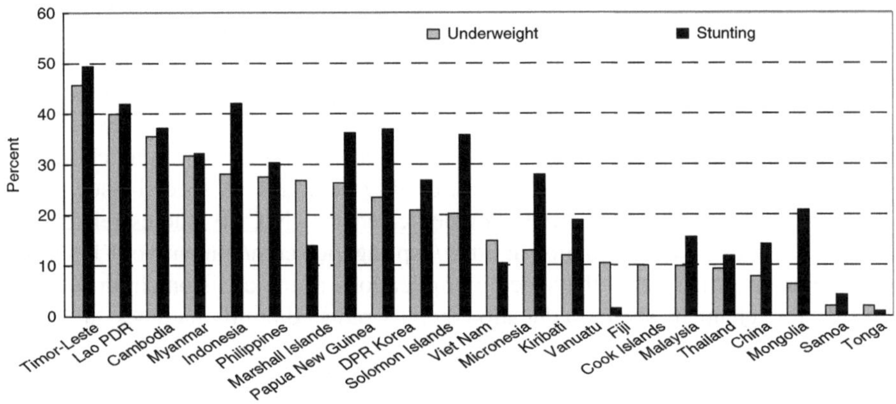

Fig. 3.5 Percentage of children stunted or underweight in East Asia and the Pacific (*Source*: UNICEF 2007)

the most pernicious result of under nutrition, occurring before children are 2 years old but with permanent effects on their physical and intellectual development. Poor households in the region spend up to 75–80 % (ADB 2008) of their income on food. So lowered purchasing power due to higher food prices (on average still much higher than their pre-crisis levels, with food prices continuing to inch up again), reduced incomes, and higher fuel/commodity prices could worsen this existing situation for children. Adverse coping strategies employed by families due to this may end in permanent repercussions such as taking children out of school or cutting down on their intake of nutritious foods which may lead to stunting in the future (Figs. 3.4 and 3.5).

The above indicators also provide an insight into the implications that the crisis can have on child poverty. Unlike income poverty, child poverty is defined by the severity of deprivation that children face in their access to various services. The UN General Assembly defines children living in poverty as children who

Example of 4 children Access to:	A	B	C	D
• Water	√	NO	√	√
• Sanitation facilities	√	√	NO	NO
• Health	√	√	NO	NO
• Nutrition	√	√	√	√
• Shelter	√	√	√	√
• Education	√	√	√	NO
• Information	√	√	√	√
• Poor: At least one right not satisfied	√	NO	NO	NO

Fig. 3.6 Child poverty linked to multiple dimensions of deprivations

are "deprived of nutrition, water and sanitation facilities, access to basic health services, shelter, education, participation and protection, and while a severe lack of goods and services hurts every human being, it is most threatening and harmful to children, leaving them unable to enjoy their rights, to reach their full potential and to participate as full members of society."

Being multidimensional in nature, a lack of income is only one of its aspects. So stunting, for example, which is caused by long-term insufficient nutrients and frequent infections, is strongly correlated to nutrition deprivation. This is one example that illustrates how the impressive reductions in income poverty rates in EAPR have not fully translated into better results for children. There are other similar examples of progress lagging (in comparison to the income growth or even success in income poverty reduction) in increasing the proportion of people with access to cleaner water and better sanitation, especially in rural areas, both of which are vital to the health and nutrition of children (Fig. 3.6).

Mendoza (2009) neatly captures how the economic crisis can transmit through different channels to children. An economic crisis transmits through different channels to households and children. Shocks to the global economy can affect national economies through decreased foreign aid and/or private investments. It can also affect international trade in goods and services. As a result, a nation's economy may suffer a slowdown that may result in constrained government spending on social services, job losses, and austerity overall. The macroeconomy ultimately impacts individual households and therefore children at the microlevel. A feedback loop is created when deprived children become vulnerable to health or behavioral problems, and family productivity declines at the macro level due to increased care and attention needed within the household. This affects the nation's economy and thus do increased deprivations caused by these transmission channels have the potential to exacerbate child poverty in the region.

As the region contemplates rebalancing economic growth, it is time to give thought to doing so in favor of efforts that align economic growth with progress for children through boosting sector specific, targeted policies. Only supporting and sustaining economic growth will not be sufficient to do this and reduce child poverty rates. This must be borne in mind when enacting fiscal responses to stimulate economies.

Vietnam's experience is illustrative of this point. Two decades of rapid economic growth and progressive state policies have contributed to significant declines in income poverty there. But child poverty in Vietnam today is almost certainly more prevalent and severe than is commonly believed (UNICEF Viet Nam 2008). This is because existing methods and techniques used to measure child poverty in Vietnam, focusing on children living in households defined as poor according to the national monetary poverty line, are inadequate and have limitations. In the context of the current global economic crisis, the government of Vietnam is putting in place new measures designed to reduce poverty and protect the most vulnerable groups from the worst impacts of the crisis; however, these measures are relying on traditional monetary methods of calculating poverty, meaning that they are not capturing the specificities of child poverty fully. Newer policies and programs to respond and mitigate the impact of the economic crisis need to better reflect the deprivations faced by children, who are the most vulnerable.[1]

But unlike the weak correlation between adult income poverty and child poverty, there is a strong link between reductions in child poverty rates and adult poverty rates because children who grow up in poverty are more likely to be poor in adulthood as well. Investing in reducing or eliminating child poverty now is therefore the smartest investment in reducing overall poverty and contributing to socioeconomic growth (UNICEF Viet Nam 2008).

Government Fiscal Responses

Governments across the region were quick to act on the threats posed by the multiple crises, especially the global economic crisis. At least eight countries have enacted some form of fiscal stimulus – differing in size, share of tax cuts versus expenditure increases, provision for public versus private financing, and whether

[1]It must be noted that although the economic policies enacted in Vietnam due to the crisis may not have been as child-sensitive as they could, from a longer term perspective, the government of Vietnam has taken the findings and recommendations from the national child poverty report it commissioned very seriously.

spending is limited to 2009 or extends to 2010 – which was aimed at boosting flagging economic growth and was also intended to counter social impacts. A fiscal expenditure package of CNY 4 trillion or US$ 585 billion (13 % of GDP or 5 % of GDP per year) that China announced in November 2008 and revised in 2009 is the largest. Indonesia, Malaysia, the Philippines, Thailand, Vietnam, and some Pacific Island countries (Northern Mariana Islands and American Samoa) too have announced fiscal measures to reverse the economic slowdown many countries in the region, having the fiscal space to implement spending measures. The significant foreign reserves accumulated by these countries after 1997/1998, which have not been drawn upon in any significant manner yet, too bolster the case for such spending with a long-term vision for social protection. But the possibility of falling ODA threatens funding for social protection programs in fiscally strapped LICs.

Although there are a few countries that have chosen to focus mostly on infrastructure and tax cuts, most countries in the region have set aside substantial portions of their stimuli programs for social spending.

China's fiscal expenditure package had provisions for expenditures in the social sector. It was adjusted in March 2009, significantly increasing the allocation on social spending. Low-income housing was set to receive CNY 400 billion (from 280 billion originally) and healthcare and education were set to receive CNY 150 billion (from 40 billion). Thailand too had notable provisions for social spending in its stimulus program drawing on the positive decisions made to maintain social spending as much as possible during the 1997 crisis. The US$ 3 billion supplementary budget announced in January 2009 included investments in upgrading rural schools and health facilities as well as a one-time allowance for low-income people in the formal sector. Thailand's provision of free basic education and healthcare to poor families should also help mitigate some of the worst impacts of falling household incomes. But it is important to ensure that fiscal budget cuts do not affect existing policies, particularly the provision of free universal healthcare. The stimulus programs in Malaysia and the Northern Mariana Islands also contained allocations for increased social sector expenditures.

Despite many positive examples, some of the stimulus packages still had huge chunks set aside for infrastructure projects or tax cuts, with little or no spending in the social sector. For instance, Indonesia's stimulus consists of significant spending on infrastructure (IDR 12.2 trillion) and tax breaks (43 trillion), while relatively little is devoted to spending on the social side. This is surprising considering its experiences during the 1997 crisis. The Philippines, which has been bracing itself for a difficult period primarily due to an anticipated 8 % decline in remittances (which accounts for over 10 % of its GDP), too appears to have targeted its stimulus mostly on infrastructure and tax cuts.

While infrastructure projects do create jobs, their effects are not apparent immediately. This is not enough to prevent poor families from embracing harmful coping strategies when crises strike. Social spending on healthcare and education, on the other hand, boosts economic recovery and also serves as safety nets that help prevent the immediate adoption of adverse coping strategies such as children being taken out of school and poorer families reducing visits to healthcare facilities.

Supply side spending on hospitals and schools also helps maintain the quality of social services during times of crisis. In a region that is marked by significant inter- and intracountry disparities, ensuring that children from poor, vulnerable families have unhindered access to quality education and healthcare during a crisis is vital. Spending on social protection in a region where there are high rates of precautionary savings due to a traditional lack of safety nets is also a smart choice. A rapid export-led recovery from this crisis is unlikely given the slump in global demand, so warding off precautionary spending to boost domestic demand makes eminent economic sense. It is also politically expedient as there were cases of unrest caused by rising food and fuel prices in 2009, which the lingering effects of the food price rises and economic shock might heighten.

Overall, the fiscal responses being enacted by governments in EAPR during the crisis have devoted a notable amount of spending on healthcare, education, and other types of social spending. This is a positive development as is the fact that even sans the stimuli packages, governments have taken steps to protect the poor and vulnerable. Maintaining regular social sector expenditure consistently is an example of this. Maintaining such commitments during the crisis to protect the achievement of the MDGs is crucial and should be applauded.

Other Government Responses

A number of common trends are visible in the other government responses to the crises, which began in early 2009. Many of these efforts gained further momentum after a high-level regional conference on the impact of the economic (and food price) crisis on children that was organized by the UNICEF EAP Regional Office (EAPRO) in partnership with the Lee Kuan Yew School of Public Policy and the Ministry of Foreign Affairs, Singapore, in January 2009. 150 leading policymakers (including more than a dozen ministers or vice-ministers, of whom four were ministers or vice-ministers of finance), academics, and practitioners from East Asia and the Pacific attended this conference. Drawing on lessons from 1997, its outcome was an enhanced understanding of the need to proactively take action to prevent the economic crisis from transmitting a full-blown social crisis, particularly to children.

Real-Time Monitoring and Surveillance

The lack of data on social indicators from the 1997 crisis, as confirmed in Singapore, was a timely rejoinder which helped governments realize the importance of tracking developments in the social sector during the current crises. UNICEF supported the initiation of some efforts as food prices shot up in 2008. Others began with the onset of the economic crisis. But countries that began with monitoring initiatives at that time have largely continued with these efforts as the economic crisis developed.

UNICEF has supported governments in ensuring that social indicators, particularly those that measure the impact on children, are included in many of these efforts.

In February 2009 EAPRO's Social Policy and Economic Analysis Section produced a concept note on monitoring the impact of the crisis on children in real time. Consisting of simple but effective indicators – to be collected in sentinel sites – as proxies for measuring educational attainment, health status of children, and commitment to social sector expenditures by governments, this idea was shared with governments and UNICEF offices throughout the region. It was presented at conferences in Lao PDR and Indonesia and shared with governments in Mongolia, the Pacific Island countries (PICs), and Cambodia, among others. It has been received positively by government counterparts who have requested UNICEF's technical assistance in devising country-specific methodologies to monitor vulnerabilities precipitated or exacerbated by the crisis on children and women.

A number of efforts have resulted from such requests:

Indonesia

In 2008, UNICEF and the World Food Programme (WFP) successfully helped the government develop and pilot a system to monitor the impact of high food prices at the household level in Greater Jakarta, East Java, Nusa Tenggara Timur (NTT), and Nusa Tenggara Barat (NTB). The government appreciated this system and adopted its methodology. In June 2009, a Food and Nutrition Security Monitoring System (FNSMS) at the household level was established in Indonesia.

Currently, the FNSMS pilot is being implemented by the Food Security Offices of four provinces (East Java, Nusa Tenggara Timur or NTT, Central Sulawesi, and West Kalimantan provinces), covering 20 more vulnerable districts (5 per province) selected based on the 2005 Indonesia Food Insecurity Atlas.

The pilot is jointly supported by UNICEF, WFP, and ILO. It also benefits from technical advice from the National Statistics Agency (BPS), SEAMEO TROPMED, University of Indonesia and Bogor Agriculture University.[2]

The FNMS produced its first bulletin in June to July 2009 and some of its noteworthy findings were as follows:

- Overall, 14 % of all surveyed households were food insecure, 30 % vulnerable, and 56 % food secure. More food insecure households were found in rural (20 %) than in urban areas (8 %).
- 56 % of all households (rural, 52 %; urban, 60 %) experienced difficulties in the previous 3 months, mostly due to the lack of cash, high food prices, health expenditures, agriculture/fishing-related difficulties, debt payment, and the increased cost of social events.

---

[2]http://www.unglobalpulse.org/projects/rivaf-research-study-impact-global-economic-and-financial-crisis-vulnerable-people-five-

- Because food insecurity was associated with underlying factors such as irregular and low remuneration cash income, low livestock, and assets, the situation was likely to be chronic rather than transitory.
- Households mostly adopted temporary, short-term coping strategies which were, so far, at an acceptable and non-depleted level to acquire food while seeking to protect their livelihoods. They mainly sought additional jobs, changed consumption pattern, and relied on credit to get food.

Lao PDR (LPDR)

The government of Lao PDR (LPDR) expressed its determination to take proactive measures to minimize the potential impacts of the economic crisis (UNICEF Lao PDR 2009) on children after the national consultation the UNICEF LPDR convened on 20 February 2009 as a follow-up to the regional UNICEF conference. At this meeting chaired by the Ministry of Planning and Investment (MPI), the government of Laos recognized the importance of establishing an early warning system that enables rapid detection of deterioration of social outcomes to respond quickly.

UNICEF was requested to provide technical support in facilitating the concerned ministries in achieving the above goal. It followed up by producing a concept note on monitoring the impact of the crisis on children in LPDR in the areas of health, education, and child protection using sentinel sites.

This note, which has been endorsed by the government, proposes that information be routinely collected on a weekly basis at grassroots level, in schools and health centers, which can be more systematically and more frequently passed upwards through the system and reviewed centrally. The Ministry of Industry and Commerce is already collecting consumer price data, including food prices, in eight sentinel markets in different areas of LPDR. This is compiled by the Department of Statistics every month and could serve as a useful alarm signal that nutritional status needs to be investigated in case of another food price spike or a significant deterioration of household income.

While the health and education monitoring methodology is being finalized, the child protection section, working with a local NGO called Friends International, has already collected some primary data from a focus group of street youths and parents to assess the impact of the food price and financial crises on this vulnerable segment of the population. Sentinel monitoring is within the capacities of sectoral ministries and would not incur additional costs. Technical support for establishing the surveillance system and drafting of the operation manual is being provided by UNICEF.

Mongolia

Mongolia's effort to initiate a real-time monitoring scheme has been led by its Deputy Prime Minister (DPM), an attendee at UNICEF's January 2009 Singapore Conference. UNICEF is providing technical and financial support in the development of the indicators, qualitative and quantitative information collection, and assisting with the scheme's development and monitoring implementation. The regional concept note was modified to make it more suitable to Mongolia's unique situation. The pilot – which was completed in December 2009 – was run from the DPM's office. The cabinet secretariat has been charged with the role of coordinating this effort among the ministries involved, namely, the Ministry of Health, Ministry of Education, Culture and Science, the Ministry of Social Welfare and Labour, and the Ministry of Justice and Home Affairs.

The pilot focused on two major channels of data collection. First, the sentinel sites selected (15 sites covering 250–280 households) consolidated information on the indicators selected through existing administrative systems. Mongolia's administrative data is very thorough, which rendered the establishment of a separate mechanism for primary data collection unnecessary. Second, a pulse survey of households explored the impact of the crisis on some 200 households vis-à-vis changes in their incomes, food intake, status of loans, changes in health and education expenditures, etc. This has been complemented by focus group discussions with children and young people as well as in-depth interviews with key informants such as relevant policymakers and service providers.

The sentinel sites themselves were chosen based on UNDP's poverty mapping. The poorest provinces and districts were selected in each of the country's five regions, including Ulaanbaatar. In each selected district/province, a sentinel school, dormitory, FGP and/or health center, police station, and convenience store/kiosk were identified. The 15 indicators monitored, classified by category, are as follows:

1. *Health*: Number of outpatients; number of children under age of one who had decrease in their weights; number of children aged 13 with decreased MUAC and number of people newly diagnosed with mental disorders
2. *Education*: Attendance among children of the 1st, 5th, and 7th grades; number of children living in dormitories who had visits to and/or from their households and/or received food, money, and others from their households
3. *Changes in livelihoods*: Number of people newly registered as unemployed; number of people who approached their respective administrative centers for certification to obtain small bank loans; number of people residing at garbage sites
4. *Protection*: Number of crimes; number of domestic violence cases
5. *Market price of some food and nonfood items*: Retail price of meat; retail price for flour (sort II); fuel price (АИ-80); price of sheepskin; goat down price

The results from the pilot are currently being translated before they can be analyzed to assess how to move forward.

The Pacific Island Countries (PICs)

UNICEF supported the initiation of the real-time monitoring efforts underway in the PICs. A number of key ministers and vice-ministers from the PICs – including the Finance Ministers of Kiribati and Vanuatu – had attended the Singapore Conference and expressed their interest to undertake a scheme to monitor the cumulative effects of the crises on the well-being of children and women. The PICs bore the brunt of the food price and fuel crises due to high transport costs and a sharp spike in the price of imported food, whose consumption has increased due to changing diet patterns.

Responding to government requests, UNICEF alongside other UN and regional agencies helped start the real-time social impact monitoring of the current economic crisis to identify the most vulnerable children and women before they are exposed to further risks. Eight PICs – Fiji, Solomon Islands, Tonga, Vanuatu, Kiribati, Federated States of Micronesia (FSM), and the Republic of Marshall Islands (RMI) – are partaking in this (FSM and RMI will join in 2010). A monitoring framework was proposed to identify adverse changes happening at the community level with a focus on the most susceptible groups across health, food and nutrition, education, and other social dimensions.[3]

The strategy has involved establishing 2–3 sentinel monitoring sites in the most vulnerable areas of each country covered including both urban and rural settings. Within each different sentinel site, services and communities will be assessed. The impact on education and health services and incidence of crime and violence will be monitored through facility based surveys and key informant interviews at schools, hospitals, health centers/clinics, pharmacy outlet, food markets, and police posts serving the concerned communities together with administrative data already collected at the national level. The impact at the household and the communities will be assessed through simple monitoring instruments such as small-scale pulse household survey and Focus Group Discussions (FGDs) which covers 30 households within the most vulnerable communities served by the facilities. Therefore, 60–90 households per country will be monitored throughout the cycle of data collections, which will be conducted on a quarterly basis and last at least for 2 years throughout 2009–2011.

The process is also nationally led. Sentinel site selection is driven by a National Steering Committee (NSC) headed by government focal ministries. Vulnerable areas in countries are defined locally and determined by comparative concentrations of some of those already considered to be facing hardship across most Pacific Island countries: (1) the young, (2) the old, (3) people living with disabilities, (4) those who had no source of regular income, (5) those with no access to adequate land on

[3]For more details, see Annex 1, UNICEF (2009).

which to grow food for consumption and/or sale, (6) households headed by women and the elderly.[4]

Initial results from Tonga are suggestive of the difficulties faced by PIC families and children: for instance, 60 % of those interviewed in the first round there suggested that it has become more difficult for them to pay school-related expenses compared to the year before. 77 % of households also said that they face greater difficulty in meeting daily expenditures compared to the same time the previous year. To cope, 75 % of them sought support from friends and relatives and 23–24 % of them used savings or sold/pawned household valuables to meet expenses.

The first round of data collection in most PICs has been completed by the end of February 2010. In addition to Tonga, Tuvalu, the Solomon Islands, Tuvalu, and Vanuatu too have issued preliminary results for this round. The second round of data is set to be gathered in July 2010 (with two further rounds scheduled in 2011).

Vietnam

The UNICEF Country Office is providing support in the Rapid Impact Monitoring (RIM) that has been in operation since mid-2009. It is being led by the Vietnam Academy of Social Sciences (VASS), which developed a concept note in April 2009 – with substantial inputs from UNICEF and UNDP – with four key objectives:

- Obtain information on the social impact of the crisis by examining how it is affecting employment and, beyond, how it is hitting people's livelihoods and (intra) household welfare.
- Learn about coping strategies by those groups of the population hit by the crisis.
- See whether existing government safety nets are able to cope with and address the new needs to social assistance emerging as a result of the crisis.
- Help in the formulation of policy initiatives that can effectively respond to new needs emerging as the crisis hits and unfolds in Vietnam.

This built upon the rapid assessments that VASS had undertaken in February and March–April 2009, supported by Oxfam GB, Action Aid, and the World Bank. The VASS concept note helped expand the scope of these assessments using a more comprehensive approach and selection of sentinel sites, hence increasing the exercise's ability to detect the social impacts of the crisis.

The RIM exercise is being undertaken in ten selected sentinel sites across the country. The sample includes five sites in rural areas and five in urban or peri-urban areas. The ten locations also cover two industrial zones (one in the North, one in the South), two urban areas with a high concentration of construction workers

[4]UN Joint Initiative on Global Economic Crisis Sentinel Site Monitoring in the Pacific Island Countries – Orientation, Training and Standardization Workshop Manual. http://www.unicef.org/pacificislands/9596_13613.html

(Hanoi and Ho Chi Minh City), a rural/coastal tourism site, a craft village, a rural site with substantial out-migration, a rural site with agricultural production for export, an "average" rural location, and a rural site with a high concentration of poor households.

The RIM exercises will be repeated at regular intervals. This is expected to help policymakers identify trends and emerging issues among affected groups, especially in terms of how the crisis impacts them, how workers and households cope with the impacts, how they are supported in their response, etc. It is also complementary to other layers of crisis monitoring information.[5]

Two rounds of rapid impacts monitoring (RIM) were conducted during the March to early May and August to September 2009 periods, respectively, to collect up-to-date information about the impact of the ongoing global economic crisis on firms, workers, and households, in order to provide timely inputs into the policymaking processes.

The final report detailing the findings from these two rounds of RIM has not been shared yet. But a preliminary copy has revealed a very impressive rebound in the labor market, which is beyond expectations of not only analysts, but of firms themselves as well. In the first round of RIM conducted in March and April 2009, unemployment or underemployment in the form of rotating shifts or short working hours was common, particularly among low-skilled workers. The opposite was observed in the second round: shortage of low-skilled labor prevails, be they migrant or non-migrant workers. Many export-oriented manufacturing firms are facing difficulties with recruitments for meeting new orders, which are now on the rise.

The importance of such data collected from lightweight monitoring initiatives that are not time and resource heavy cannot be overstated. There are two reasons for this. First, all information collected in real time will be useful in contributing to evidence-based efforts to assist governments in creating effective social protection measures that shield children from the worst effects of the crises. Second, in many cases, the International Financial Institutions have undertaken monitoring efforts that focus narrowly on macroeconomic impacts and their implications. It is important that indicators measuring outcomes for children are included in such efforts.

National Meetings to Build Consensus on Responses

Meetings, consultations, and conferences at the national level have been organized to mobilize and give momentum to policy responses that address social impacts of the crises.

---

[5]Concept note on undertaking a series of Rapid Impact Monitoring (RIM) exercises of the impact of the global financial crisis in Vietnam – more details at http://www.childimpact.unicef-irc.org/documents/view/id/64/lang/en

A conference in Indonesia on "Monitoring the Impact of the Global Economic Crisis on the Poor and Vulnerable in Indonesia" was jointly organized by BAPPENAS, UNICEF, UNDP, ILO, and WFP in March. In Thailand, UNICEF, UNDP, and the World Bank partnered with the National Economic and Social Development Board to organize a workshop in March 2009 on the Impact of the Financial Crisis in Thailand.

The Lao PDR conference in February 2009 was notable for reasons mentioned earlier and a similar opportunity was made use of in Myanmar when a Social Sector Analysis Workshop for senior government officials was conducted there at the end of July 2009.

The subregional conference in Vanuatu in February 2010 deserves particular mention due to the unique sources of vulnerabilities and manner in which Pacific Island nations have been affected by the crisis.

Conclusion

Despite the swift and severe impact of the global economic crisis on EAPR, which compounded the effects of other external shocks, many countries have been able to respond to the threats posed by these crises. But there are a number of low-income and commodity-exporting countries from the region that have been most affected by the shocks and have minimal fiscal cushions to mount robust responses. Attention must be paid to such countries in particular.

In the midst of all of this, it must be remembered that children face more severe risks than adults during economic crises. Unlike adults, they face increased risks of dying. While adults face risk of hunger, children face risk of permanent stunting. While adults face risk of temporary unemployment, children risk dropping out of school permanently (Patel 2009b). Progress in reducing income poverty is not sufficient in doing the same for child poverty. Governments must bear this in mind when they fashion responses to the crisis.

References

Asian Development Bank. (2008). *Key indicators for Asia and the Pacific 2008*. Manila: The Asian Development Bank.

Asian Development Bank. (2010, April). *Asian development outlook 2010: Macroeconomic management beyond the crisis* (Asian development outlook series). Manila: The Asian Development Bank. http://www.adb.org/sites/default/files/ADO/2010/PRC.pdf.

Bhutta, Z. A., Bawany, F. A., Feroze, A., Rizvi, A., Thapa, S. J., & Patel, M. (2009, April). Effects of the crises on child nutrition and health in East Asia and the Pacific. *Global Social Policy, 9*(Special Issue), 119–143.

Economist Intelligence Unit (EIU). (2009). *Country reports*. London: The Economist Intelligence Unit. http://www.eiu.com.

International Monetary Fund. (2010). *World economic outlook April 2010*. Washington, DC: International Monetary Fund.
Mendoza, R. (2009). Aggregate shocks, poor households and children: Transmission channels and policy responses. *Global Social Policy, 9*(Special Issue), 55–78.
Patel, M. (Ed.) (2009a). Children and the economic crisis in East Asia. *Global Social Policy, 9*(Special Issue). Thousand Oaks, CA: Sage Publications.
Patel, M. (2009b). Economic crisis and children: An overview for East Asian and the Pacific. *Global Social Policy, 9*(Special Issue), 33–54.
PricewaterhouseCoopers (PWC). (2010, January 21). Shift in world economic power means a decade of seismic change. *PricewaterhouseCoopers News Release*. http://www.pwc.com.br/pt/sala-de-imprensa/assets/release-pib-2030-uk.pdf.
The Economist. (2009). From slump to jump. *The Economist*. http://www.economist.com/node/14133744?story_id=14133744. Accessed 5 Aug 2009.
The Financial Times. (2009, February 10). Unlucky numbers. *The Financial Times*.
The Financial Times. (2009, September 10). Asia economic weather map. *The Financial Times*.
UNCTAD. (2009, March). *UNCTAD policy brief: Keeping ODA afloat*. Switzerland: UNCTAD Press.
UNICEF EAPR. (2007). *East Asia & Pacific in 2015: Implications for future UNICEF advocacy and action for children*. Draft report. Bangkok: UNICEF East Asia and Pacific Regional Office.
UNICEF. (2009, July). *Protecting Pacific children and women during food and economic crises*. Word edition one for advocacy, debate and guidance. http://www.unicef.org/pacificislands/Pacific_GEC_children_and_women_final_edition_one.pdf
UNICEF Cambodia. (2008). *Cambodia anthropometrics survey*. Phnom Penh: UNICEF Cambodia
UNICEF Lao PDR. (2009, February). *Potential impacts of the global financial crisis on children in Lao PDR and options for responses*. Paper presented at the Conference on Impact of the Economic Crisis on Children, Lee Kuan Yew School of Public Policy, Singapore, 6–7 January 2009.
UNICEF Viet Nam. (2008). *Children in Viet Nam – Who and where are the poor? The development and application of a multidimensional approach to child poverty*. Hanoi: UNICEF Viet Nam and MOLISA.
World Bank. (1993). *The East Asian miracle: Economic growth and public policy* (Vol. 1 of 2). A World Bank Policy Research Report. Washington, DC: Published by the Oxford University Press for the World Bank. http://documents.worldbank.org/curated/en/1993/09/698870/east-asian-miracle-economic-growth-public-policy-vol-1-2-main-report.
World Bank. (2008). *Global economic outlook 2009*. Washington, DC: World Bank.
World Bank. (2009a). *East Asia: Battling the forces of global recession*. Washington, DC: World Bank.
World Bank. (2009b). *Global monitoring report 2009*. Washington, DC: World Bank.
World Bank. (2009c). *Global development finance 2009*. Washington, DC: World Bank.
World Bank. (2010a). *East Asia: Emerging stronger from the crisis*. Washington, DC: World Bank.
World Bank. (2010b). *Global monitoring report 2010*. Washington, DC: World Bank.

Chapter 4
The Long Reach of Early Childhood Poverty

Greg J. Duncan and Katherine Magnuson

Introduction

Using a poverty line of about $22,000 for a family of four, the US Census Bureau counted more than 15 million US children living in poor families in 2009.[1] Poor children begin school well behind their more affluent age mates and, if anything, lose ground during the school years. On average, poor US kindergarten children have lower levels of reading and math skills and are rated by their teachers as less well behaved than their more affluent peers (Fig. 4.1). Children from poor families also go on to complete less schooling, work less, and earn less. Understanding the origins and persistence of these differences in fortunes is a vital step for ensuring the prosperity of future generations.

Our focus is on the causal role of low income in childhood for attainment and health later in life. Poverty is associated with a cluster of disadvantages that may be detrimental to children, such as low levels of parental education and living with a single parent. To determine how children would be affected by a policy that increased family incomes but did nothing else, we focus on distinguishing the effects of family income from those of other sources of disadvantage. In policy terms, this approach will enable us to answer the following question: To what extent are

[1]http://www.census.gov/hhes/www/cpstables/032010/pov/new01_100_01.htm

G.J. Duncan (✉)
School of Education, University of California, Irvine, CA, USA
e-mail: gduncan@uci.edu

K. Magnuson
School of Social Work, University of Wisconsin, Madison, WI, USA
e-mail: kmagnuson@wisc.edu

W.J.J. Yeung and M.T. Yap (eds.), *Economic Stress, Human Capital, and Families in Asia: Research and Policy Challenges*, Quality of Life in Asia 4,
DOI 10.1007/978-94-007-7386-8_4, © Springer Science+Business Media Dordrecht 2013

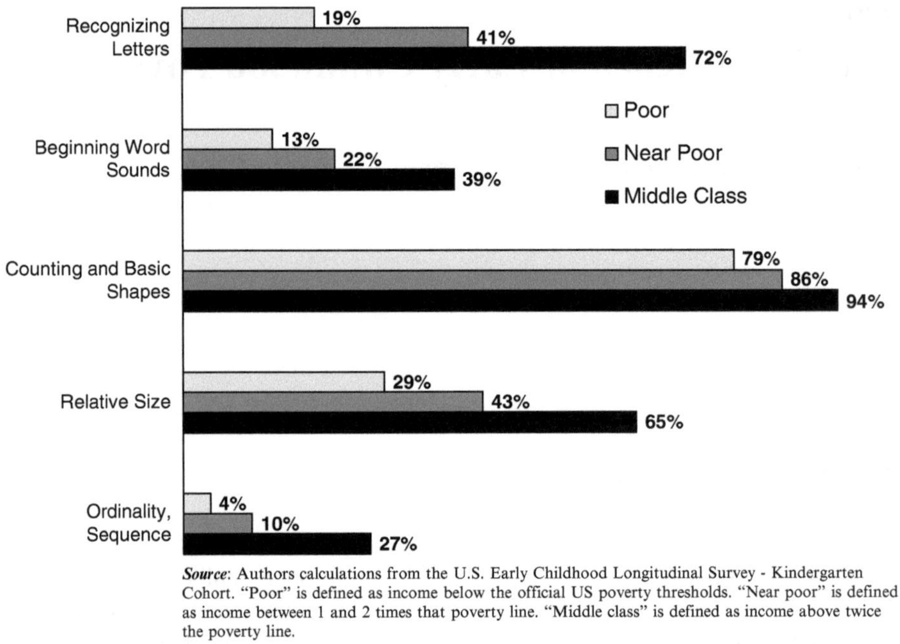

Fig. 4.1 Rates of kindergarten proficiencies for poor, near poor, and middle-class children (*Source*: Authors calculations from the US Early Childhood Longitudinal Survey – Kindergarten Cohort. "Poor" is defined as income below the official US poverty thresholds. "Near poor" is defined as income between 1 and 2 times that poverty line. "Middle class" is defined as income above twice the poverty line)

successes in adulthood affected by a policy such as a child allowance that provides the parents of poor children with more income, but does not directly change any other characteristic of their parents or family environments?

Social scientists have been investigating links between family poverty and subsequent child outcomes for decades. As in many research areas, early empirical studies were typically based on point-in-time cross-sectional data. The creation of nationally representative longitudinal data sets in the late 1960s and 1970s enabled researchers to test more refined and dynamic models of links between children's poverty experiences and later outcomes, which predicted, for example, that persistent poverty is more harmful than transient poverty. Remarkably, large-scale random-assignment social experiments that manipulated family income were conducted in the United States in the 1970s; however, most of them focused on the question of how additional income affected adult work effort rather than on child well-being.

Almost universally neglected in the poverty indicators and impacts literatures are careful thought about the *timing* of economic hardship across childhood and adolescence. Emerging research in neuroscience and developmental psychology suggests that poverty early in a child's life may be particularly harmful. Not only does the astonishingly rapid development of young children's brains leave them sensitive (and vulnerable) to environmental conditions, but the family context (as opposed to schools or peers) dominates young children's everyday lives.

After a brief review of possible mechanisms and both experimental and non-experimental evidence linking poverty with childhood outcomes, we highlight emerging research based on newly available data providing both poverty measures as early as the prenatal year and adult outcomes measured in the fourth decade of life. We conclude with thoughts about how policy attention might focus on deep and persistent poverty occurring early in childhood.

Poverty in the United States and Elsewhere

Social scientists disagree about how poverty should be defined and measured. Some scholars focus on income, others on indicators of material hardship; both approaches have merit. Townsend described poverty as income insufficient to enable individuals to "play the roles, participate in the relationships, and follow the customary behavior which is expected of them by virtue of their membership of society" (Townsend 1992: 10) and directed his research toward determining income levels that correspond to low scores on a deprivation index. Other researchers have defined poverty in terms of deprivation indicators such as lack of access to a telephone and appliances, or wearing used rather than new clothing, regardless of income level (see, e.g., Mack and Lansley 1985).

The official US definition of poverty is based on a comparison of a household's total income with a threshold level of income that varies with family size and inflation. Most cross-national work also bases poverty definitions on insufficient family income, but typically defines poverty thresholds as some fraction (e.g., 40 % or 50 %) of a country's median income. Drawing the poverty line at 50 % of median disposable income (about $29,000 for a family of three in today's dollars) classifies 16 % of the US population as poor (Fig. 4.2).[2] Poverty rates are considerably smaller in the United Kingdom and continental Europe and lowest in Scandinavian countries. Poverty rates in the two Asian countries that participate in the Luxembourg Income Study program – Taiwan and South Korea – are in between the United States and most other Western countries.

Poverty rates for children are considerably higher. Nearly one-quarter of US children are classified as poor using the 50 % of median standard (Fig. 4.3).[3] While higher than any of the countries in the study, the US rate is only a few points above rates in the United Kingdom, Canada, and Poland (comparable data on Asian countries are not available). More striking are the cross-country differences

[2]These data are drawn from Kim and Choi (2008).

[3]These data are drawn from Gornick and Jantti (2010).

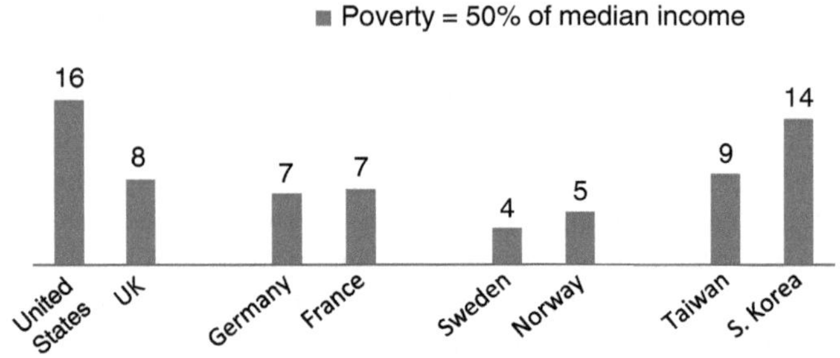

Fig. 4.2 Poverty rates for individuals (*Source*: Kim and Choi 2008)

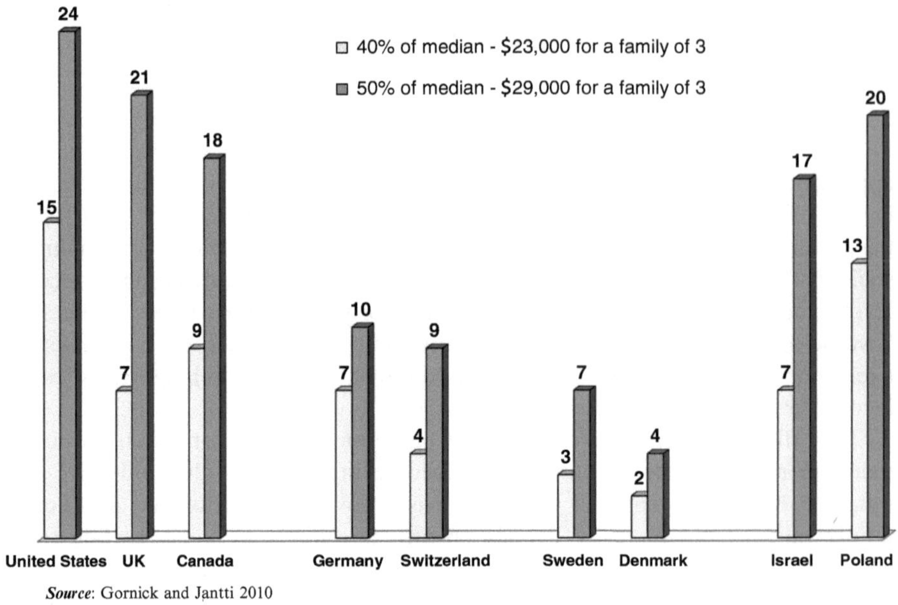

Fig. 4.3 Poverty rates for individuals (*Source*: Gornick and Jantti 2010)

when the poverty threshold is set at a more spartan 40 % of median disposable income (about $23,000). The 15 % US rate is more than half again as high as any country other than Poland. Thus deep poverty for US children is considerably more pervasive than among children in most Western industrialized countries.

Income-based poverty standards are less relevant and more difficult to measure in developing countries. Gordon et al. (2003) provide estimates of poverty in major regions of the world using a deprivation-based definition of poverty. They define levels of "severe deprivation of basic human need" for food, safe drinking water, sanitation facilities, health, shelter, education, information, and access to services. Based on survey data on children living in 46 countries in developing countries across the globe, they calculate the fraction of deprived children in each of these areas as well as fractions of children who are deprived in at least one of the areas.

Most striking are the large fractions of children living with at least one source of deprivation, which Gordon et al. (2003) estimate to constitute nearly half of all rural children and 12 % of all urban children – over a billion children worldwide. Children living in rural areas are consistently more deprived than children living in urban areas. Deprivation rates range widely, with the highest levels in sub-Saharan Africa where 78 % of rural children live with at least one source of deprivation while 25 % or a quarter of all urban children do so. Close behind are children in South Asia whose deprivation rates are at 70 % for rural children and 22 % for their urban counterparts. In the Middle East and North Africa, more than half (57 %) of rural children live with at least one source of deprivation, while in Latin America 41 % of them do so. Fewer urban children in both regions suffer deprivation – 9 % of those in the Middle East and North Africa and 6 % of those in Latin America. The lowest deprivation rates are found in East Asia and the Pacific, though even in these areas 9 % of rural children and 3 % of urban children live with at least one source of deprivation.

Why Poverty May Hinder Development

What are the consequences of growing up in a poor household? Economists, sociologists, developmental psychologists, and neuroscientists emphasize different pathways by which poverty may influence children's development. Economic models of child development focus on what money can buy (see, e.g., Becker 1981). They view families with greater economic resources as being better able to purchase or produce important "inputs" into their young children's development (e.g., nutritious meals, enriched home learning environments and child care settings outside the home, safe and stimulating neighborhood environments) and, with older children, higher-quality schools and post-secondary education.

Psychologists and sociologists point to the quality of family relationships to explain poverty's detrimental effects on children. These theoretical models point out that higher incomes may improve parents' psychological well-being and family processes, in particular the quality of parents' interactions with their children (Chase-Lansdale and Pittman 2002; McLoyd 1990; McLoyd et al. 1994). A long line of research has found that low-income parents, as compared with middle-class parents, are more likely to use an authoritarian and punitive parenting style and less likely to provide their children with stimulating learning experiences in the home. Poverty and economic insecurity take a toll on a parent's mental health, which may be an important cause of low-income parents' non-supportive parenting (McLoyd 1990). Depression and other forms of psychological distress can profoundly affect parents' interactions with their children (Zahn-Waxler et al. 2002).

Why Early Poverty May Matter the Most

We argue that the *timing* of child poverty matters and that for some outcomes later in life, particularly those related to achievement skills and cognitive development, poverty *early* in a child's life may be particularly harmful. Emerging evidence from human and animal studies highlights the critical importance of early childhood for brain development and for establishing the neural functions and structures that will shape future cognitive, social, emotional, and health outcomes (Sapolsky 2004; Knudsen et al. 2006). Two recent neuroscience studies show strong correlations between socioeconomic status and various aspects of brain function (Farah et al. 2006; Kishiyama et al. 2009).

Cuhna and his colleagues propose an economic model of development in which preschool cognitive and socio-emotional capacities are key ingredients for human capital acquisition during the school years (Cunha et al. 2005). In their model, "skill begets skill" and early capacities can affect the likelihood that later school-age human capital investments will be successful and productive. This model predicts that economic deprivation in early childhood creates disparities in school readiness and early academic success that widen over the course of childhood.

Support for the idea that children's early years are a fruitful time for intervention to improve educational and achievement outcomes for low-income and disadvantaged children comes from a number of intensive programs aimed at providing early care and educational experiences for high-risk infants and toddlers. The best known are the Abecedarian program, which provided a full-day, center-based, educational program for children who were at high risk for school failure, starting in early infancy and continuing until school entry, and the Perry Preschool program, which provided 1 or 2 years of intensive center-based education for preschoolers (Karoly 2001). Both of these programs have been shown to generate impressive long-term improvements in subsequent education, crime, and employment that are strongly associated with poverty.

Methods for Assessing Causal Impacts of Poverty

Regardless of the timing of low income, isolating its causal impact on children's well-being is very difficult. Poverty is associated with other experiences of disadvantage, rendering it difficult to know if it is poverty per se that really matters or other related experiences, for example, low maternal education or being raised in a single-parent family. The best method to identify how much money itself really matters is an experiment that compares families who receive some additional money to those who are otherwise similar, but do not receive such money.

The only large-scale randomized interventions to alter family income directly were the US Negative Income Tax Experiments, which were conducted between 1968 and 1982 with the primary goal of identifying the influence of guaranteed income on parents' labor force participation. Researchers found that elementary school children in the experimental group (whose families enjoyed a 50 % boost in family income from the program) exhibited higher levels of early academic achievement and school attendance than the control group (Maynard and Murnane 1979). No test score differences were found for adolescents, although youth in the experimental group did have higher rates of high school completion and educational attainment. This suggests that higher income may indeed cause higher achievement, although even in this case it is impossible to distinguish the effects of income from the possible benefits to children resulting from the reductions in parental work effort that accompanied the income increases.

Providing income support to working poor parents through wage supplements has been shown to improve children's achievement, according to data from experimental welfare reform evaluation studies undertaken during the 1990s. One study analyzed data from seven random-assignment welfare and antipoverty policies, all of which increased parental employment, while only some increased family income (Morris et al. 2001). Preschool and elementary school children's academic achievement was improved by programs that boosted both income and parental employment, but not by programs that only increased employment. The school achievement of adolescents did not appear to benefit from either kind of program.[4] A separate analysis of the data on younger children suggests that a $3,000 annual income boost is associated with about one-fifth of a standard deviation gain in achievement test scores (Duncan et al. 2011).

These findings suggest that income may play a causal role in younger children's achievement, although it should be kept in mind that the beneficial welfare reform programs increased both income and parental employment. Combining these results with those from the 1970s experiments reviewed above, it is apparent that income effects on younger children's achievement emerge when policies increase parental employment as well as when they decrease employment, which suggests that the income boost may have been the most active ingredient in the beneficial impacts.

Convincing evidence can sometimes be derived from nonexperimental studies that take care to ensure they are comparing families who differ in terms of income, but are otherwise similar. One such study took advantage of the fact that between 1993 and 1997, the maximum US Earned Income Tax Credit, which provides a credit to working poor families, increased by more than $2,000 for a family with two children (Dahl and Lochner 2008). This generous increase in tax benefits enabled the authors to compare the school achievement of children before and after the increase in the tax credit. They found improvements in low-income children's achievement in middle childhood that coincided with the policy change. A second, Canada-based study found similar results when it took advantage of variation across Canadian provinces in the generosity of the National Child Benefit program to estimate income impacts on child achievement (Milligan and Stabile 2008).

---

[4]Though leveraging experimental data, the analysis itself is not an experiment as families were not randomly assigned across types of treatments.

Linking Early Poverty to Adult Outcomes

None of this past income literature has been able to relate family income early in a child's life to adult attainments, largely because data on both early childhood income and later adult outcomes had not been collected in one study. However, recent research has made this link using data from the Panel Study of Income Dynamics, which has followed a nationally representative sample of US families and their children since 1968 (Duncan et al. 2010).

The study is based on children born between 1968 and 1975, for whom adult outcomes were collected between ages 30 and 37. The study measured income in every year of a child's life from the prenatal period through age 15. This enabled Duncan and colleagues to measure poverty across several distinct periods of childhood, distinguishing income early in life (prenatal through fifth year) from income in middle childhood and adolescence. The simple associations between income early in life and adult outcomes are striking (Table 4.1). Compared with children whose families had incomes of at least twice the poverty line during their early childhood, poor children completed two fewer years of schooling, earned less than half as much, worked 451 fewer hours per year, received \$826 per year more in food stamps as adults, and are nearly three times as likely to report poor overall health. Poor males are more than twice as likely to be arrested. For females, poverty is associated with a more than fivefold increase in the likelihood of bearing a child out of wedlock prior to age 21.

Building on these simple associations, Duncan and colleagues estimate a series of regressions shown in Table 4.2. The first row shows correlations between each adult outcome and 5-year average childhood income (Model 1).[5] The directions of all of

Table 4.1 Adult outcomes by poverty status between the prenatal year and age 5

	Income below the official US poverty line	Income between one and two times the poverty line	Income more than twice the poverty line
	Mean or %	*Mean or %*	*Mean or %*
Completed schooling	11.8 year	12.7 year	14.0 year
Earnings (\$10,000)	\$17.9	\$26.8	\$39.7
Annual work hours	1,512	1,839	1,963
Food stamps	\$896	\$337	\$70
Poor health	13 %	13 %	5 %
Arrested (men only)	26 %	21 %	13 %
Nonmarital birth (women only)	50 %	28 %	9 %

Note: Earnings and food stamp values are in 2005 dollars
Source: Duncan et al. (2010)

[5]In fact, the natural logarithm of income is used for these correlations. Using income rather than log income assumes that a \$1,000 increment to a poor family's annual income has the same

Table 4.2 Unadjusted and adjusted correlations between childhood income and adult outcomes

	Income measure	Schooling (years)	Annual earnings	Annual work hours	Food stamps	Poor health	Arrested	Nonmarital birth
Model 1: Bivariate associations	Prenatal to age 15 average family income	.41**	.38**	.22**	−.38**	−.18**	−.15**	−.34**
Model 2: Associations adjusted for differences in family background	Prenatal to age 15 average family income	.22**	.37**	.20**	−.24**	−.08*	−.13†	−.18**
Model 3: Associations with childhood stage-specific income, adjusted for differences in family background	Family income averaged over:							
	Prenatal to age 5	.10*	.27**	.20**	−.08†	.07	−.11	.02
	Age 6–10	−.04	.06	−.03	−.12*	−.05	.11	.07
	Age 11–15	.18**	.08	.06	−.06	−.11†	−.17†	−.27**

"Background controls" consist of birth year, race, sex, whether the child's parents were married and living together at the time of the birth, mother's age at birth, region, number of siblings, parent schooling, parent test score, cleanliness of the house, parent's expectations for child, parent achievement motivation, parent locus of control, and parent risk avoidance. All incomes are in natural logarithm form, but all of the table entries reflect standard deviation changes in a given outcome associated with a one standard deviation increase in log income

Source: Based on Duncan et al. (2010)

Note: $^{**}p < .01$; $^{*}p < .05$; $^{\dagger}p < .10$

the correlations are as expected – positive for "good" outcomes and negative for "bad" ones – and statistically significant for each outcome. The largest correlations, all in the .3–.4 range, are found for schooling, adult earnings, and nonmarital births.

In the second row, these correlations are adjusted for an extensive set of background control variables (listed at the bottom of Table 4.2), all of which are measured either before or near the time of birth (Model 2). This effort to separate income from other related disadvantages and characteristics of poor children finds that most correlations are reduced by the introduction of these statistical controls. This, in turn, suggests that often a substantial portion of the simple correlation between childhood income and most adult outcomes can be accounted for by the disadvantageous conditions associated with birth into a low-income household.

But what about the timing of poverty? To better understand if poverty in early childhood itself is particularly important in a final set of analyses, Duncan and colleagues replaced the average childhood income measure used in Model 2 with three stage-specific measures of log income. As before, adjustments are made for the effects of the extensive list of background controls. If childhood income mattered equally across all three stages, the three correlations should be roughly the same size and about one-third the magnitude of the Model 3 correlations.

In the case of adult earnings and work hours, early childhood income appears to matter much more than later income. The adjusted correlation for work hours and the prenatal to age 5 log average income (.20) is every bit as large as the coefficient on all-childhood log average income (Model 2), suggesting little role for income beyond age 5. Early income also appears to matter for completed schooling, but in this case adolescent family income has a considerably larger standardized coefficient. In contrast, the strong association between overall childhood income and health and nonmarital birth, seems to be largely attributed to income during adolescence, rather than earlier in childhood.

More detailed analyses carried out by Duncan and colleagues found that for families with average early childhood incomes below $25,000, a $3,000 annual boost to family income was associated with a 17 % increase in adult earning (Fig. 4.4). Results for work hours are broadly similar to those for earnings – a highly significant estimated impact of early childhood but not later childhood income. In this case, a $3,000 annual increase in the prenatal to age 5 income of low-income families is associated with 135 additional work hours per year after age 25. In contrast, increments to early childhood income for higher-income children were not significantly associated with higher adult earnings or work hours.

Further work showed that adult attainment measures – earnings, work, the absence of receipt of welfare income, and "on-time" completed schooling – were

---

beneficial effect on a child's adult outcomes as a $1,000 increment to an affluent family's income. The logarithmic transformation assumes equal percentage effects. So, for example, the logarithmic model presumes that a 50 percent (and $5,000) increase in average childhood income from $10,000 to $15,000 has the same effect as the 50 percent (but $50,000) increase from $100,000 to $150,000. The log income models fit the data considerably better than the income models.

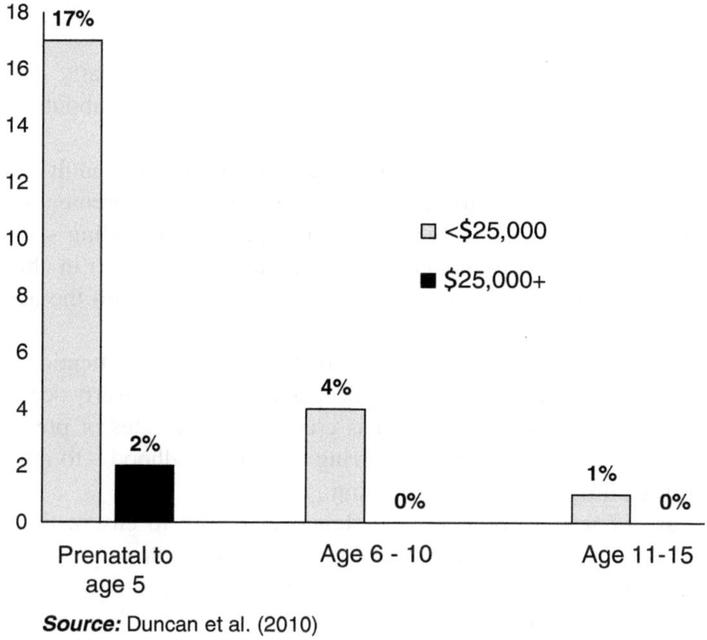

Fig. 4.4 Percentage increases in adult earnings associated with a $3,000 annual increase in childhood income (*Source*: Duncan et al. 2010)

generally quite responsive to income increases in early childhood. In contrast, most adult behavior and health measures were more likely to be responsive to income increases later in childhood as well, although the patterns were not nearly as consistent as those found for the attainment measures.

Some Policy Implications

Our review points to early childhood as a particularly sensitive period in which economic deprivation may compromise children's life achievement and employment opportunities. Of greatest conceptual interest is the remarkable sensitivity of developing brain structures and functions as well as the growing list of brain functions that differ between children raised in high and low socioeconomic circumstances. From the social sciences comes convincing evidence linking early poverty with both child achievement and adult employment. The achievement studies employ unusually rigorous methods for estimating causal relationships between income early in life and achievement test scores. The effect sizes estimated in these studies are broadly similar, with $3,000 annual income increases sustained for several years appearing to boost children's achievement by roughly one-fifth of a standard deviation.[6]

In the early grades, children's achievement increases by nearly one standard deviation per year, so 20 % of a standard deviation amounts to about a 2 months' advantage.

Very recent research has linked poverty early in childhood to adult earnings and work hours. Although not as strong methodologically as the aforementioned quasi-experimental studies of child achievement, the study's key finding – that income early in childhood appears to matter much more than income later in childhood for a range of employment outcomes – is strikingly consistent with the achievement studies.

Taken together, this research suggests that greater policy attention should be given to remediating situations involving deep and persistent poverty occurring early in childhood. In terms of indicators, it is crucial to track rates of poverty among children – especially deep poverty occurring early in childhood – to inform policy discussions regarding children's well-being.

In the case of welfare policies, we should take care to ensure that sanctions and other regulations do not deny benefits to families with very young children. Not only do young children appear to be most vulnerable to the consequences of deep poverty, but mothers with very young children are also least able to support themselves through employment in the labor market.

More generous would be income-transfer policies that provide more income to families with young children. In the case of work support programs like the Earned Income Tax Credit, this might mean extending more generous credits to families with young children. In the case of child tax credits, this could mean making the credit refundable and also providing larger credits to families with young children.

Interestingly, several European countries gear time-limited benefits to the age of children in their assistance programs. In Germany, a modest parental allowance is available to a mother working fewer than 20 h per week until her child is 18 months old. France guarantees a modest minimum income to most of its citizens, including families with children of all ages. Supplementing this basic support is the *Allocation de Parent Isolé* (API) program for lone parents with children under age 3. In effect, the API program acknowledges a special need for income support during this period, especially if a parent wishes to care for very young children and forgo income from employment. The state-funded child care system in France beginning at age 3 alleviates the problems associated with a parent's transition into the labor force.

In emphasizing the potential importance of policies to boost income in early childhood, we do not mean to imply that focusing on this area is the only policy path worth pursuing. Obviously investments later in life and those that provide direct services to children and families may also be well advised. Economic logic requires a comparison of the costs and benefits of the various programs that seek to

---

[6]These effect sizes are based on the full samples used in Milligan and Stabile (2008) and the low-income subsample used in Dahl and Lochner (2008).

promote the development of disadvantaged children throughout the life course. In this context, expenditures on income-transfer and service-delivery programs should be placed side by side and judged by their benefits and society's willingness to pay for the outcomes they produce, relative to their costs.

Acknowledgment An earlier version of this paper was prepared for the *International Conference on Economic Stress, Human Capital, and Families in Asia: Research and Policy Challenges*, which took place June 3–4, 2010, at the National University of Singapore. We greatly appreciate the helpful comments and other assistance from Jean Yeung and Tom Boyce.

References

Becker, G. (1981). *A treatise on the family*. Cambridge, MA: Harvard University Press.

Chase-Lansdale, P. L., & Pittman, L. (2002). Welfare reform and parenting: Reasonable expectations. *The Future of Children, 12*, 167–185.

Cunha, F., Heckman, J. J., Lochner, L., & Masterov, D. (2005). Interpreting the evidence on life cycle skill formation. In E. Hanushek & F. Welch (Eds.), *Handbook of the economics of education* (pp. 697–812). Amsterdam/London: North-Holland.

Dahl, G., & Lochner, L. (2008). *The impact of family income on child achievement* (NBER Working Paper No. 14599). Cambridge, MA: National Bureau of Economic Research.

Duncan, G., Ziol-Guest, K., & Kalil, A. (2010). Early childhood poverty and adult attainment, behavior and health. *Child Development, 81*(1), 306–325.

Duncan, G., Morris, P., & Rodrigues, C. (2011). Does money matter? Estimating impacts of family income on young children's achievement with data from random-assignment experiments. *Developmental Psychology, 47*(5), 1263–1279.

Farah, M. J., Shera, D. M., Savage, J. H., Betancourt, L., Giannetta, J. M., & Brodsky, N. L. (2006). Childhood poverty: Specific associations with neurocognitive development. *Brain Research, 1110*, 166–174.

Gordon, D., Nandy, S., Pantazis, C., Pembertonj, S., & Townsend, P. (2003). *Child poverty in the developing world*. Bristol: The Policy Press.

Gornick, J., & Jantti, M. (2010). Child poverty in upper-income countries: Lessons from the Luxembourg income study. In S. B. Kamerman, S. Phipps, & A. Ben-Arieh (Eds.), *From child welfare to child well-being: An international perspective on knowledge in the service of making policy* (pp. 339–370). A special volume in honor of Alfred J. Kahn. Dordrecht: Springer.

Karoly, L. (2001). Investing in the future: Reducing poverty through human capital programs. In S. Danziger & R. Haveman (Eds.), *Understanding poverty in America: Progress and problems* (pp. 314–346). Cambridge, MA: Harvard University Press.

Kim, J., & Choi, Y. (2008). *Private transfers and emerging welfare states in East Asia: Comparative perspectives* (Luxembourg Income Study Working Paper No. 507). Luxembourg.

Kishiyama, M., Boyce, W., Jimenez, A., Perry, L., & Knight, R. (2009). Socioeconomic disparities affect prefrontal function in children. *Journal of Cognitive Neuroscience, 21*(6), 1106–1115.

Knudsen, E., Heckman, J., Cameron, J., & Shonkoff, J. (2006). Economic, neurobiological, and behavioral perspectives on building America's future workforce. *PNAS, 103*, 10155–10162.

Mack, J., & Lansley, S. (1985). *Poor Britain*. London: George Allen and Unwin, Ltd.

Maynard, R., & Murnane, R. (1979). The effects of a negative income tax on school performance: Results of an experiment. *Journal of Human Resources, 14*(4), 463–476.

McLoyd, V. (1990). The impact of economic hardship on black families and children: Psychological distress, parenting and socioeconomic development. *Child Development, 61*, 311–346.

McLoyd, V. C., Jayaratne, T. E., Ceballo, R., & Borquez, J. (1994). Unemployment and work interruption among African American single mothers: Effects on parenting and adolescent socioemotional functioning. *Child Development, 65*, 562–589.

Milligan, K., & Stabile, M. (2008). *Do child tax benefits affect the wellbeing of children? Evidence from Canadian child benefit expansions* (NBER Working Paper No. 14264). Cambridge, MA: National Bureau of Economic Research.

Morris, P., Huston, A., Duncan, G., Crosby, D., & Bos, H. (2001). *How welfare and work policies affect children: A synthesis of research*. New York: MDRC.

Sapolsky, R. (2004). Mothering style and methylation. *Nature Neuroscience, 7*, 791–792.

Townsend, P. (1992). *The international analysis of poverty*. Hemel Hempstead: Harvester-Wheatsheaf.

Zahn-Waxler, C., Duggal, S., & Gruber, R. (2002). Parental psychopathology. In M. H. Bornstein (Ed.), *Handbook of parenting* (2nd ed., Vol. 4, pp. 95–328). Mahwah: Lawrence Erlbaum Associates, Inc.

Part II
Women, Children and Economic Stress

Chapter 5
The 1997 Economic Crisis, Changes in the Pattern of Achieved Fertility and Ideal Number of Children in Korea

Doo-Sub Kim

Introduction

Over the past decade, economic depression and labor market insecurity have been accompanied by a remarkable demographic transition in East and Southeast Asian societies. Korea, for example, has witnessed a drastic decline in the level of fertility after the 1997 Asian economic crisis. The total number of births in 2010 was estimated at 470,171 revealing a 29.7 % reduction from 668,344 births in 1997. The total fertility rate (TFR) was recorded at 1.23 in 2010, down from 1.52 in 1997 (Statistics Korea 2011). The TFR of Korea is currently at the lowest level in the world except for Hong Kong, Macau, and Taiwan (Population Reference Bureau 2009). Similar phenomena of rapid fertility decline have also been observed in Japan, Singapore, and Taiwan.

Most demographers did not foresee the steepest fertility declines in human history in these societies. There is no doubt, however, that the 1997 economic crisis marked an important turning point in the process of fertility transition of Korean society. Korean fertility has shown the most drastic declines during the past decade and has eventually fallen down to merely half of the replacement level. Labor market deregulation and high unemployment associated with a poorly performing economy have made many young people delay or avoid marriage and childbearing. The negative effects of economic recession and increased insecurity in the labor market on the level of fertility have also been substantial among those in their forties (Kim 2009).

Up to the mid-1980s, there was an enormous amount of theoretical and empirical research on socioeconomic differentials in Korean fertility (Kim et al. 1974; Cho et al. 1982; Kwon 1982; Kim, D. S. 1987; Kim, I. K. 1987). In contrast, only a few

D.S. Kim (✉)
Department of Sociology, Hanyang University, Seoul, South Korea
e-mail: duskim@hanyang.ac.kr

W.J.J. Yeung and M.T. Yap (eds.), *Economic Stress, Human Capital, and Families in Asia: Research and Policy Challenges*, Quality of Life in Asia 4,
DOI 10.1007/978-94-007-7386-8_5, © Springer Science+Business Media Dordrecht 2013

studies have been conducted during the past decades to explore the changing pattern of socioeconomic differentials in the transition to an ultra-low fertility context (Eun 2003; Kim 2005, 2007, 2009; Kim et al. 2006; Yoo 2006). As yet, we do not have satisfactory explanations for the nature of the recent transition to ultra-low fertility or the extent of the fertility impact of the recent economic recession among different socioeconomic groups. Nor is it clear what causal mechanisms have operated in changing the pattern of achieved and desired fertility.

The main purpose of this study is to explore the effects of the 1997 Asian economic crisis on the level of achieved and desired fertility and the pattern of socioeconomic differentials. This chapter explores recent changes in the level of fertility and ideal number of children according to the socioeconomic status of the couple. Attention is given to the construction of a theoretical model of differential fertility. Utilizing data from *the 2006 Korean National Fertility, Family Health and Welfare Survey*, this study focuses on a comparative analysis of children ever born (CEB) and the post-1998 CEB of married women. For the second round of comparative analysis, the study population is split into two groups, i.e., those married before 1997 and those married for the first time after the economic crisis. The level of fertility and ideal number of children as well as the pattern of socioeconomic differentials of the two groups are compared.

Trends in Fertility-Related Indicators After the 1997 Asian Economic Crisis

There is no doubt that the 1997 Asian economic crisis has exerted a profound impact on all spheres of Korean society, and fertility is not an exception. High unemployment due to increased insecurity in the labor market and expansion of poverty after the 1997 crisis have influenced the timing and magnitude of marriage and childbearing. The singulate mean age at marriage (SMAM) of women rose from 25.5 in 1996 to 28.9 in 2010. Korea also witnessed rapid downward trends in the number of marriages and the crude marriage rate after reaching a peak of 434,911 and 9.4 per thousand, respectively, in 1996. As of 2010, the counterpart figures were estimated to be 326,104 and 6.5 per thousand, respectively. In contrast, economic hardship after the 1997 crisis has expedited family dissolution. The number of divorces was estimated as 166,617 in 2003, up from 79,895 in 1996. During the same period, the crude divorce rate increased rapidly from 1.7 to 3.4 per thousand (Statistics Korea 2011).

Delay in the timing of childbearing has become prominent after the 1997 crisis. The mean age at first birth rose from 26.9 in 1997 to 30.1 in 2010. The mean age at second birth also rose from 29.1 to 32.0 during the same period. A marked downward trend in fertility rate for the prime reproductive age group has been observed. The fertility rate for women aged 25–29 declined 8.9 % during the 2 years immediately after the 1997 crisis and 50.7 % during the period 1997–2010 (Statistics Korea 2011).

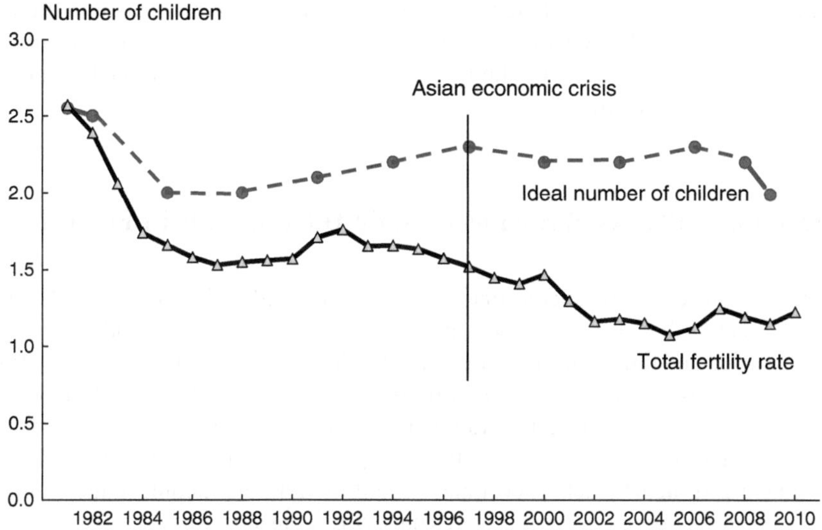

Fig. 5.1 Trends in total fertility rate and ideal number of children, Korea, 1981–2010 (*Sources*: Statistics Korea 2011; KIHASA 1982, 1988, 1994, 2000, 2009)

Figure 5.1 shows a marked downward trend TFR since 1981. TFR dropped from 2.57 births per woman in 1981 to a replacement level of 2.1 by 1983. The fertility transition has continued to accelerate after the 1997 economic crisis, even though slight upturns were noticed in 2000, 2006, and 2007. These minor upturns were mainly due to the superstitious beliefs of many Koreans on the auspiciousness of these specific birth years according to the animal cycle of the lunar calendar. In 2005, TFR was estimated at 1.08, the lowest recorded in the history of Korea. The pace of TFR decline in Korea was even faster than in Japan (United Nations 2011).

In a series of *Korean National Fertility Surveys* conducted by the KIHASA, attitudinal questions have been addressed to the wife regarding the ideal number of children: "What do you think is the ideal number of children for a family to have?" Attempts have been made to analyze the INC in comparison with actual fertility. Some demographers have used INC statistics as a guide in projecting the future fertility of the cohorts considered.

As shown in Fig. 5.1, INC reveals a different pattern of change from that of TFR. Both INC and TFR were estimated to be as high as 2.6 in 1981. After a substantial drop during the first half of the 1980s, INC has maintained a relatively stable level between 2.2 and 2.3. In contrast to TFR declines, no significant change in INC is observed after the 1997 economic crisis. It is also clear in this figure that INC has always been higher than actual fertility, measured as TFR, and the gap between the two has been widening since 1982.

This implies that Korea's descent to ultra-low fertility during the past decade has not been accompanied by major changes in values and norms related to family size.

Rather, it can mostly be attributed to factors related to economic hardship after the 1997 crisis. Detailed discussion on changes and differentials in achieved fertility, measured in CEB, and INC by the major educational and occupational groups are provided in a later section.

Changing Patterns of Socioeconomic Differentials in Fertility

Interest in the effect of socioeconomic status on fertility is not recent. Malthus believed that higher income induces people to get married earlier and abstain less while married and thus, leads to a large increase in family size (cited in Becker 1960: 212). Numerous studies have resulted in the construction of theoretical models for the analysis of fertility. In turn, studies have applied these conceptual models to empirical data from various sources. Beginning in the late 1950s, based on concepts of demand and factors such as cost and benefit of children, income, education, and other indicators of socioeconomic status have been considered as the most important determinants of fertility. Many economists have analyzed demand for children based on family income from a microeconomic perspective and have contributed to our understanding of differential fertility (Leibenstein 1957, 1975, 1977, 1981; Becker 1960; Freedman 1963; Mincer 1963; Easterlin 1969, 1975; Willis 1973; Cain and Weininger 1973; Andorka 1978; Mueller and Short 1983). It was argued that education directly contributes to fertility reduction by shaping certain attitudes, values, and beliefs toward a smaller family (Mueller 1972; Cochrane 1979; Choe and Retherford 2009). Education also affects other variables that have direct or indirect effects on fertility. It has been widely accepted that a woman's education is positively related with family income and tends to delay age at marriage.

Classic studies conducted in various countries have shown a generally negative relationship between indicators of socioeconomic status and fertility. Becker (1960) argued that a rise in income would lead to higher quality elasticity of children and more effective contraception and contribute to fertility reduction. Many economists maintain that income, other things being equal, is positively related with fertility (Becker 1960; Namboodiri 1970). Achieved fertility, desired fertility, and ideal family size were found to decrease with increased education regardless of residence and work experience (Yaukey 1963; Chung et al. 1972; Speare et al. 1973; Freedman et al. 1974).

During the past half a century, however, various results have been found in empirical studies that attempt to relate socioeconomic status to fertility at the micro and macro level. After reviewing differential fertility in Western countries, Wrong (1958) argued that three different types of relation between socioeconomic status and fertility represent different stages in a process of transition from the inverse pattern. The negative and linear pattern of the relationship yields first to a reverse *J*-shaped curve, which is later succeeded by a *U*-shaped pattern. Ultimately, relatively stationary populations with low fertility are characterized by the emergence of a positive relation between socioeconomic status and fertility (Wrong 1958).

Based on his comparative analysis using US and Korean data, Kim D. S. (1987) argued that a cubic relationship between socioeconomic status and fertility can be generalized across the development level of countries. As socioeconomic status rises at a low level, fertility tends to rise. Then the relationship becomes negative as socioeconomic status rises further to a certain point, after which a rise of fertility occurs again for the highest socioeconomic group. However, it was suggested that the range of the fertility curve is dependent on the socioeconomic level of a specific country. The high and low limits of socioeconomic status would move rightward in more developed countries and move leftward in less developed countries. This leads to conjecture that the pattern of socioeconomic differentials in a specific country would follow such a process of evolution in the course of socioeconomic development (Kim, D. S. 1987).

The present study attempts to decompose fertility into three factors: demand for children, fertility regulation, and fecundity. It is designed to examine the effect of socioeconomic status on each of these three component factors. A modified microeconomic model of demand for children is applied into the theoretical framework. As socioeconomic status rises, opportunity cost and desire for relative goods that have negative effects on demand for children also increase. In addition, economic utility of children as a source of income and as a source of security after the parents' retirement declines as socioeconomic status rises. These factors raise the relative cost of children and thus make the couple lower their demand for children to maximize their economic and noneconomic utility. Without being constrained by these factors, however, a couple in the highest socioeconomic group can afford to have more children, and demand for children increases again as socioeconomic status rises above a certain point.

Socioeconomic status also influences fertility regulation. Contraceptive knowledge and services become more available and acceptable as socioeconomic status rises. Therefore, a couple can regulate their fertility more effectively and have lower unwanted fertility. It is assumed in this study that nutritional and health factors do not raise or impede fecundity substantially regardless of socioeconomic status. From this theoretical background, as indicated by the curve of CEB in Fig. 5.2a, a quadratic relationship between socioeconomic status and fertility is hypothesized in this chapter. Among those in the low and middle socioeconomic groups, the relationship between socioeconomic status and CEB is negative. For the highest socioeconomic group, CEB is likely to be positively related with socioeconomic status.

It is postulated in this chapter that a reverse *J*-shaped pattern of the relationship between socioeconomic status and fertility was succeeded by a slightly positive relationship, in general, in the process of transition to ultra-low fertility after the 1997 economic crisis. For the highest socioeconomic group, however, the relationship is likely to become a slightly negative one: fertility is likely to decline slightly as socioeconomic status rises above a certain point of high family income, education of wife, or occupational prestige of husband. A new model of hypothesized relationship between socioeconomic status and fertility for an ultra-low fertility context is presented in Fig. 5.2b.

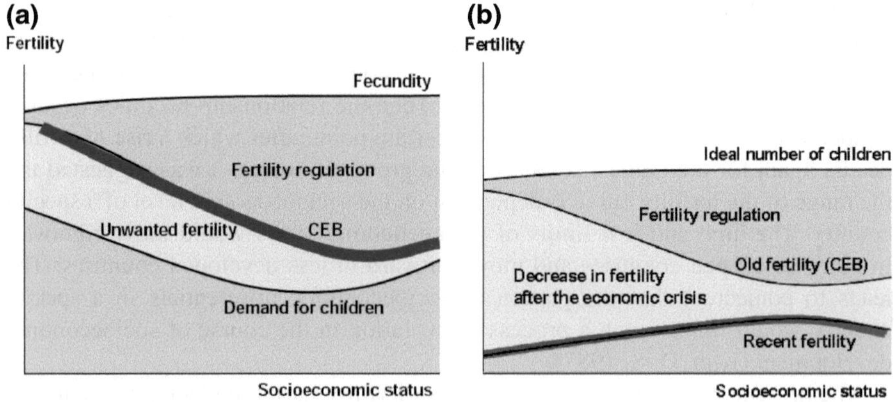

Fig. 5.2 Hypothesized relationship between socioeconomic status and fertility. (**a**) The old model. (**b**) A new model for an ultra-low fertility context

It is assumed that decrease in fertility after the 1997 economic crisis has been most drastic among those in the low socioeconomic group with a high level of fertility and relatively slow for those with a low level of fertility. A remarkable increase in unemployment, layoffs, and part-time and temporary jobs during the past decade has played a decisive role in delaying marriage and widening the birth interval particularly among those with low socioeconomic status. The relative deprivation of those in the low socioeconomic group becomes greater in the process of increasing inequality. In particular, the psychological burden of child education expenditures has become much more serious among metropolitan residents. Thus they tend to emulate the status-related and child-rearing expenditures of those with higher socioeconomic status rather than have more children. With a bad economy and serious job insecurity after the crisis, they have not had many choices other than drastically reducing their level of fertility (Kim 2009).

Increasing inequality has also led those in the highest socioeconomic group to be exposed to and spend more on status-related and status-differentiating expenditures, which compete with children for the couple's income, and reduce their family size. Compared to those in the next group in the socioeconomic hierarchy, they have responded more sensitively to fears of social slippage and labor market insecurity combined with an unpredictable economic recovery. Thus, a negative association between socioeconomic status and fertility may appear among those in the highest socioeconomic group. As a result, level of fertility is likely to be highest among those with upper-middle socioeconomic status, followed by those with the highest socioeconomic status, and finally those with the lowest status.

Hypotheses

Based on the theoretical concerns and findings from previous studies, several hypotheses are proposed in this chapter. The first hypothesis is drawn from the old model shown in Fig. 5.2a, and the next three hypotheses are from a new model shown in Fig. 5.2b for an ultra-low fertility context:

1. Those with low and middle socioeconomic status are likely to have fewer CEB as socioeconomic status rises. For the highest socioeconomic group, CEB is likely to rise slightly as socioeconomic status rises.
2. In an ultra-low fertility context, the relationship between socioeconomic status and the level of recent fertility is slightly positive. For the highest socioeconomic group, the level of recent fertility is likely to decrease slightly as socioeconomic status rises.
3. In an ultra-low fertility context, INC is not likely to be affected substantially by socioeconomic status.
4. Decrease in fertility after the economic crisis has been most drastic among those with the highest level of fertility and relatively slow for those with a lower level of fertility.

Data and the Study Population

The main data set to be used for the analysis is from *the 2006 Korean National Fertility, Family Health and Welfare Survey*. This study focuses on 4,739 women aged 25–44 and currently married at the time of this survey. The number of CEB and the post-1998 CEB are estimated in order to analyze recent changes in the level of fertility and the pattern of socioeconomic differentials in fertility. For the second round of comparative analysis of fertility, the sample of this study is divided into two groups. The first group contains 2,829 women who married before 1997 or who remarried regardless of their timing of marriage. The second group includes 1,910 women who married for the first time in 1997 or thereafter. The ideal numbers of children as well as the pattern of socioeconomic differentials in CEB for these two groups are also compared. It is assumed that the second group reveals a pattern of socioeconomic differentials in CEB similar to the pattern of the post-1998 CEB in the first round of analysis: both reflect reproductive behavior during the period from 1997 to 2006. The basic demographic profiles of the study population are presented in Table 5.1.

The mean CEB of women aged 25–44 and currently married is estimated at 1.8. When the sample is divided into two subgroups, the counterpart figures for Group A (women married before 1997 or remarried) and Group B (women married for

Table 5.1 Demographic profile of the study population

	Currently married (aged 25–44)					
	Group A		*Group B*			
	Married before 1997		First married in or after 1997		Total	
	Mean	*N*	Mean	*N*	Mean	*N*
CEB	2.0	2,829	1.3	1,910	1.8	4,739
Post-1998 CEB	0.4	2,829	1.3	1,910	0.8	4,739
Ideal number of children (INC)	2.3	2,802	2.2	1,895	2.2	4,697
Husband's age	42.9	2,829	34.9	1,910	39.7	4,739
Wife's age	39.6	2,829	32.3	1,910	36.7	4,739
Husband's age at marriage	27.6	2,829	29.7	1,910	28.5	4,739
Wife's age at marriage	24.3	2,829	27.0	1,910	25.4	4,739

the first time in 1997 or thereafter) are 2.0 and 1.3, respectively. The mean post-1998 CEB for the whole sample is 0.8, and 0.4 and 1.3 for Group A and Group B, respectively. Table 5.1 shows that the level of desired fertility is higher than that of achieved fertility. The mean value of INC is calculated as 2.2, substantially higher than the mean CEB. In contrast to the pattern of CEB, no significant difference in INC is observed between the two groups. The mean age of husbands and wives is found to be 8.0 and 7.3 years higher, respectively, in Group A. In contrast, husbands and wives in Group B turn out to have gotten married at older ages of 2.1 and 2.7 years, respectively, compared to their counterparts in Group A.

Though specific statistics are not presented in this chapter, the distinctive socioeconomic characteristics of the two groups can be summarized as follows. Women in Group B are relatively younger than those in Group A, and thus their level of educational attainment is significantly higher. Around 55.6 % of wives and 64.4 % of husbands in Group B received college education. Only 1.1 % of wives and 0.9 % of husbands are found to have received middle school education or lower. These are substantially lower than the counterpart figures of 8.4 % and 7.1 % for Group A.

Distribution of the husband's occupations in the two groups also reveals a pattern consistent with that of educational attainment. In Group A, craft workers compose the largest occupational subgroup (31.6 %), followed by service workers (19.6 %) and professionals (18.4 %). The occupational pattern is quite different in Group B, where the largest occupational groups are professionals (27.3 %), craft workers (24.2 %), service workers (19.6 %), and clerical workers (18.0 %). The proportion of wives who did not work at the time of the survey is 44.9 % for Group A and 62.4 % for Group B. As for working wives, service workers constitute the largest group of 22.5 % for Group A, while the proportion (15.6 %) of professionals is found to be the largest for Group B.

Distinctive Patterns of CEB and the Post-1998 CEB

It was postulated in this study that the 1997 economic crisis affected the causal mechanisms of Korean fertility a great deal, and thus the pattern of socioeconomic differentials in fertility during the past decade became significantly different from that of the old pattern. In other words, the patterns of socioeconomic differentials in CEB and the post-1998 CEB would not be similar to each other. It is clear in Fig. 5.3a that CEB and the post-1998 CEB according to wife's education reveal contrasting patterns. As wife's education goes up to a certain level, the CEB of the blue dotted line tends to decline. Though the difference turned out to be very small, college graduates reveal higher CEB than those of the next group in the hierarchy. The pattern is found to be consistent when CEB is analyzed according to husband's education.

In Fig. 5.3a, the post-1998 CEB according to wife's education shows a contrasting pattern. As the level of wife's education rises, the post-1998 CEB tends to increase. However, college graduated women are more likely to have slightly less children than the next group in the hierarchy. The contrasting patterns of CEB and the post-1998 CEB imply that, after the 1997 crisis, fertility decline has been most remarkable among less educated couples and relatively moderate for the highly educated. The pace of fertility decline during the past decade has been negatively associated with the level of fertility. Thus Korea's descend to ultra-low fertility can mostly be attributed to drastic reduction of fertility among the least and less educated couples.[1] It is also apparent in Fig. 5.3a that the level of INC is substantially higher than the level of achieved fertility and that it does not vary significantly according to wife's education.

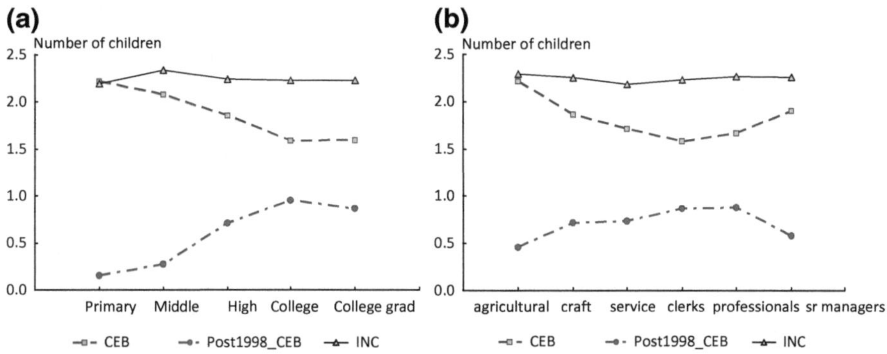

Fig. 5.3 CEB, the post-1998 CEB and INC by wife's education and husband's occupation. (**a**) By wife's education. (**b**) By husband's occupation

[1]According to results from the 2010 census, the proportion of population (aged 30 or higher) with middle school education or lower was estimated as 23.9 % and those with high school education, 37.3 % (Statistics Korea 2011).

To strengthen the above findings, analysis of differential fertility according to husband's occupation was conducted. Assuming that the sequence of occupational categories on the *X*-axis of Fig. 5.3b reflects prestige hierarchy with the highest score on the right end, the pattern of differential fertility according to husband's occupation is consistent with the one in Fig. 5.3a. The mean CEB for husbands with agricultural occupations and simple labor jobs turns out to be the highest, while husbands with clerical jobs reveal the lowest CEB. As occupational prestige goes up and moves rightward along the *X*-axis of Fig. 5.3b, CEB shows a declining pattern. However, legislators and senior managers with the highest prestige show a significantly higher mean CEB than those with the next prestigious group of occupations.

The pattern of the post-1998 CEB according to husband's occupation in Fig. 5.3b appears to contrast remarkably with that of CEB. As the level of occupational prestige goes up, the post-1998 CEB tends to increase. However, legislators and senior managers with the highest prestige are more likely to have fewer children than the next group in the prestige hierarchy. Analysis of the recent decrease in fertility according to husband's occupation reveals a similar pattern to the one in Fig. 5.3a. After the 1997 crisis, fertility decline has been most drastic among those with the highest level of fertility and relatively slow among those with lower fertility. Figure 5.3b indicates that the decline has been most substantial for husbands with agricultural occupations and simple labor jobs and relatively less substantial for husbands with clerical jobs. Figure 5.3b also shows that the ideal number of children maintains a higher level than CEB and the post-1998 CEB and that there is no significant relationship between ideal number of children and occupational prestige.

Regression Analysis

To double-check the data supporting the abovementioned arguments on the pattern of socioeconomic differentials in fertility, this study conducted a series of regression analyses. In order to examine nonlinear relationships between independent and dependent variables, linear and quadratic terms of education years of wife were introduced into the regression analysis. First, the variable of wife's years of education was standardized in such a way that the resulting mean was zero and the resulting standard deviation was one. Then, the quadratic term was created by taking the squared value of the standardized variable. One of the advantages of this transformation is that colinearity between the linear and quadratic terms is substantially reduced, while the correlation coefficients with other variables are not affected by this transformation.[2] Table 5.2 presents the results from regression analyses of education variables to CEB, the post-1998 CEB, and INC.

Model 1 in Table 5.2 yields a significantly negative coefficient for the linear term of wife's education. Though it does not hold statistical significance, the quadratic

[2]For detailed discussion on this technique of transformation and its applications, see Kim D. S. (1987: 154–159).

Table 5.2 Regression analysis to examine the nonlinear relationship between wife's education and fertility

	Dependent variable		
	CEB	Post-1998 CEB	INC
	[Model 1]	[Model 2]	[Model 3]
	b/beta	b/beta	b/beta
Education_yr_wife_std	(−)**	(+)**	(−)
Education_yr_wife_std_sq	(+)	(−)**	(+)
F-ratio	83.59**	74.28**	0.61
No. of cases	4,733	4,733	4,691

Notes:
1. Considering that this analysis was conducted to examine the shape of curvilinear relationship between the independent and the dependent variables, and that the independent variables were measured in a standardized form, this table presents just signs rather than real numbers of regression coefficients
2. (Education_yr_wife_std) is a standardized variable of education years of wife; (Education_yr_wife_std_sq) is a squared variable of (Education_yr_wife_std)
3. $*p < 0.05$; $**p < 0.01$

term of wife's education turns out to be positive. The signs of the regression coefficients for these terms support the pattern of CEB in Figs. 5.2a and 5.3a. In Model 2, the positive regression coefficient for the linear term and the negative regression coefficient for the quadratic term are found to be statistically significant and apparently support the nonlinear pattern of the post-CEB in Figs. 5.2a and 5.3a. The consistent level of INC regardless of wife's education is also confirmed by the results summarized in Model 3 in Table 5.2. The linear and quadratic terms of wife's education do not reveal any significant pattern of relationship with INC, and this regression model does not hold statistical significance.

In sum, it can be concluded based on these observations that the pattern of fertility indicators, that is, CEB, the post-CEB, and INC, in Fig. 5.3a, b matches the postulated differentials in Fig. 5.2 and supports the main hypotheses of this study.

Decrease in Fertility After the 1997 Economic Crisis

This study conducted another round of analysis to test the hypothesis that decrease in fertility after the economic crisis has been most drastic among those with the highest level of fertility and relatively slow for those with a lower level of fertility. In this analysis, decrease in CEB after the economic crisis was estimated by taking the difference in CEBs of those married before 1997 (Group A) and of those married for the first time in 1997 or thereafter (Group B), with the level of wife's education controlled. The recent decrease in INC was also estimated separately for each level of wife's education by taking the difference in the INCs of the two groups.

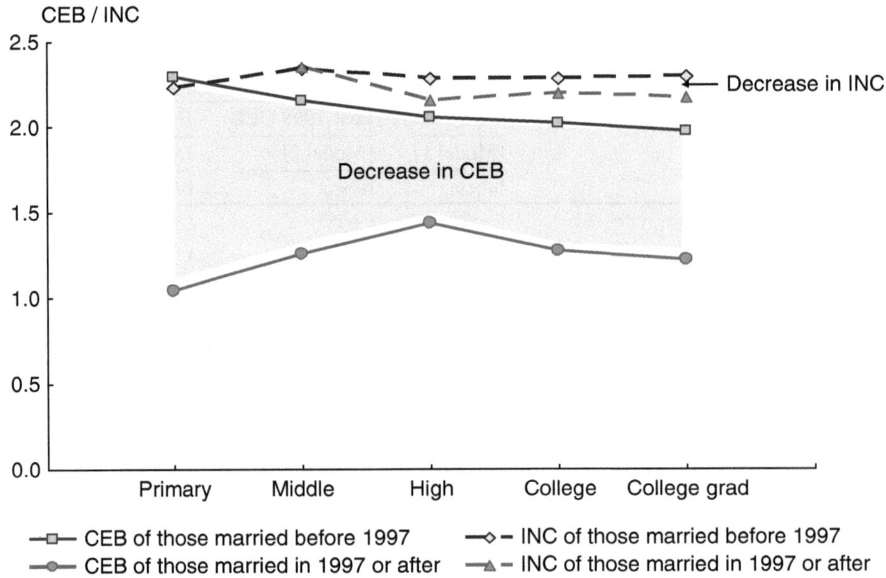

Fig. 5.4 Recent decreases in CEB and INC by wife's education

Figure 5.4 shows the recent changes in CEB and INC according to the level of wife's educational attainment. It is not surprising to find that the recent decrease in CEB has been substantial, while the decrease in INC is found to be at the minimal level. Despite a drastic decline in achieved fertility during the past decade, the desired level of fertility has not dropped seriously.

It is also indicated in Fig. 5.4 that the INC of the two groups maintains a similar level regardless of wife's education. In contrast, CEB of those married before 1997 reveals a generally negative relationship with wife's education. A slight upturn of CEB among those with the highest education is not observed in this figure. Among those married for the first time in 1997 or thereafter, however, the relationship between the two variables appears to be a reverse *V*-shaped pattern. Though the peak is positioned a bit leftwards, this pattern of the relationship resembles the one in Fig. 5.2b.

It is clear in Fig. 5.4 that the amount of the recent decrease in CEB varies according to wife's educational attainment. The decrease in CEB after the economic crisis has been most substantial among the less educated and least substantial among those who received high school education (Kim 2007, 2009).[3]

It can also be stated that decrease in fertility after the economic crisis has been most drastic among those with the highest level of fertility and relatively slow for those with a lower level of fertility. In this analysis, the correlation coefficient

[3]It should be noted that the proportion of those with middle school education and below is very small among those married in or after 1997. It was found, however, that a series of tests of statistical significance support this argument.

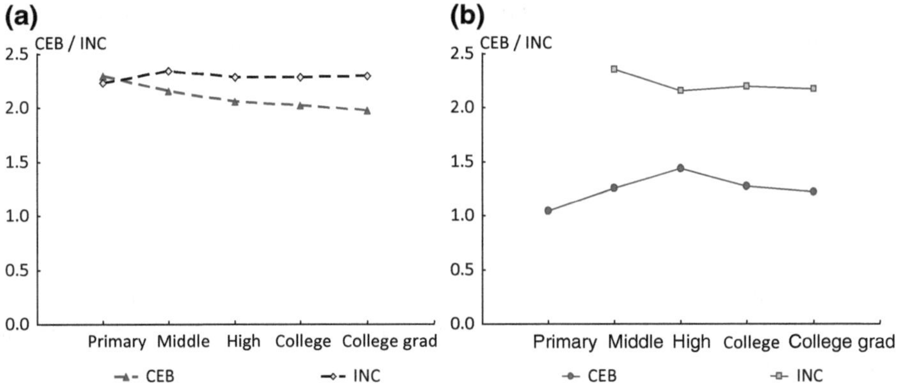

Fig. 5.5 Gap between INC and CEB by wife's education. (**a**) Those married before 1997. (**b**) Those married in 1997 or after

between CEB and the recent decrease in CEB was measured as high as 0.58. The counterpart figure between the post-1998 CEB and the recent decrease in CEB was calculated at −0.63. Both correlation coefficients were statistically significant at the 0.01 level.

As a result of the recent decrease in fertility, the gap between INC and CEB has tended to become wide. Figure 5.5a does not disclose a meaningful gap between INC and CEB for those who married before 1997. Their level of CEB is found to be relatively high and very close to that of INC. Thus the gap between the two does not appear to be dependent on the level of wife's education. Though the level of CEB turns out to be slightly higher than that of INC among those who received only primary education, this was calculated based on a relatively small number of 50 cases, so it cannot be strongly generalized.

For those who married for the first time in 1997 or thereafter, the gap between INC and CEB appears to be substantially wider as shown in Fig. 5.5b. The narrowest gap of the average 0.71 is found among wives with high school education. Results from the *F*-ratio test imply that the gap between INC and CEB does not vary significantly for other levels of wife's education. Due to the very small number of cases, the mean INC for wives with primary education is not presented in Fig. 5.5b.

Though results are not presented here, another round of analysis on the gap between INC and CEB according to husband's occupation was conducted in this study. For those who married before 1997, the gap was not found to be substantial regardless of husband's occupation. For those who married for the first time in 1997 or thereafter, the gap for husbands with agricultural occupations and simple labor jobs turned out to be the widest, while craft workers revealed the narrowest gap. In general, the pattern of the gap was found to be similar to the one in Fig. 5.5, but less apparent. It can be attributed mainly to the fact that each occupational category of this analysis includes various kinds of occupations, and thus the order of occupational categories adopted in this analysis does not correspond strictly to the hierarchical order of occupational prestige. It can also be pointed out that occupation variable is not widely used as an independent variable in the analysis of fertility using cross-sectional data, due to its relatively unstable nature over time.

Concluding Remarks

The objective of this study has been the analysis and the comparison of socioeconomic differentials of recent Korean fertility. The investigation was stimulated by three major considerations. First, the changing pattern of relations between socioeconomic status and fertility is one of central issues in the study of fertility. In an effort to explore the effects of the 1997 Asian economic crisis on the level of achieved fertility and on the pattern of socioeconomic differentials, the present chapter conducted a comparative analysis of CEB and the post-1998 CEB of married women. The level of fertility as well as the pattern of socioeconomic differentials for those married before 1997 and for those married for the first time in 1997 or thereafter is also compared.

Secondly, the data set used for this study includes attitudinal questions, addressed to the wife, regarding the total number of children expected and the number regarded as ideal. The gap between the number of children a couple currently has and the number regarded as ideal is likely to indicate the potential for population policy programs on the basis of present attitudes. Attempts have been made to use findings on the ideal size of completed family as a guide in projecting the future fertility once the economic crisis is overcome. The present chapter incorporated the concept of INC into analysis of socioeconomic differentials in fertility.

Finally, even in the context of ultra-low fertility, socioeconomic status as reflected in wife's educational attainment and husband's occupation has been found to be significantly correlated with various measures of fertility and change in fertility. However, demographers have been less successful in building theoretical frameworks of differential fertility based on new pattern of empirical findings after the 1997 Asian economic crisis. After reviewing the existing theoretical and empirical literature, several hypotheses concerning fertility patterns and differentials were proposed in this chapter. To provide a broader basis for generalization of empirical findings of this chapter, these hypotheses were tested using other data sets from the 2005 census and birth registration of recent years in addition to the main data set of this chapter. Due to space limitations, confirming findings based on other data sets are not presented in this chapter.

Results of analysis reveal that the economic crisis affected the causal mechanisms of Korean fertility significantly. CEB and the post-1998 CEB show contrasting patterns according to the socioeconomic status of the couple. In the ultra-low fertility context after the economic crisis, the relationship between socioeconomic status and the level of fertility is found to be positive. As the level of the wife's education or husband's occupational prestige goes up, CEB tends to increase slightly. For the highest socioeconomic group, however, the level of recent fertility tends to decrease slightly as socioeconomic status rises. College graduates show slightly lower CEB than those of the next group in the hierarchy. This pattern is found to be consistent for husband's education as well as other indicators of socioeconomic status. This implies that changes in reproductive behavior after the economic crisis have been most drastic among those with a high level of fertility and among those who received middle school education or lower. It is also indicated that the level of fertility of couples who graduated from college or with higher education decreased more sensitively than those in the next group in the educational hierarchy. This pattern turns out to be consistent when husband's occupation is used as an indicator of socioeconomic status.

It is found that the level of INC does not show contrasting patterns according to mother's education or husband's occupation. During the past decade, the economic crisis has not changed the level and pattern of socioeconomic differentials in INC seriously. As a result of the recent decrease in fertility, the gap between INC and CEB has tended to become wide. For those who married before 1997, the gap between INC and CEB was not found to be meaningful and did not appear to be dependent on the level of wife's education or socioeconomic status of the couple. For those who married for the first time in 1997 or thereafter, the gap between the two turned out to be widest among those with the lowest socioeconomic status and narrowest among those with middle or upper-middle status.

As Kim (2009) argued, with the poor economy and serious job insecurity after the 1997 economic crisis, couples with low socioeconomic status have not had many choices other than to reduce their family size. Greater relative deprivation due to increasing socioeconomic inequality has made them emulate the status-related and child-rearing expenditures of those with higher socioeconomic status rather than have more children. Increasing socioeconomic inequality has also led couples with the highest socioeconomic status to spend more on status-differentiating expenditures to fulfill their aspirations. This is particularly true for child education expenditures among Seoul and other metropolitan residents who have been exposed and receptive to status-related and status-differentiating expenditures, causing them to reduce their level of fertility drastically.

Empirical findings of this chapter offer two broad strands of lessons for future research and population policies. First, if the current situation continues, it is postulated that the pattern of socioeconomic differentials in fertility is likely to be substantially different in the future. In spite of the amount of literature on fertility determinants and differentials, there is a dearth of understanding when it comes to the context of ultra-low fertility. This chapter was part of an attempt to highlight the significance of this issue in an ultra-low fertility context and to provide guidance for future scholarly endeavor.

Second, findings of socioeconomic variations in the pace of fertility decline and differences in the gap between the achieved and desired fertility according to couple's socioeconomic status provide an important additional basis to policy makers for focusing pro-natal programs on least educated couples and other selected target groups. To enhance effectiveness in boosting fertility, policy directions and action programs should be established based on results from refined analyses of changes in recent fertility. Priority should also be given to selected groups that show a wider gap between achieved and desired fertility.

The next step resulting from this chapter would be theorization efforts based on the new pattern of socioeconomic differentials in the context of ultra-low fertility. Before the findings of this chapter can be generalized, however, further research is needed to provide a broader basis for assessing the fertility differentials explored in this chapter. One of the promising directions of future research is to apply the theoretical framework set out here to other countries that experienced a similar economic crisis in the late 1990s. This expansion may provide further insights into the pattern of socioeconomic differentials in fertility.

References

Andorka, R. (1978). *Determinants of fertility in advanced societies*. New York: The Free Press.

Becker, G. S. (1960). An economic analysis of fertility. In National Bureau of Economic Research (Ed.), *Demographic and economic change in developed countries* (pp. 209–231). Princeton: Princeton University Press.

Cain, G. G., & Weininger, A. (1973). Economic determinants of fertility: Results from cross-sectional aggregate data. *Demography, 10*(2), 205–223.

Cho, L. J., Arnold, F., & Kwon, T. H. (1982). *The determinants of fertility in the Republic of Korea* (National Research Council, Report No. 14. Committee on Population and Demography). Washington, DC: National Academy Press.

Choe, M. K., & Retherford, R. D. (2009). The contribution of education to South Korea's fertility decline to "lowest-low" level. *Asian Population Studies, 5*(3), 267–288.

Chung, B. M., Palmore, J. A., Lee, S., & Lee, S. J. (1972). *Psychological perspective: Family planning in Korea*. Seoul: Hollym Corporation.

Cochrane, S. H. (1979). *Fertility and education: What do we really know?* Baltimore: Johns Hopkins University Press.

Easterlin, R. A. (1969). Towards a socioeconomic theory of fertility: A survey of recent research on economic factors in American fertility. In S. J. Behrman, L. Corsa Jr., & R. Freedman (Eds.), *Fertility and family planning: A world view* (pp. 127–156). Ann Arbor: University of Michigan Press.

Easterlin, R. A. (1975). An economic framework for fertility analysis. *Studies in Family Planning, 6*(3), 54–63.

Eun, K. S. (2003). Understanding recent fertility decline in Korea. *Journal of Population and Social Security*, Supplement to Volume 1. Tokyo: National Institute of Population and Social Security. Research. http://www.ipss.go.jp/index-e.html. Accessed 15 Apr 2010.

Freedman, D. (1963). The relation of economic status to fertility. *American Economic Review, 53*(3), 414–426.

Freedman, R., Coombs, L., Chang, M., & Sun, T. H. (1974). Trends in fertility, family size preferences and practices of family planning: Taiwan, 1965–73. *Studies in Family Planning, 5*(9), 270–288.

KIHASA. (1982, 1988, 1994, 2000, 2009). *The Korean national fertility survey*. Seoul: Korea Institute for Health and Social Affairs.

Kim, D. S. (1987). *Socioeconomic status, inequality and fertility*. Seoul: Population and Development Studies Center, Seoul National University.

Kim, D. S. (2005). Theoretical explanations of rapid fertility decline in Korea. *The Japanese Journal of Population, 3*, 2–25.

Kim, D. S. (2007). *The "IMF economic crisis" and changes in Korean fertility (in Korean)*. Seoul: Jipmoon dang.

Kim, D. S. (2009). The 1997 Asian economic crisis and changes in the pattern of socioeconomic differentials in Korean fertility. In G. Jones, P. Tay Straughan, & A. Chan (Eds.), *Ultra-low fertility in Pacific Asia: Trends, causes and policy issues* (pp. 110–131). Oxon: Routledge.

Kim, I. K. (1987). *Socioeconomic development and fertility behavior in Korea*. Seoul: Population and Development Studies Center, Seoul National University.

Kim, M. I., Rider, R. V., Harper, P. A., & Yang, J. M. (1974). Age at marriage, fertility planning practices, and other variables as correlates of fertility in Korea. *Demography, 11*(4), 641–656.

Kim, T. H., Lee, S. S., & Kim, D. H. (2006). Fertility differentials by demographic and socioeconomic characteristics: Analysis of Korean population census data (in Korean). *Korea Journal of Population Studies, 29*(1), 1–23.

Kwon, T. H. (1982). Differentials in Korean fertility. In Y. Chang et al. (Eds.), *Society in transition: With special reference to Korea, essays in memory of Har Young Lee*. Seoul: Seoul National University Press.

Leibenstein, H. (1957). *Economic backwardness and economic growth*. New York: Wiley.

Leibenstein, H. (1975). The economic theory of fertility decline. *Quarterly Journal of Economics, 89*(1), 1–31.

Leibenstein, H. (1977). Beyond economic man: Economics, politics and the population problem. *Population and Development Review, 3*(3), 183–199.

Leibenstein, H. (1981). Economic decision theory and human fertility behavior: A speculative essay. *Population and Development Review, 7*(3), 381–400.

Mincer, J. (1963). Market prices, opportunity costs and income effects. In C. Christ (Ed.), *Measurement in economics: Studies in mathematical economics and econometrics in memory of Yehuda Grunfeld*. Stanford: Stanford University Press.

Mueller, E. (1972). Economic motives for family limitation. *Population Studies, 24*(3), 383–404.

Mueller, E., & Short, K. (1983). Effects of income and wealth on the demand for children. In R. A. Bulatao & R. D. Lee (Eds.), *Determinants of fertility in developing countries, Vol. 1: Supply and demand for children* (pp. 590–642). New York: Academic.

Namboodiri, N. K. (1970). On the relation between economic status and family size preferences when status differentials in contraceptive instrumentalities are eliminated. *Population Studies, 24*(2), 233–239.

Population Reference Bureau. (2009). *2009 World population data sheet*. Washington, DC: Population Reference Bureau.

Speare, A., Jr., Speare, M. C., & Lin, H. S. (1973). Urbanization, non-familial work, education and fertility in Taiwan. *Population Studies, 27*(2), 323–334.

Statistics Korea. (2011). *Korea statistical information system (KOSIS)*. On-line Government Statistics Database. Daejeon: Statistics Korea. http://kosis.kr/index.jsp/. Accessed 28 Oct 2011.

United Nations. (2011). *World population prospects: The 2009 revision*. Population database, United Nations Population Division. New York: United Nations. http://esa.un.org/wup2009/unup/index.asp?panel=1. Accessed 28 Oct 2011.

Willis, R. J. (1973). A new approach to the economic theory of fertility behavior. *Journal of Political Economy, 81*(2), S14–S64.

Wrong, D. H. (1958). Trends in class fertility in western nations. *Canadian Journal of Economics and Political Science, 24*(2), 216–229.

Yaukey, D. (1963). Some immediate determinants of fertility differences in Lebanon. *Marriage and Family Living, 25*(Feb), 27–33.

Yoo, S. H. (2006). On regional fertility differentials: understanding the causal mechanisms of low fertility in Korea (in Korean). *Population and Society, 2*(2), 53–76.

Chapter 6
Abandoned or Abandoning Men: Economic Stress, Gender Relations, and Migration of Filipinas to Singapore

Janet M. Arnado

Economic Stress and Gender Woes as Motives for Migration

Globalization processes have promoted gendered labor migration, which has simultaneously liberated and subjugated Filipino women. Globalization has provided them with economic liberation through vast opportunities to work in the economic north. On the other hand, their subjugation is reproduced as the kinds of jobs made available to them are racialized and feminized, and thus poorly paid. Filipinas' plight as domestic workers in other Asian countries has been beset with hardships: their labor and reproductive rights are often clipped by the state (Constable 2002; Asis et al. 2004; Devasahayam 2006), and their time and space are often controlled by their employers (Lan 2006). In addition, prolonged separation from their families poses relational problems (Arnado 2010). In spite of this bleak picture, labor migrants have employed various coping strategies to survive (see for example, Yeoh and Huang 1998; Lan 2003).

What pushes women to work abroad, leaving behind their families? Family economic stress, influenced by macroeconomic processes, is a well-documented labor migration push factor. Second on the list is unhappy or abusive gendered relationships. While not always the case, unhappy marital relationships are linked to economic stress, which in this context refers to the loss of job, income, and assets, as well as the "experience of material hardships" (Yeung, Chap. 1, this volume).

Research has demonstrated that economic stress impacts negatively on marital quality. Unstable work, for instance, results in "feelings of economic pressure that, in turn, are related to higher rates of depression for both mothers and fathers" (Parke et al. 2004) and "greater hostility in the marriage" (Kinnunen and Pulkkinen 1998). Economic stress also leads to gender-based violence (Falkingham 2000;

J.M. Arnado (✉)
Research Institute for Gender and Women, Inc., Malaybalay City, Philippines
e-mail: janetarnado@gmail.com

W.J.J. Yeung and M.T. Yap (eds.), *Economic Stress, Human Capital, and Families in Asia: Research and Policy Challenges*, Quality of Life in Asia 4,
DOI 10.1007/978-94-007-7386-8_6, © Springer Science+Business Media Dordrecht 2013

Henry-Lee et al. 2003). In Tajikistan, recent research shows that "nearly half of women thought that economic stress had led to more arguments and tensions within the household and 36 % of women reported an increase in violence against women, mainly linked to the frustrations that men felt with unemployment and the lack of income" (Falkingham 2000: xii–xiii).

In the Philippines, families largely deal with economic stress by sending family members to work abroad and surviving with their remittances, as the country has not been able to recover from its economic downturn that began in the 1970s. Labor export has long become a national strategy, with overseas work remittances increasing annually despite the global financial crisis, thus keeping the economy resilient.[1] No less than the former Philippine President Gloria Arroyo admitted in 2001 that jobs were difficult to find and the national economy relied on the remittances from overseas workers (APMMF n.d.). The Philippines has about eight million overseas Filipinos (CFO 2008), roughly about 10 % of its population. This figure is significantly higher compared to the total migrant population which is only about 2 % of the world's population (Faist 2000).

With increased global opportunities for women's reproductive labor in wealthy countries, Filipinas have joined men in their quest for greener pastures through international labor migration. Traditionally viewed as the "light of the home," Filipinas have courageously left their families behind to become "reluctant breadwinners" (Parrenas 2005). Motivations for women's labor migration have been overwhelmingly pointed at economic hardship, but economic stress is a complex condition worthy of deeper analysis, in this case, a gender analysis. Many studies have identified the interaction between economic stress and strained gender relations between heterosexual couples in the household. For example, economic stress results in or exacerbates people's indulgence in vices and violence, challenging the mental and emotional well-being of those concerned.

This study delves into pre-migration gender and class dynamics within the Filipino family. It examines the gender dimensions of the causes and consequences of economic stress that eventually encourage women to migrate for work overseas, specifically in Singapore. In particular, this chapter analyzes how major life events (i.e., death of a husband, marital dissolution, loss of a job) and sustained conditions of poverty promote emotional distress and impact gender relations and family well-being. Within the context of global structural processes that push women to work overseas, this chapter focuses on household-level factors.

The chapter is based on Jean Yeung's (Chap. 1, this volume) framework of economic stress in which objective economic stress factors generate subjective economic strain among family members, who cope using various strategies available to them. One of these strategies which is the focus of this study is overseas labor migration, leaving family members behind. The impact of economic stress on poor

[1]Remittances to the Philippines have increased to 9.3 % from a year earlier (Bloomberg 15 Dec 2010). The Philippines is one of the four biggest recipients of remittances worldwide (Inquirer.net, 9 November 2010).

Filipinos is not as dramatic as the global financial crisis experiences of Taiwanese families who lost income, property, and jobs because of the recent global recession (see summary of presentation by Wang and Chen in Yeung, 2010). Neither can it be compared with the devastation caused by the natural calamities, such as the 2004 tsunami that affected almost a million people in Asia (see summary of Frankenberg's presentation in Yeung, 2010). Rather, what poor Filipinos experience is a prolonged state of poverty which is exacerbated by another economically debilitating event.

Examining women's situated positions and gender relations prior to their migration provides insights into the gendered processes that had resulted in their departures. This project contributes to studies that examine family economic stress as a pre-migration characteristic of the Filipina labor migrants' households. It attempts to "disentangle the specific experience of women" (Bujis 1993) in various marital statuses. This microlevel analysis provides in-depth and contextual information absent in macro theories of migration. This analysis also considers Filipino women migrants as heterogenous; thus, I selected cases from women with different marital statuses, such as the married, separated, widowed, and never-married. This analysis of the gender and economic stresses of women prior to their migration would contribute an added dimension to existing literature on social adjustment of labor migrants in the receiving country, as women migrants' coping difficulties may not only be caused by the sociocultural conditions in their new place of residence but also by the gendered and economic stresses prior to their move.

Notes on Methods

I draw my analysis from my ethnographic fieldwork in Singapore over the period 2006–2007, involving in-depth interviews with 43 Filipina domestic workers and participant observation of Filipina domestics in public places. Details of my methodology are available in my previous work on global households (Arnado 2009, 2010). For this chapter, I particularly choose cases or narratives where the gender dimension significantly interacted with class issues. This chapter neither intends to generalize nor show a trend among informants in the study. It is an analysis of how gender interacts with poverty to push women to migrate using cases from my ethnographic study of 43 informants.

Motives for Migration

Motivation is a significant facet of migration, influenced by the macro dynamics of push and pull factors, as well as the micro processes at the household and individual levels (Kothari 2002). Microlevel economic explanation of migration is based on the assumption that "people are rational and that they try to '*maximize their individual utility* or, put in another way, *their individual quality of life.*' The potential mover (migrant) is conceived as a '*utility maximizer*'" (Faist 1997: 249). According to Fischer and others (1997: 52), at the microlevel of decision-making, individuals consider the following factors in their decision to migrate or to stay. These include the fulfillment of (1) existential needs, (2) needs for security, (3) needs for social integration and acceptance, and (4) needs for self-fulfillment. The discussion in this chapter is contextualized in this microlevel framework of decision-making, with a gender lens.

Motivations for labor migration among women may be due to two-pronged stress: economic based and gender based. Scholars examining the link between gender and migration have identified gender-based motives for migration, such as escaping from "gender discrimination or constraining gender norms" (Jollie and Reeves 2005). Among Jollie and Reeves' examples are the following: women wanting to earn more and have more economic independence instead of staying put; young men leaving the country to escape being forced to become soldiers; women migrating to escape sexual violence and abuse, sometimes related to a conflict situation; single women, widows, and divorcees migrating to escape social stigma; and young women migrating to escape restrictions on their freedom, pressure to marry, or to remain chaste until marriage.

Economic factors are a well-expressed motive for migration. Lindio-McGovern (2003: 518) discusses the motives of Filipinas who move to Italy:

> ...the Filipino domestic workers in Italy were propelled by economic need in seeking overseas work. The Filipino domestic workers who had jobs before they came to Italy frequently cited insufficient income (*hindi sapat ang kita*) as the main reason for emigrating. Those who were unemployed before they came to Italy cited the difficulty of finding a job in the Philippines and deciding to try one's luck (*makipagsapalaran*) abroad as the main reason for emigrating.

Clearly, Filipino domestics in Europe migrate for existential or economic reason. Another dimension, however, which is often overlooked is what Fischer and others call the "need for security," particularly from their spouses. Anderson indicates that in addition to economic need, Filipinas also migrate to run away from abusive husbands (Anderson 2001). Anderson writes: "The difficulties of marital relationships can be seen from the fact that only six out of 83 women sent back money to their husbands alone, and most sent back to other women, to mothers, daughters, and sisters" (p. 28).

Women and girls have used labor migration as a convenient excuse for running away from their boyfriends, husbands, and fathers (Parrenas 2001; Arnado 2003). Similarly, single mothers, or those abandoned by men, have resorted to working as cheap laborers in other countries as a means to raise their children. Family economic stress is a common pattern pushing Filipinas to migrate for work (Lan 2000; Parrenas 2001; Arnado 2003; Asis et al. 2004). In addition, strained gender relations are another motivation for labor migration. However, the gender issue has been placed on the sideline or assumed in the economic argument of many analytical frameworks that examine household-level deciding factors for labor migration.

Hondagneu-Sotelo (1992: 393) argues that patriarchy is a "fluid and shifting set of social relations in which men oppress women, in which different men exercise varying degrees of power and control, and in which women collaborate to resist in diverse ways." Filipino women's decisions to migrate are vivid ways of either resisting men's "varying degrees of power and control," especially when they are under economic stress.

Abandoned or Abandoning Men via Labor Migration

In reflecting on the ways by which gender is constituted in women's motivations to migrate to Singapore, I have noted two gender-related patterns that interacted with economic stress: some women were abandoned by men, and others wanted to run away from men. Jollie and Reeves' (2005) identification of gender motivation, as discussed above, focused on women's migration as a mechanism of abandoning men. They did not consider women migrating because of men's abandonment. In the following cases, I show stories of women in different circumstances, dealing with their economic lives with and without men. I will provide narratives of women abandoned by men, such as widowed and separated women. I will also detail stories of women – runaway brides and married women – who abandoned men through labor migration. Finally, complex stories of single women tell tales of men's abandonment as well as abandonment of men.

Male Abandonment and Women's Migration

The following cases provide stories of how the disappearance of the male breadwinner in the family creates not only economic stress but also psycho-emotional distress on women. In the midst of their grief, formerly contented housewives wasted no time in looking for jobs overseas when their male providers became unable to perform their role as "pillars of the home."

Case 1. Widowed Women: Stories of Pamela and Narda

52-year-old Pamela Jamero is a mother of seven children, left behind by her policeman husband who died in a shootout in 1987. Faced with the sole responsibility of raising her children, she left for Singapore 2 years later, to afford the cost of raising them. When she left, her eldest child was only 11 years old, while the youngest was 2 years old; now they all have college degrees.

Her siblings and other relatives took care of her children during the first 8 years when she did not go home in order to save money for remittances. In lieu of vacation, her benefits were converted to the cash equivalent of a roundtrip plane ticket and 2 weeks' salary every 2 years. With the money that she had saved, she was able to build a house for her children.

Like Pamela, Narda Bracero became a widow with three children in her 20s. Her husband's demise turned her life upside-down. She was 19 years old when she got married in 1995. With only a high school diploma at hand, she remained at home to become a full-time homemaker while her then 23-year-old husband, Ted, supported the family with his home-based barbershop.

In 2003, Ted died from a heart attack. At that time, Narda was breastfeeding her youngest child. In her distress, she refused to eat, thus making breastfeeding a difficult process (see also, Arnado 2010). Narda did not have the luxury of grieving over her husband as she suddenly faced single parenthood and became the breadwinner. Compounding these new burdens, Narda was disturbed by a growing number of men in her village who showed interest in her as she was a young widow. She avoided these men by not going out of her house for an extended period of time. She thought it would be most convenient if she went abroad to support her children and avoid relationships with men.

A year later she was already in Singapore, having left her children with her parents. Sudden changes in her life made it difficult for her to adjust to the new environment, culture, and work conditions. In her two and half years in Singapore, she has had three employers.

Case 2. Separated Women: The Stories of Isabela Roa and Hana Catre

Isabela Roa is 43 years old. Hers is an appropriate case study which shows the already desperate conditions of Filipinas before they migrated to Singapore. Isabela had been involved tragically with two men. At age 19, she married a drug addict who beat her up when under the influence of drugs. They broke up within 4 years and their two children lived with her husband. In the 1990s while she was working as a cashier in a restaurant, she was raped by an avid admirer, who eventually became her live-in partner for 10 years, and she bore him two sons. Like the first, her second relationship was chaotic as her partner (who was married to another woman) was lured into drugs like her first husband. He was accused of murder and jailed for 10 months, leaving Isabela and the children with nothing. Unable to bear the stresses in her life, she attempted suicide but survived.

When her partner was released from jail, he continued using drugs and beat her up. Isabela also caught him with another woman. They separated after this event. At this time, their house was also demolished by the government and she and her youngest son had to literally live on the street for a month. To support themselves, she would accept odd jobs selling compact discs, sweeping the street, and doing laundry and domestic work, leaving her children with neighbors and family members. Her work downgraded from office clerk, cashier, and sales lady to domestic work. She kept getting into debt until she could not get out of it any more. All avenues that she tried failed. When an opportunity came for her to work in Singapore, she did not hesitate to take it, not fearing what lay ahead.

Another story is that of 42-year-old Hana Catre whose marriage to Ariel only lasted for 2 years. Ariel left her when their son, Louie, was less than a year old. Working as a substitute teacher for 8 years, Hana never found a permanent teaching job because she failed in the teacher's board examination. To augment her meager salary of P100 per day, she would cook and sell food for the school canteen. Her small business helped her earn P2000 every month, but she needed to earn more to provide a comfortable life for her son. In 2000, her opportunity to move to Singapore came, when a friend based in Singapore had a Singaporean boyfriend with connections to a recruitment agency. Despite her son's protestation of having only one parent left, she migrated to Singapore leaving Louie with her sister.

Abandoning Men Through Labor Migration

Unhappiness in marriage due to their husband's extramarital relations or gender violence push women to migrate overseas. This will then lead to the paradoxical issue posed in the title of this chapter: are women abandoning men through the guise of labor migration or are they migrating because they have been abandoned by men?

Case 3. The Runaway Brides: The Stories of Flora and Trinidad

27-year-old Flora Gallardo from Quezon City went through a difficult life: a product of a broken family, a victim of a cycle of abuse, a runaway bride, and a runaway maid. Her father died when she was four; her mother remarried and sent her to her grandmother's house. A few years later, her mother took her back, and her stepfather physically abused her.

After only 8 years of schooling, Flora quit school to work. She became a maid and then a factory worker, where she met her husband who was 10 years her senior and had a college degree. She married and became a housewife at the age of 17 and bore him two children. There was no household financial difficulty at the time Flora decided to work in Singapore. Her husband had a stable work, her children went to a private school, and they owned the house they were living in.

"Having fallen somewhat out of love" with her husband was Flora's primary motive for leaving the country in 2005. Because she was a product of a broken family, she did not want to break up her own. She thought that overseas work would be a better arrangement than marital breakup. She needed space from her spouse and overseas work sounded like a good excuse.

Like Flora, 27-year-old Trinidad Acurantes also went to Singapore to run away from her husband. When I asked why, she answered, "because my husband could not love me." I later learned that her husband was beating her up. She has two children with him: 7 and 9 years old. The youngest was 2 years old when she left for Singapore. Her husband could support the family with his job as an electrician but she could no longer bear him hurting her, which began when she was pregnant with their first child.

In 2000, she packed her things to work in Singapore. She worked for Chinese-Singaporean employers for 5 years and left when her male employer sexually abused her. At first he would ask her to give him a massage when his wife was not around. Then later, he started to fondle her private parts. She gave him a warning but when he persisted, she decided to cut short her contract and returned to the Philippines. Her female employer had no idea what had happened.

She stayed in the Philippines for 4 months. Again, her husband beat her up. From Trinidad's point of view, her husband was not happy when he could not hurt her. She ran away to her mother's place while the children remained with their father. It was not fruitful to stay in the Philippines so she went back to Singapore.

Case 4. Married Women: The Stories of Emma and Marlene

Many married informants did not reveal any gender issues with their spouses. In these cases, their move was simply driven by economic stress and opportunities available to women. 27-year-old Emma Dadole was a housewife before her stint in Singapore, relying on the earnings of her spouse who worked as a driver. When he lost his job, the family had a hard time coping with their needs. This prompted Emma to take up the invitation of her sister to work in Singapore. Similarly, 50-year-old Marlene Dacudao went to Singapore in 1992 because her husband's occupation as a farmer could not support the educational needs of their three children. Her husband, Eddie, took care of their children with the help of his three sisters who were never married and stayed in the neighborhood. Eddie did farming on a one-hectare maize plantation and later drove a tricycle, which Marlene bought, to supplement their income.

Case 5. Single Women: The Stories of Caroline Luna and Sharon Tangcongco

Even with a college degree, 32-year-old Caroline Luna decided to become a domestic worker in Singapore, as a stepping-stone for her planned move to Canada. Her father died when she was 10 years old and her mother raised her and her four siblings. Her mother was even more generous as she also adopted another child while raising her own. In 1999, her mother suffered a stroke and had to be taken care of. The two girls in the family absorbed the burden of care, with the eldest taking physical care of her mother while Caroline shouldered their financial needs. As her brothers already had families of their own, they were exempted from the obligation of caring for their mother.

At one point her eldest sister wanted to get married. Caroline agreed as long as she took their mother with her. The boyfriend, however, disagreed, so Caroline discouraged her sister from marrying. "If he cannot accept our mother, he does not love you enough," Caroline told her sister, who eventually decided against marrying her boyfriend.

Her mother died a few months prior to the interview. Even with her mother gone, Caroline's family responsibility continues as her mother left the now-10-year-old adopted child who stays with her sister under her financial care. This child has become her inspiration and resolve to live.

Hailing from Laguna, Sharon Tangcongco is the second of seven children. Throughout her life, she knew her father to be an alcoholic who would beat them with a branch of the coconut tree when he was drunk. He would also scare them with a knife. To save themselves, Sharon and her siblings often jumped out of the window whenever they heard their father approaching their house.

Her father, a farmer, was very strict with them. At six p.m., their house door was already closed; they were not allowed to go outside to play. Her father made an impact on Sharon's life, influencing many of her decisions. He did not provide education for his daughters beyond elementary school, feeling it was unnecessary because they would just marry, making his investment fruitless. The other reason which he did not reveal was their very limited resources that will not afford education to all seven children. Thus, males were given priority. Because of such situation, her eldest sibling left their family at a young age, looking for better opportunities for herself.

Because of her negative experience with her father, she has not been interested in men and marriage. In 1990, a friend working in Singapore recommended Sharon to her employers who then sent an air ticket and paid for the other fees. She sends the money she earns to her nieces and nephews in the Philippines.

Analysis: Economic Stress, Gender Woes, and Migration

As shown in the cases presented above, the chapter considered the multifaceted lives of women in various marital statuses or relationships with men – widowed, separated, ever-married, runaway bride, and never-married. Abandoned by men whether voluntarily or involuntarily, the widows and separated women took the risk of leaving their children behind despite their condition as already single parents. The breadwinning role, it seems, took priority over their reproductive role towards their children. Pushed by economic needs brought by their husbands' deaths, widowed women, Pamela and Narda, who used to be contented homemakers, were out of the country within 2 years of their husbands' deaths.

Separated from their spouses with the children under their care, Isabela and Hana, likewise had to make both ends meet. Their situation is similar to the widows'; the difference being that the men's abandonment of their families was voluntary in nature. The life of Isabela, for example, depicted trouble in her two relationships with men. In the midst of economic hardship, she was raped, beaten up, and abandoned. Isabela's migration was more of a survival while Hana's was for a "better life."

The other set of narratives deals with women abandoning men. In this case, when men did not abandon women, it was the latter who did the abandoning in various ways. The least radical form is physical abandonment of their families by married women to pursue economic goals in Singapore while keeping psycho-emotional bonds with their husbands stable. In this situation, migration was primarily prompted by economic needs, and the women were recipients of opportunities to migrate.

A more radical yet subtle form is that of runaway brides: unhappily married women who were uncertain about breaking up with their husbands, as shown in the stories of Flora and Trinidad. Interestingly, the concept of love was a main factor in Flora's and Trinidad's decisions to migrate. In Flora's case, she fell out of love with her spouse, in part because of very early marriage and her full-time role as a housewife for years. In Trinidad's situation, it was because her husband was not capable of loving her, and showing this "dis-love" through gender-based violence. Flora wanted to run away to have some space to think her marriage over; Trinidad to save herself from violence.

For the never-married women, the gender factor is contextualized in their family of orientation. Their move was motivated by their obligation to support their family of orientation. In Caroline's case, the motive was to financially provide for her family – the needs of her mother as well as her sister who acted as her mother's caregiver and sacrificed an opportunity of marriage to attend to family obligation. The story of Sharon, on the other hand, tells a life of a poor family where the limited resources were distributed by gender to the disadvantage of female offspring. The dominant man in her life was her father, who despite his death several years ago, continues to influence her life choices. Sharon was exposed to domestic violence as a child, with her alcoholic father as the perpetrator. Sharon has remained single and enjoys her financial freedom. The image of her father has discouraged her from entering into a marital relationship where she would be bound to serve a man all her life.

This chapter argues that the interaction of family economic stress, strained gender relations, and global structural opportunities push women to migrate for work. The economic stress may be caused by the husband's loss of a job or it may be that the economic stress is felt only by the woman/wife who has been serving as housewife for a long time and needs some kind of economic independence. This economic stress is strongly intertwined with gender relations at home, as shown in Flora's case.

Another form where gender and economic stress are intertwined is that of disintegrated relationships, such as death of a spouse/father, marital separation, or alcoholism, where women are abandoned emotionally and economically. This is very stressful on women's part as they have to confront psycho-emotional and economic issues at the same time.

In the cases presented above, several micro conditions encouraged women to move and to escape or survive economic stress, marital trouble, gender violence, and spousal/parental death. One form of stress gave rise to another. For example, economic stress pushed men to beat their wives (as shown in other studies too) and engage in vices such as drugs and alcohol, which exacerbated their propensity to abuse their wives and children, and in one case also resulted in imprisonment. Economic stress and domestic violence affected marital relations as well as parent-child relationships. These women wrestled with the impact of economic stress on their gendered relationships. These hardships were so difficult to bear that one of them had attempted suicide in the Philippines.

Poverty at home has often been used as the primary motivating factor for migration, but most people in "chronic poverty" have remained nonmigrants (Kothari 2002). Many have wondered why Filipinas leave their families to work overseas as domestic helpers, despite the threat to their lives/safety. Several news stories tell of violence inflicted on domestic workers by their employers in other countries. Yet these women would rather face such uncertainty in a foreign land because of destitution at home.

The enormous hardship they went through in the Philippines provided them the courage to explore Singapore even with very little information about the country. The economic strains pushed these women to the edge, even deviating from the traditional gender ideology of women as the "light of the homes" and caregivers. They described their journey into the unknown as "kapit sa patalim" (grasping a double-edge sword), "bahala na" (come what may), and "panimpalad" (finding one's destiny) (Arnado 2010). Their lives back home were very difficult; life in Singapore could not be worse, they would explain to me. "I already got partly wet, I will just make myself fully wet" was a similar disposition shared by my informants, believing that they would not "die twice." They also wanted to prove to themselves that something good could arise from their experiences. Whatever the difficulty in a foreign land, they believed they could hurdle it.

This chapter argues that abandoning husbands is a hidden motivation behind labor migration for some women, whereas the expressed motive is a quest for material well-being. By hiding the real motive, the marriage is still kept intact at least in the eyes of children and the social world. In some cases, the migrant hopes that by temporarily leaving her spouse, their relationship will be renewed, romance rekindled, and things will turn out for the better.

Several noneconomic benefits of labor migration can be drawn when one suffers from strained gender relations or male abandonment whether voluntary or involuntary. One, labor migration offers numerous opportunities for women trapped in unhappy relations with men. Two, it forms a coping mechanism for women abandoned by men, as it provides economic relief as well as space for emotional recovery. The new place allows them to escape from spaces that remind them of their husbands, spaces that would relieve the hurt and pain.

Sometimes there is no clear-cut distinction as to who abandons whom; it can be mutual in that when women are abandoned, they also abandon in return. Such is the case of one informant. When she learned of her husband's extramarital affairs, she withheld her remittances from him.

Summary and Conclusions

Jean Yeung (Chap. 1, this volume) has pinpointed how macroeconomic stressors "filter down through households to affect the economic and socio-psychological wellbeing of individuals." In addition to economic stress, this chapter has also examined their impact on gender relations. The chapter has examined Filipino women's labor migration as an adaptation strategy to overcome economic hardship and strained gendered relations in their families, resulting in increased and more stable income, accumulation of property, and physical and emotional space from fathers, boyfriends, or husbands. It cited detailed stories or narratives that demonstrated the varying impacts of poverty on them as women. Migration has long been considered a gendered phenomenon. Where women only used to follow men where they go, women have been on the move on their own for years now, sometimes leaving their families behind. Without a gender analysis of migration motives of women labor migrants, escape from gender issues in relationships or abandonment by men will remain a secondary motive of migration viewed as not integral to economic stress.

I have noted in my previous work that long-term overseas work poses significant risks to family stability (Arnado 2010). Prolonged absence of migrant workers from their families often creates marital trouble, with husbands engaging in extramarital affairs. As "transient wives" these migrant workers appear to tolerate their husbands' relationships with other women, but actually punish these men by depriving them of remittances. In this chapter, I found that the marital conditions of some labor migrants may already be in trouble prior to their decisions to move and that their migration decision was in fact motivated by an already strained gender relationship. Some women would like to leave in the hope that space or distance may help in fixing the problem, and when this problem can no longer be fixed, they leave in the hope that migration may lessen the impact of marital separation, particularly on the children.

With the Philippine government's dependency on remittances, labor will continue to dominate as the Philippine's export commodity in the future. Filipino family members will continue to be separated and rely on technological devices to communicate. Abused women may find solace in other countries or they may be trapped in the cycle of violence in the hands of their employers. Never-married women may find a harder time changing their marital status, given the sexual, time, and space restrictions in their workplaces in Singapore.

In the light of these findings, policy recommendation is directed at the strengthening of psychosocial support for labor migrants in the countries of destination as well as in the Philippines prior to their move and upon their return. The Philippine reintegration program, which is primarily geared towards economic reintegration, should strengthen its scope on family reintegration, particularly on rebuilding marriages and parent-child relationships, by tapping socio-civic and religious institutions. In addition, technological support can be provided in the form of incentives or discounts on the use of information and communication technologies, such as international calls and internet, to left-behind families to allow constant communication with their transnational mothers and wives, mending wounds, deepening relationships, and allowing global householding.

References

Anderson, B. (2001). Just another job? Paying for domestic work. *Gender and Development, 9*(1), 25–33.

Arnado, J. M. (2003). *Mistresses and maids: Inequality among third world women wage earners*. Manila: De La Salle University Press.

Arnado, J. M. (2009). Localizing the global and globalizing the local: Global households of Filipina transmigrant workers and Singapore employers. In D. Heng & S. M. K. Aljunied (Eds.), *Reframing Singapore: Memory, identity, trans-regionalism* (pp. 229–246). Amsterdam: Amsterdam University Press.

Arnado, J. M. (2010). Performances across time and space: Drama in the global households of Filipina transmigrant workers. *International Migration, 48*(6), 132–154.

Asia Pacific Mission for Migrant Filipinos (APMMF). (n.d.). *The role and process of remittances in the labor export industry in the Philippines*. Kowloon: APMMF.

Asis, M. M. B., Huang, S., & Yeoh, B. S. A. (2004). When the light of the home is abroad: Unskilled female labor migration and the Filipino family. *Singapore Journal of Tropical Geography, 25*(2), 198–215.

Bloomberg. (2010, December 15). Philippine remittances climb on rising overseas jobs. *Bloomberg*. http://www.bloomberg.com/news/2010-12-15/philippine-remittances-climb-on-rising-overseas-jobs-update1-.html

Bujis, G. (Ed.). (1993). *Migrant women: Crossing boundaries, changing identities*. Oxford: Berg.

CFO (Commission on Filipino Overseas). (2008). *Stock estimate of overseas Filipinos as of December 2008*. Philippines: Commission on Filipino Overseas.

Constable, N. (2002). Sexuality and discipline among Filipina domestic workers in Hong Kong. In F. V. Aguilar (Ed.), *Filipinos in global migrations: At home in the world?* (pp. 237–268). Quezon City: Philippine Social Science Center.

Devasahayam, T. W. (2006, April 10–11). Is sex on the agenda?: Singapore NGOs constructing Filipina migrant domestic worker sexuality. In *International workshop on sexuality and migration in Asia*. Singapore: National University of Singapore.

Faist, T. (1997). From common questions to common concepts. In T. Hammar, G. Brochmann, & K. Tamas (Eds.), *International migration, immobility and development: Multidisciplinary perspectives* (pp. 247–276). Oxford: Berge.

Faist, T. (2000). *The volume and dynamics of international migration and transnational social spaces*. Oxford: Oxford University Press.

Falkingham, J. (2000). *Women and gender relations in Tajikistan*. Manila: Asian Development Bank.

Fischer, P., Martin, R., & Straubhaar, T. (1997). Should I stay or should I go? In T. Hammar, G. Brochmann, & K. Tamas (Eds.), *International migration, immobility and development: Multidisciplinary perspectives* (pp. 49–90). Oxford: Berg.

Henry-Lee, A., Bailey, W., & Branche, C. (2003). Conflict, gender relations and the health of women in two low-income communities in Jamaica. In S. Arber & M. Khlat (Eds.), *Social and economic patterning of health among women* (pp. 357–374). Paris: CICRED.

Hondagneu-Sotelo, P. (1992). Overcoming patriarchal constraints: The reconstruction of gender relations among Mexican immigrant women and men. *Gender and Society, 6*(3), 393–415.

Inquirer.net. (2010, November 9). *OFW remittances to PH is '4th largest in the world'—WB report*. Manila: Philippine Daily Inquirer. http://newsinfo.inquirer.net/topstories/topstories/view/20101109-302313/OFW-remittances-to-PH-is-4th-largest-in-the-worldWB-report

Jollie, S., & Reeves, H. (2005). *Gender and migration: Overview report*. Brighton: Institute of Development Studies.

Kinnunen, U., & Pulkkinen, L. (1998). Linking economic stress to marital quality among Finnish marital couples: Mediator effects. *Journal of Family Issues, 19*(6), 705–724.

Kothari, U. (2002). *Migration and chronic poverty* (Chronic Poverty Research Centre Working Paper Series 16). Manchester: Chronic Poverty Research Centre, Institute for Development Policy and Management, University of Manchester.

Lan, P.-C. (2000). Global divisions, local identities: Filipina migrant domestic workers and Taiwanese employers. PhD dissertation, Northwestern University, Evanston.

Lan, P.-C. (2003). "They have more money but I speak better English!" Transnational encounters between Filipina domestics and Taiwanese employers. *Identities-Global Studies in Culture and Power, 10*, 133–161.

Lan, P.-C. (2006). *Global Cinderellas: Migrant domestics and their newly-rich employers in Taiwan*. Durham: Duke University Press.

Lindio-McGovern, L. (2003). Labor export in the context of globalization: The experience of Filipino domestic workers in Rome. *International Sociology, 18*, 513–534.

Parke, R. D., et al. (2004). Economic stress, parenting and child adjustment in Mexican-American and European American families. *Child Development, 75*(6), 1632–1656.

Parrenas, R. S. (2001). *Servants of globalization: Women, migration and domestic work*. Stanford: Stanford University Press.

Parrenas, R. S. (2005). *Children of global migration: Transnational families and gendered woes*. Stanford: Stanford University Press.

Yeoh, B. S. A., & Huang, S. (1998). Negotiating public space: Strategies and styles of migrant female domestic workers in Singapore. *Urban Studies, 35*(3), 583–602.

Yeung, W. J. (2010, June 3–4). *Report on the international conference on economic stress, human capital and families in Asia: Research and policy challenges*. Singapore: Asia Research Institute/National University of Singapore. Available at: http://www.ari.nus.edu.sg/docs/downloads/Reports-and-Proceedings/EconomicReport.pdf

Chapter 7
Economic Insecurity and Husband-to-Wife Physical Assault in Hong Kong: The Role of Husband's Power Motive

Adam K.L. Cheung and Susanne Y.P. Choi

Introduction

Domestic violence against women is a serious social issue. Husband-to-wife physical violence not only leads to various physical and mental health problems for the victims (Campbell 2002; Ellsberg et al. 2008) but also adversely affects the quality of the couple's relationship and significantly elevates the risk of union and marital dissolution (DeMaris 2000). Behind closed doors, home can be a dangerous place for many women and a place where these women face violence at the hands of the person they love and trust (Straus et al. 1980). High prevalence rates of husband-to-wife physical assault are documented in human societies across cultures, including both Western and non-Western societies (Garcia-Moreno et al. 2006; Kaukinen 2004; Parish et al. 2004; Straus and Gelles 1995). In China, for example, a nationally representative sample reveals that 34 % of women had ever been hit by a spouse during the current relationship (Parish et al. 2004).

Indeed, previous representative surveys show that spousal violence has also been common in Hong Kong. Approximately 10 % of married women in Hong Kong were physically assaulted by a spouse during the preceding year (Tang 1999a), and approximately 15 % of married or cohabiting women had been either physically or sexually assaulted by their intimate partner (Chan 2005), a higher prevalence rate of husband-to-wife violence than in some Western countries. Recent studies show that the 1-year prevalence rate of husband-to-wife violence was about 3.3 % in Canada (Kaukinen 2004) and 7.4 % in the United States (Salari and Baldwin 2002). Yet, the

A.K.L. Cheung (✉)
Asia Research Institute, National University of Singapore, Singapore
e-mail: Adam.kalok@gmail.com

S.Y.P. Choi
Department of Sociology, The Chinese University of Hong Kong, Hong Kong
e-mail: choiyp@cuhk.edu.hk

W.J.J. Yeung and M.T. Yap (eds.), *Economic Stress, Human Capital, and Families in Asia: Research and Policy Challenges*, Quality of Life in Asia 4,
DOI 10.1007/978-94-007-7386-8_7,

prevalence rate of husband-to-wife violence in Hong Kong is lower than the rates from some developing countries (Haj-Yahia 2000; Xu et al. 2005; Yount and Carrera 2006; Yount and Li 2010).

Although husband-to-wife violence is common in many societies, previous research suggests that the risks of violence are not evenly distributed throughout the society. Previous research demonstrates that the risk, severity, and frequency of domestic violence vary considerably across social classes (Schumacher et al. 2001; World Health Organization 2005). Low socioeconomic status is found to be a consistent risk marker for husband-to-wife physical assault in many societies around the globe (e.g., see Haj-Yahia 2000; Hoffman et al. 1994; Hotaling and Sugarman 1986). This finding has important sociological implications, especially in times of rising income inequality and poverty.

During the 1990s and the early years of the new millennium, a series of events and phenomena (such as the Asian financial crisis, the burst of the IT bubble, the outburst of SARS, and the subsequent industrial restructuring) adversely affected the economic security for many households in Hong Kong. The unemployment rate in Hong Kong increased dramatically from 1.8 % in 1991 to 5.1 % in 2001 and climbed to a record high of 7.9 % in 2003 after the outbreak of SARS. Underemployment rate doubled from 1.6 to 3.5 % between 1996 and 2003 (Hong Kong Census and Statistics Department 2007). The adverse effects were particularly visible for some groups of men who were unskilled and from the lower class. Both unemployment rate and underemployment rate for men were higher than the rates for women. Also, a sharper rise of the unemployment rate for men was recorded in the years after the Asian financial crisis. With this background in mind, two relevant but unanswered questions for family sociologists are posed: Does men's economic insecurity affect the prevalence rate of husband-to-wife violence in Hong Kong? If so, what is the possible mechanism linking up husband-to-wife violence with men's economic insecurity?

Some recent works have begun to assess the mediation mechanism between economic resources and domestic violence with empirical data (e.g., DeMaris et al. 2003; Fox et al. 2002; Hoffman et al. 1994). In the literature, there are works (e.g., Anderson 1997; Goode 1971; McCloskey 1996) suggesting that the husband's economic insecurity is related to violence because men, in times of economic hardship, desire to have more decision-making power in the relationship and to control their wives as their dominance in the relationship is challenged. However, this mediation hypothesis is seldom formally tested with empirical data, especially in a non-Western context.

This study aims to fill this gap by assessing whether the husband's economic insecurity exerts its influence on the risk of husband-to-wife physical assault in a Chinese context. In particular, a special focus is put on the mediating role of husband's power motive, which is defined as his desire for more decision-making power in the relationship. Using couple-level data from a household survey in Hong Kong ($N = 871$), the current study finds that the husband's desire to have more power in the relationship is positively associated with husband-to-wife physical assault, controlling for other covariates. Meanwhile, husband's power motive is a function of his economic insecurity. Mediation analysis in this study shows that a couple's income difference, the husband's full-time employment status, and his financial stress exert significant indirect effects on the risk of violence through the husband's power motive.

Theoretical Framework: Husband's Economic Insecurity and Domestic Violence

Resource Theories and Husband-to-Wife Violence: The Role of the Power Motive

Resource theory is one of the most cited theories in studies explaining the relationship between economic resources (or the lack of resources) and domestic violence. Different versions of resource theory have been proposed in the literature. The classical/absolute resource theory of family violence originally proposed by Goode (1971) posits that the husbands with few resources, compared with the husbands with abundant resources, are more likely to use violence. Goode (1971) conceptualizes marriage as an exchange relationship and proposes that violence and force are alternative forms of resources to use in this exchange relationship. Resources such as income and educational attainment are useful for men to gain and maintain decision-making power in the relationship. However, when husbands do not have adequate resources to gain what they consider to be enough power in the relationship, force and violence are the ultimate resources for maintaining the power in that relationship. Therefore, it is hypothesized that husbands from lower class are more likely to use violence against their wives because they have few resources to employ in the relationship. This hypothesis, suggesting a negative association between the husband's economic resources and the use of violence, is confirmed by empirical studies in some Western contexts (Cubbins and Vannoy 2005; Fergusson et al. 1986; Fox et al. 2002) and non-Western contexts (Haj-Yahia 2000; Hoffman et al. 1994; Yount 2005).

In addition to the absolute resource theory, other versions of resource theory have been proposed (e.g., Hornung et al. 1981) in which the focus of the theory is shifted from the husband's absolute resources to a pattern of relative resources (such as income difference or income ratio) between husband and wife. Violence is interpreted as a way for husbands to regain power from their resourceful wives (Anderson 1997; McCloskey 1996). It has been found that violence occurs primarily in a status reversal situation or status inconsistency in which wives contribute more resources than their husbands (Kaukinen 2004). Macmillan and Gartner (1999) have found that wives are at greater risk when they are employed while their husbands are unemployed. Similar findings in favor of relative resource theory are found in other studies examining couples' differences in education and income level (Anderson 1997; Fox et al. 2002; Haj-Yahia 2000).

Regardless of absolute or relative resource theory, researchers have assumed that men with few resources or fewer resources than their wives desire to have more power in the relationship that finally leads to domestic violence. This argument is a mediation hypothesis assuming that the husband's lack of economic resources, regardless absolutely or relatively, strengthens men's desire to have more decision-making power, which in turn provides the motivation for men to use physical violence. However, there is a common problem in most of these studies that the husband's power motive is usually excluded in the empirical analysis. Whether husbands who abuse their wives actually want to have more decision-making power has often been ignored in empirical studies that reference resource theories.

However, the assumption of these studies has its foundation in another line of studies that focuses on men's power motive and partner violence. It has been proposed that violence is initiated by men who feel that they should be in control of the relationship but are unable to assume that power (Babcock et al. 1993). Some studies have shown that the husband's need for power is positively associated with wife assault. Dutton and Strachan (1987) find that wife assaulters have a higher power motivation than satisfactorily married men. Mason and Blankenship (1987) also show that men with a strong power motive are more likely to initiate partner violence. In a study of family homicide, Websdale (2010: 35) argues that violence is not an expression of power but that violence "signifies an absence of it and an attempt to obtain it." This argument is echoed by the findings that female dominance in the relationship is often found associated with higher risk of husband-to-wife violence (Babcock et al. 1993; Coleman and Straus 1986; Hindin and Adair 2002). Studies focusing on the husband's perceived power have also found that the risk of husband-to-wife violence is higher when husbands feel powerless (e.g., Sagrestano et al. 1999). To explain the relationship between power arrangement and violence, Sagrestano et al. (1999: 67) argue that "husbands compensate for their lack of power or need for power by engaging in violence against their wives as a form of control." Altogether, these findings provide empirical support for the argument on the relationship between the power motive and the risk of husband-to-wife violence suggested in the resource theories.

However, in the above empirical studies that reference resource theories, only objective economic resources indicators have been used to predict the risk of violence. The role of husband's financial stress is seldom discussed in the literature of resource theories. The husband's perceived economic well-being is not considered as a key factor that affects his power motive and his tendency to use violence in the relationship. With reference to family stress theory, however, it is known that perceived economic well-being is a strong predictor of family well-being (Fox and Chancey 1998). Recently, theoretical discussion in the family violence literature has also emphasized financial stress as the mechanism that mediates the effects of economic conditions on domestic violence (DeMaris et al. 2003; Fox et al. 2002). Yet, these studies mainly focus on the direct effect of financial stress on domestic violence. The husband's power motive is absent in these studies in connecting the relationship between financial stress and husband-to-wife violence. By excluding power motive in their analysis, they implicitly assume that the husband's financial

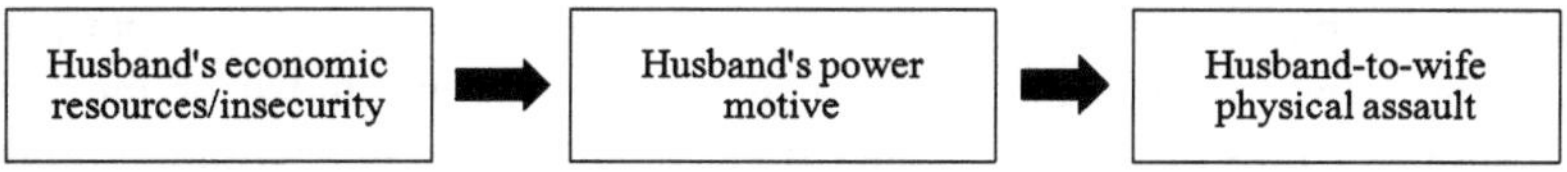

Fig. 7.1 The relationships among husband's economic resources, his power motive, and husband-to-wife physical assault

stress and his power motive are not related. Husband-to-wife violence is treated as a direct outcome of stress. The current study questions this assumption and additionally examines the role of power motive in mediating the relationship between husband's financial stress, as an indicator of his perceived economic insecurity and his use of violence. It is hypothesized that an economically distressed husband will desire for more decision power in the household, to compensate his loss of self-esteem and control of his own economic condition.

Summarizing the above discussion, we have derived the following hypotheses in the current study. With reference to absolute and relative resource theories, we hypothesize that the husband's resource indicators such as his income, employment, education, and his income level relative to his wife's, are negatively associated with his desire to have more decision-making power in the relationship. A resourceful husband is less likely to have a strong power motive in the relationship. His financial stress is, however, positively associated with his desire for more decision-making power.

Hypothesis 1a: *The husband's economic resources indicators are negatively associated with his power motive.*

Hypothesis 1b: *The husband's financial stress is positively associated with his power motive.*

With reference to the literature related to power motive and domestic violence, we hypothesize that husbands who desire for more decision-making power in the relationship are more likely to act violently toward their wives.

Hypothesis 2: *The husband's power motive is positively associated with husband-to-wife physical assault.*

Combining the hypotheses, we posit that the husband's economic insecurity exerts indirect effects on the risk of husband-to-wife physical assault by strengthening the husband's power motive. The mediation mechanism between economic insecurity and husband-to-wife physical assault is shown in Fig. 7.1.

Economic Resources and Husband-to-Wife Violence: Other Possible Explanations

Although the husband's lack of economic resources is shown as a consistent risk marker of domestic violence in many studies, the resource theory is not necessarily supported. The power motive is not the only plausible explanation of the relationship between a husband's resources and his use of violence against a partner. The association between resources and violence may be confounded or mediated by other factors such as husband's gender traditionalism and an egalitarian household arrangement within the household.

Some previous works (Dobash and Dobash 1979; Smith 1990; Yllo 1993) have suggested that husbands' gender traditionalism is a cause of husband-to-wife violence. They hypothesize that men with traditional gender attitudes and sex-role beliefs are more likely to act aggressively toward their disobedient wives, compared with men who are relatively more egalitarian (Crossman et al. 1990; Harris et al. 2005; Smith 1990; Yllo 1993). Some studies find significant effects of husbands' gender-role attitudes on wife assaults and injurious violence against wives in some contexts including the United States (Atkinson et al. 2005; Salari and Baldwin 2002), Canada (Smith 1990), South Africa (Jewkes et al. 2002), and China (Xu et al. 2005). However, a person's exposure to egalitarian gender-role ideology is partly determined by his social class and educational background (for a review, see Davis and Greenstein 2009). Therefore, some previous works hypothesize that gender-role ideology may play an important role in the relationship between husband's economic resources and domestic violence (Gelles 1974; Jewkes 2002). This alternative mechanism should be controlled for, in order to separate the effect of husband's economic resources on power motives and violence.

Besides, previous research have also shown that couples with an egalitarian power arrangement experience the lowest rate of violence (Choi and Ting 2008; Hindin and Adair 2002; Lenton 1995; Straus et al. 1980; Tang 1999b). Meanwhile, this power arrangement is more likely for couples from better social backgrounds who have higher education and income levels. In this study, shared power arrangement is also included as a control variable in the analysis.

Hong Kong as a Chinese Society

The above hypotheses are derived from the theories that are mainly developed in the Western context. However, the relationships between economic resources and family outcomes are not necessarily the same for all societies (e.g., see Rodman 1972). The relationship between husband's economic resources and the power motive can be a function of how universal it is that men play the role as a breadwinner in the household and dominate the relationship in a particular social context. Meanwhile, the relationship between the power motive and the use of violence may also depend on how legitimate it is considered in the society for men to use violence in a relationship. Therefore, the impacts of husband's economic insecurity on the risk of domestic violence may vary greatly across different social contexts. However, the applicability of the resource theory in Chinese societies is seldom empirically tested. In this study, we examine the above hypotheses in the context of Hong Kong Special Administrative Region of the People's Republic of China.

In Hong Kong, men are still expected to be the breadwinner of a household. In 2008, for example, a representative sample survey revealed that only 38 % of the sampled respondents would accept a status reversal situation in which women work outside the home while men stay at home to take care of the family (Chow and Lum 2008). Indeed, the image as a breadwinner is central for the male gender role in Hong Kong. A recent study by Choi and colleagues for the Equal Opportunities Commission in Hong Kong finds that paid employment is considered as the most important element in the construction of men's self-identity in Hong Kong, regardless of the respondents' background (Choi et al. 2012a). Economic insecurity such as job and income loss can be particularly stressful and frustrating for men.

However, the economic conditions have been changing fast in the recent years. Economic restructuring and globalization have led to social polarization in the income and occupational structure of the city (Chiu and Lui 2004). For example, the Gini index for Hong Kong was 53.3 in 2007, a figure which is much higher than other developed countries (World Bank 2008). In particular, men are more vulnerable to the shrinkage of the manufacturing sector and are more likely to suffer from structural unemployment (Tai 2012). Therefore, it is argued that the recent economic changes in Hong Kong have caused enormous stress or even "pain" for some groups of men (Choi et al. 2012a). As a result, some men in Hong Kong are "increasingly worried about their vanishing power" (Choi et al. 2012a: 47).

Meanwhile, in times of marital conflict, wife beating is acceptable in the traditional culture in the Chinese context and is still considered a private issue by many people in Hong Kong nowadays (Cheung et al. 1997; Liu and Chan 1999; Tang and Lai 2008). Although Hong Kong is a modern city that was ruled by the British for over a century, traditional Chinese culture still has a great influence in the society. A study reveals that attitudes toward violence against women in Hong Kong are not substantially different from other Chinese societies, such as mainland China and Taiwan (Tang et al. 2002a). Another study focusing on the social construction of women as legitimate victims of violence in Hong Kong, mainland China, and Taiwan also has similar findings. The belief that victims precipitate the violence they face is still widely held in all three Chinese societies, and it is common to attribute the responsibility to the victims in case of wife abuse (Tang et al. 2002b). This belief is also prevalent among police officers and social service providers, many of whom still believe that "wife abuse is a private matter and men should not be arrested if they only hit their wives" (Tam and Tang 2005: 36). In addition, in Chinese societies, family problems are mostly kept within the family because exposing such a problem to outsiders would lead to loss of face (Sullivan 2005). With all these background in mind, this study explicitly examines the impact of husband's economic insecurity on domestic violence, with a special focus on the role of husband's power motive in the relationship, as informed by the resource theory.

Methods

Data Source

Data analyzed in this study are from a research project "Hurting Each Other: Marital Inequality, Social Capital and Spousal Aggression in Hong Kong." As a part of the project, a household survey was conducted in a northwestern district of Hong Kong in 2007. The sampling frame for the survey was the Frame of Quarters maintained by the Hong Kong Census and Statistics Department. The Frame of Quarters is continuously updated by the government and contains the most complete and up-to-date register of residential addresses in Hong Kong. From this register, a probability sample of addresses was selected and contacted for face-to-face interviews. The survey was titled as "A Study of Family Relations" because of the sensitivity of the topic. The data collection approach for this survey adopted the procedure implemented in an earlier household survey of family violence by the Hong Kong Social Welfare Department (Chan 2005). Both members of the couples were interviewed, but they were interviewed separately in different time slots to ensure that the interviews were conducted on a one-to-one basis and that the respondents would not know what their spouses were asked and how they had answered. The interviews were conducted by well-trained interviewers on a face-to-face basis. However, sensitive questions were listed in a separate, self-administered questionnaire. The respondents were told that the interviewers could not know the answers given by the respondents in that separate questionnaire. After completion, the self-administered questionnaires were placed into a sealed envelope in front of the respondents to further ensure confidentiality. This measure was designed to protect the respondents' privacy and to maximize the respondents' trust in the interviewers to encourage the respondents' disclosure. More detailed description of the survey administration of this study has been included in Choi et al. (2012b).

Our units of analysis are on a couple level, with each case representing a couple with certain husband and wife characteristics. In total, 871 couples (1,742 respondents) completed the survey, constituting a response rate of 72 %, which is slightly lower than the response rate of another household survey of family violence in Hong Kong by the Social Welfare Department (Chan 2005). Nonresponses included refusals (addresses with eligible couples who refused to participate, 12.7 %) and noncontacts (addresses with eligible couples but no successful contact could be made during the survey period, 14.6 %) but excluded non-approachable addresses (vacant addresses) and inappropriate households (nonresidential addresses and no couple living in the household).

Dependent Variable: Husband-to-Wife Physical Assault

Husband-to-wife physical assault is the primary concern of this study. It is measured with items from the Revised Conflicts Tactics Scale (CTS2, developed by Straus et al. 1996). CTS2 is the most commonly used and standardized survey items to measure domestic violence in the family violence literature. Different from some early studies, which consisted of only a single global question to measure domestic violence (e.g., *Did your partner beat you in the past year?*), CTS2 uses multiple behavior-specific items to capture the prevalence rate of violence. With multiple behavior-specific items, it is believed that recall bias and differences in subjective understanding of the definition of abuse among respondents could be minimized (Smith 1994). The Chinese translation of the CTS2 used in this study was previously validated with a general population survey in Hong Kong (Chan 2005).

Physical assault is measured by the items from the minor physical assault subscale (i.e., throwing something, pushing, grabbing, shoving, slapping, and spanking), the severe physical assault subscale, and injuries subscale of the CTS2 (which include kicking, biting, hitting with fist, hitting or trying to hit with something, beating up, threatening with a gun or knife, or causing burns, sprains, bruises, small cuts, and injuries requiring medical attention and hospitalization). For each CTS2 item, the respondents were asked to indicate how often they had done a specific aggressive behavior to their spouse in the past year and how often their spouse had done the same to the respondents in the past year. The response for each item ranged from "never" (scored 0) to "3 or more times" in the last year (scored 3). There was a considerable discrepancy in the reporting of husband-to-wife physical assault by husbands and wives in the data. For a more accurate prevalence estimate, responses from both husband and wife were combined to construct the outcome variable (Szinovacz and Egley 1995).

Although CTS2 indicates the frequency of the aggressive behaviors and could be used as a continuous scale, the items are more often transformed into a dichotomous measure in studies with nonclinical samples because the variable is usually concentrated at zero in the population (Cubbins and Vannoy 2005). Therefore, the outcome variable, husband-to-wife physical assault, is dichotomized into a binary variable in this study, in which "0" indicates that both husband and wife did not report any item in the subscales that had been used and "1" indicates that either the woman reported that her partner had used violence in any of the items in the subscales or that the man reported having done any of the items in the subscales or both.

Independent Variables

Economic Resource Measures

Several husband's economic resources indicators were used to measure a husband's economic insecurity. The resource indicators include the husband's monthly income level, his income level relative to spouse, a low-income status, education level, and full-time employment status. The husband's monthly income level is used to measure the absolute resource level and is recorded as a 10-category variable, ranging from "less than HK$4,000 a month" to "more than HK$40,000 a month." The husband's low-income status is a dummy variable indicating that the husband's income level is under $6,000, which is approximately equivalent to the salary of an elementary service worker in 2007 (Hong Kong Census and Statistic Department 2007). This dummy variable is created to capture the nonlinear effect of income on violence to determine whether there is a concentration of violent cases in the most economically vulnerable group of men. The relative resource level between the husband and the wife is measured by subtracting the wife's personal income level from the husband's personal income level. Husbands' education level is measured as an 8-category variable, ranging from "not received any education" to "master's degree or above." Husband's education level is treated as an economic resource in this study because it indicates the husbands' employability in the labor market. Husbands' full-time employment status is measured as a dichotomous variable in which 1 is coded when the husband was employed full time and 0 is coded otherwise.

Husbands' Financial Stress

In addition to the husband's objective economic resources indicators, his subjective economic strain is also measured as an indicator of economic insecurity in this study. Husbands were asked how often they had worried about "their income not meeting their expenditure," "debt," and how much they were satisfied "with the current household financial condition." The first two items are recorded in four-point scales ranging from "never" (scored 1) to "always" (scored 4). Their satisfaction on financial well-being is measured by a five-point scale, ranging from "very satisfied" (scored 1) to "very dissatisfied" (scored 5). All items are then standardized and summed to obtain a score to indicate the husband's financial stress. The scale is readjusted to have a range from 0 to 4.5 (Cronbach's alpha = .71).

Husbands' Power Motive

This variable is the mediating variable in this study and is measured by a three-item scale indicating whether the husband desired to have more decision-making power in the relationship. Husbands were asked by how much they desired to have "more say" in the following areas in the relationship: "financial decision," "household division of labor," and "child care." Responses for these items ranged from "not at all/never mind" (scored 1), "yes, a little bit" (scored 2), "yes" (scored 3), to "yes, very much" (scored 4). Items were summed and averaged, constructing a scale ranging from 1 to 4. Cronbach's alpha of this scale is .92, which indicates good internal consistency.

In addition to the resources indicators, the husband's financial stress, and his power motive, we controlled for several other variables, including the couple's age difference (measured in years), the husband's age (measured in years), husband's gender-role attitude, and a shared power arrangement in the household.

Gender-Role Attitude

The husband's gender-role attitude was measured with a six-item scale. Respondents were asked how much they agreed with the following items related to traditional gender-role expectations: "Men should pay for women even when they have the same income level"; "Men should go to work, and women should take care of the housework"; "Women should try harder than men to avoid premarital sex"; "It is more difficult to accept women, rather than men, getting drunk"; "It is more inappropriate for a woman than a man to use foul language"; and "Women working as truck drivers are as ridiculous as men knitting sweaters." Responses for each item range from strongly disagree (scored 0) to strongly agree (scored 4). The items were summed to obtain a score with a range from 0 to 24 in which a higher score indicates a more traditional gender attitude (Cronbach's alpha = .69).

Shared Power Arrangement

This variable is measured by a four-item scale indicating the number of household items for which the interviewed couples had "equal say" in making the final decision. The items included "What job the husband should take," "When to visit friends and relatives," "Whether the wife should work outside the home or stay at home," and "The amount of money spent on groceries." The responses for each item are "Wife made the decision totally," "Wife made the decision mostly," "We made the decision together," "Husband made the decision mostly," and "Husband made the decision totally." For each item, the couples who made the decision jointly scored 1, and scored 0 otherwise. The four items are summed to obtain a scale ranging from 0 to 4 (Cronbach's alpha = .66).

Analytic Strategy

This study tests whether there are significant direct and indirect effects of the husband's economic insecurity on the risk of domestic violence through the power motive, as suggested by resource theories. We first estimate two separate regression models for husband-to-wife physical assault (outcome variable) and the husband's power motive (intervening variable) with the same set of independent variables. Because the outcome variable is a dichotomous variable, we use logistic regression to estimate the direct effect of the husband's economic resources, financial stress, and the power motive on the log odds of husband-to-wife physical assault, controlling for other relevant covariates. The power motive, the intervening variable in this study, is a continuous variable. We use OLS regression to estimate the associations between indicators of the husband's economic insecurity and his desire to have more decision-making power, while controlling for other relevant covariates.

Many previous works have used different methods to estimate indirect effects in the context of logistic regression. Unlike OLS regression, coefficients in logistic regression across nested models cannot be compared directly unless they are y-standardized (Mood 2009). MacKinnon and colleagues (2002) suggest the product of coefficients method (multiplying the coefficients from the two equations) to estimate the indirect effects of the predictor variables on the dichotomous outcome variable because this method asymptotically yields the lowest bias in estimating the indirect effect. Therefore, the product of coefficients strategy is used to calculate the indirect effects in this study. To test the statistical significance for the indirect effects, standard errors and confidence intervals for the indirect effects are derived by bootstrapping. The approach is recommended to assess mediation hypotheses, especially for studies with a small to moderate sample size (Hayes 2009). In this study, 5,000 bootstrap replicates were drawn from the original sample, and 95 % bias-corrected confidence intervals are used to assess the sampling variability over the indirect effects. The indirect effects are said to be significant at .05 level when the 95 % bias-corrected bootstrap confidence intervals do not overlap with zero. The significance tests for indirect effects were performed through a user-written program "binary_mediation" in Stata 11.

Results

Descriptive Statistics and Bivariate Associations

Table 7.1 summarizes the characteristics of couples included in the models and indicates whether there are statistically significant bivariate associations between these characteristics and the experience of husband-to-wife physical assault in the past year. In our sample, 10.5 % of the couples reported at least one incidence of husband-to-wife physical assault during the past year, and this figure is close to the prevalence rate estimated from other representative samples in Hong Kong (Chan 2005; Tang 1999a).

The median of the husbands' education level in our sample is secondary education. Education level of those husbands who physically assaulted their wives was not significantly different from those husbands who did not physically assault their wives. Approximately 73 % of our sampled husbands were employed full time. The median of the husbands' monthly income level in the sample was HK$8,000 to HK$9,999 but about 23 % of the sampled husbands were having less than HK$6,000. Bivariate analysis shows that couples who experienced wife beating during the preceding year were couples with husbands from the low-income groups ($p < .001$) and who were not engaged in full-time employment ($p < .01$). The results echo with the findings of some previous studies which show that couples with less economic resources are more likely to suffer from domestic violence. Also, those couples who reported physical assault during the preceding year had husbands, on

Table 7.1 Descriptive statistics and bivariate association: Husband's resource-related indicators, power motive, control variables, and husband-to-wife physical assault ($n = 851$)

Variable	Whole sample ($n = 851$)	Physical assault reported ($n = 89$, 10.5 %)	No physical assault reported ($n = 762$, 89.5 %)	p-Value
Husband's age	47.161	45.629	47.340	.126
	(9.978)	(10.006)	(9.966)	
Couple's age difference	6.454	7.775	6.299	.021*
	(5.725)	(6.477)	(5.615)	
Husband's education level	3.088	3.067	3.091	.858
	(1.156)	(0.876)	(1.185)	
Husband's income level	3.633	2.933	3.715	.000***
	(2.079)	(2.344)	(2.032)	
Husband's income <$6,000 (Yes = 1)	0.229	0.416	0.207	.000***
	(0.421)	(0.496)	(0.406)	
Husband's full-time employment status (Yes = 1)	0.727	0.584	0.744	.001**
	(0.446)	(0.496)	(0.437)	
Couple's income difference	2.505	1.865	2.580	.017*
	(2.698)	(2.877)	(2.669)	
Husband's financial stress	1.721	2.302	1.653	.000***
	(0.789)	(0.903)	(0.746)	
Husband's power motive	1.453	1.850	1.406	.000***
	(0.754)	(0.883)	(0.723)	
Husband's gender-role attitude	14.408	15.090	14.328	.019*
	(2.896)	(2.640)	(2.916)	
Shared power arrangement	1.237	1.315	1.228	.500
	(1.143)	(1.174)	(1.136)	

*$p < .05$; **$p < .01$; ***$p < .001$

average, with higher scores on the financial stress scale ($p < .001$). On average, our sampled husbands earned more than their wives. Bivariate analysis shows that the couple's income difference is negatively associated with the risk of husband-to-wife physical assault ($p < .05$).

The average score for husband's power motive scale in our sample is 1.453 (SD = 0.754). The husbands' desire for more power in the household is positively and significantly related to their use of physical assault against a partner. The husbands who scored higher in the scale were more likely to use physical violence ($p < .001$).

The mean score for the gender attitude scale in our sample is 14.408 (SD = 2.896), which is above the midpoint for the scale. The husbands' gender attitude is positively associated with the use of physical violence at a significant level ($p < .05$). Couples experiencing husband-to-wife physical assault had a husband with comparatively more traditional gender-role attitude. On average, the sampled couples had a shared power arrangement for 1.2 household arrangement items. The couples experiencing assault are not statistically different from couples who did not experience assault, in terms of number of household decision items decided by the couples jointly.

Table 7.2 Logistic regression model: Husband's resource-related variables, power motive, control variables, and husband-to-wife physical assault in the past year ($n = 851$)

Variable	Logit coefficient	(S.E.)
Resource-related variables		
Husband's education	0.038	0.118
Husband's income level	0.030	0.154
Husband's low-income status	1.360*	0.639
Husband's full-time employment status	0.554	0.482
Husband's financial stress	0.688***	0.161
Couple's income difference	−0.012	0.073
Intervening variable		
Husband's power motive	0.396**	0.151
Control variables		
Husband's age	−0.066***	0.017
Couple's age difference	0.071**	0.024
Shared power arrangement	0.081	0.099
Husband's gender traditionalism	0.080	0.046
Intercept	−3.733***	1.319
(McFadden's) Pseudo-R^2	0.151	
LR Chi-sq. (df)	86.05(11)***	

*$p < .05$; **$p < .01$; ***$p < .001$

The mean age of husbands in the overall sample is approximately 47 years (SD = 9.978). On average, the age difference between husbands and wives is 6.5 years (SD = 5.725). In the bivariate analysis, the husband's age is not significantly associated with husband-to-wife physical assault. Yet, husbands who used physical violence against their wives over the past year tended to be among those couples with a larger age difference ($p < .05$).

Results from Logistic and OLS Regression Models

Table 7.2 presents the results of logistic regression predicting the log odds of husband-to-wife physical assault in the past year. The husbands' full-time employment status, income level, and education level are not significantly associated with the husband-to-wife physical assault. The couples' income difference is also not significantly associated with husband-to-wife physical assault when the intervening variable and other covariates are controlled for. However, husbands who are of low-income status are significantly at higher risk (logit coefficient = 1.360; $p < .05$), indicating that physical assault is likely concentrated at the lowest-income stratum even after controlling for other covariates. In addition to low-income status, the husband's financial stress is also positively associated with husband-to-wife physical assault (logit coefficient = 0.688; $p < .001$) when other covariates are controlled for. The risk of husband-to-wife violence is higher for those husbands who are more economically distressed.

Table 7.3 OLS regression model: Husband's resource-related variables, control variables, and husband's power motive ($n = 851$)

Variable	Coefficient	(S.E.)
Resource-related variables		
Husband's education	0.009	0.023
Husband's income level	0.184***	0.029
Husband's low-income status	0.224	0.132
Husband's full-time employment status	−0.284**	0.092
Husband's financial stress	0.355***	0.032
Couple's income difference	−0.045***	0.014
Control variables		
Husband's age	−0.001	0.003
Couple's age difference	−0.006	0.005
Husband's gender traditionalism	0.049***	0.008
Shared power arrangement	0.080***	0.020
Intercept	−0.322	0.255
R^2	0.205	
F-test	21.72 (10,840)***	

*$p < .05$; **$p < .01$; ***$p < .001$

The husband's desire for more power in the relationship is significantly associated with the outcome variable. The husbands with a stronger desire to have more decision power in the relationship are more likely to beat their wives (logit coefficient = 0.396; $p < .01$). The husbands' gender traditionalism and shared power arrangement are however not significantly associated with wife beating after controlling for other covariates.

Table 7.3 presents the results of the linear regression for husbands' desire to have more decision power in the relationship, which is a key predictor of husband-to-wife physical assault in our logistic regression model. A couple's income difference is negatively correlated with the husband's power motive, indicating that the husbands who earn less than a partner are more likely to have a stronger desire for more power in the relationship (coefficient = −0.045; $p < .001$). The husband's full-time employment is also negatively correlated with his desire to have more relationship power (coefficient = −0.284; $p < .01$). In other words, husbands who are not in full-time employment are more likely have a stronger desire for power in the relationship. Husband's financial stress (coefficient = 0.355; $p < .001$) is also a significant correlate of husband's power motive. An economically distressed husband is more likely to have a strong desire for decision power in the relationship. Other objective resource indicators, such as education level and low-income status, are not significantly correlated with the husband's desire for power after controlling for other covariates.

Besides, gender traditionalism (coefficient = 0.049; $p < .001$) and shared power arrangement (coefficient = 0.080; $p < .001$) are all positively correlated with the husband's desire for power, indicating that the husband with a traditional gender-role attitude and sharing more household decision-making power with his wife has a stronger desire for more relationship power. Yet, the husband's age and the couple's age difference are not significantly correlated with the desire for more decision-making power.

Table 7.4 Direct and indirect effects of resource-related variables on husband-to-wife physical assault

Variable	Direct effect	Indirect effect via husband's power motive
Husband's education	n.s.	n.s.
Husband's income level	n.s.	+
Husband's low-income status	+	n.s.
Husband's full-time employment status	n.s.	−
Couple's income difference	n.s.	−
Husband's financial stress	+	+

Note: Significance tests for indirect effects were based on 95 % bias-corrected bootstrap confidence intervals (5,000 replicates)

Whether the resource-related variables influence the power motive and therefore the log odds of husband-to-wife physical assault is examined through statistical tests on the products of coefficients (MacKinnon et al. 2002) with 95 % bias-corrected bootstrapping method. The results are presented in Table 7.4 above.

The husband's full-time employment status exerts a significant and negative indirect effect on domestic violence. Full-time employed husbands have a weaker desire for more relationship power and therefore are less likely to act violently toward their wives. This finding is consistent with the resource theory (Goode 1971). In other words, a husband, who cannot find a full-time job, is more violence prone because of his strengthened power motive. A couple's income difference also has a significant and negative indirect effect on the risk of violence through the husband's power motive. The husbands who earn more than their wives have a weaker desire for more than their current level of decision-making power in the relationship and therefore are less likely to use violence to satisfy their need for power. This finding is consistent with the relative resource theory (Anderson 1997). Interestingly, our analysis also shows that husband's financial stress exerts its influence on the risk of violence both directly and indirectly through strengthening the husband's power motive. Husbands are more economically distressed in times of economic hardship, and they are more violent prone because of the stress itself and also the subsequently strengthened power motive. The husband's education level and low-income status do not exert an indirect effect on violence through the desire for power.

Unexpectedly, the husband's income level has a positive indirect effect on violence when all of the covariates are controlled. Controlling for couple's income difference, gender traditionalism, financial stress, and shared power arrangement, the husband's income level is associated with his desire for decision-making power positively. This finding contradicts the prediction of classical resource theory and is not found in previous studies. A plausible explanation is that, controlling for relative income between husbands and wives, husbands with higher income may believe that they are more legitimate and therefore entitled to have more say in making household decisions. However, the effect size of this indirect effect is weak and is suppressed by the direct and indirect effects of other economic insecurity measures. Overall, economic insecurity measures altogether still increase the risk of husband-to-wife physical assault.

To summarize the relationship between resource-related variables and domestic violence, we note that the husband's education has neither a direct nor an indirect effect through the power motive on physical assault against the wives in our analysis. This finding is not surprising because the husband's education is only one of the indicators of the husband's resources, whereas this indicator is least symbolic, compared with other indicators such as income and employment, in locating one's social location and negotiating the power arrangement in a relationship in the context of Hong Kong. Education is also merely an inconsistent risk marker of husband-to-wife violence in other samples (Stith et al. 2004). The husband's full-time employment status, his income level, and the couple's income difference have no direct effect on husband-to-wife physical assault after controlling other covariates, but these variables have significant indirect effects through the power motive. We also note that physical assault against wives was more likely to happen for couples with husbands who are of low-income status. We have, however, no evidence to claim that husbands in the lowest-income stratum are more likely to beat their wives because those husbands have a stronger power motive.

Discussion and Conclusion

This study advances our empirical knowledge on the relationships among husband's economic resources, his power motive, and husband-to-wife physical assault in a Chinese context. Although the associations between husband's economic resources and husband-to-wife physical assault are well documented in the empirical literature, hypotheses about the mechanism are seldom formally verified with empirical data. This study fills this gap by providing evidence to show that husbands' power motive plays a role in associating husbands' economic insecurity with their tendency to use violence against a partner in a Chinese context. Our analysis shows that a couple's income difference, the husband's full-time employment status, and his financial stress exert indirect effects on violence through the power motive. Having a better understanding of the mechanism that explains how husband's economic insecurity affects the risk of domestic violence not only potentially helps practitioners to design better intervention programs but also lets family sociologists have a more complete picture of the interconnection between the macroeconomic environment and the family relations.

Recent economic changes in Asia, which have led to rising income inequality, emerging poverty, and structural unemployment for unskilled workers, have played an important role in shaping family dynamics in Hong Kong. As Blood and Wolfe (1960) note, the changing pattern of economic structures affects the exchange relationship between husband and wife. Nowadays, the dominance of men in the household is becoming less based on men's superior role in making financial contributions to the household. Nevertheless, the cultural scripts about the men's role as the breadwinner still prevail in the society. As suggested in a research that explores the impact of gender stereotyping of males in Hong Kong, the centrality of the role as a provider in male's identity has increased men's burden, especially in times of increasing economic vulnerability for lower-class households (Choi et al. 2012a).

Under the social context that family problems are treated as private issues in traditional Chinese culture, violence may be used as an alternative instrument to maintain power in the relationship. Atkinson and colleagues (2005) hypothesize that the family outcome is a result of the interaction between structural and cultural arrangements. If egalitarian arrangements between husbands and wives are more widely accepted, economic problems for men led by the economic changes can become less of an issue. In the literature about social polarization in the Asian economy, however, it is very often that the empowerment of women is emphasized while the "downgrade of men is largely ignored" (Tai 2012: 15). Eventually, men's economic hardship can turn to affect women's health and cause marital instability in these households.

The findings have implications for policy-makers and practitioners. The government and policy-makers should be aware of the impacts of economic restructuring on family relations. In our analysis, we show that husband's financial stress is a key predictor of violence. Policies to strengthen the social protection of those who are economically distressed and vulnerable are desirable. Besides, providing anger and stress management programs alone may not help in eliminating the relationship between husband's economic insecurity and his tendency to use violence if the husband's power motive plays an important role in turning husbands to violence in times of economic hardship. Power dynamics inside the family should also be considered when intervention programs are designed.

However, some of the findings in our analysis are unexpected ones. Our data suggest that husbands' low-income status has a direct effect on the risk of violence, but we have no evidence that it has an indirect effect through the power motive. Husband-to-wife violence is concentrated in the lowest-income stratum, and this association is statistically significant even when controlled for other covariates including the husband's financial stress, gender-role attitude, and power motive. This suggests that the specified mechanisms cannot fully explain why the men from the poorest income group are more likely to beat their wives. It is left for further research to study whether this group of husbands is more violent due to other factors such as violent subculture, alcoholism, or social isolation.

In addition, the limitations of this study should not be overlooked. There are several assumptions that are not verifiable with cross-sectional and couple-level data. Although we attempt to establish the relationship between husbands' economic insecurity, power motive, and the risk of domestic violence, our evidence based on cross-sectional data are not conclusive. Longitudinal research design is preferred in establishing the causal relationship among the variables. In addition, we did not consider the contextual effect of community-level economic deprivation on the individual-level risk of domestic violence in this study. Some previous studies suggest that community-level economic disadvantage would also adversely affect the risk of domestic violence for couples living in the economically disadvantaged neighborhoods (Benson et al. 2003; Cunradi et al. 2000). In times of economic downturn, both individual-level economic insecurity and community-level economic deprivation may both play important roles in affecting the risk of domestic violence. Readers should be aware of other channels through which economic downturn and structural changes in macro-level may affect family well-being.

Besides, in this chapter, we discuss the relationship between economic insecurity and domestic violence mainly from men's perspective. We are aware of the importance of women's economic resources and their economic contributions to the households. However, the relationship between both men's and women's economic contributions to the family and the risk of violence would be more complicated than what we can cover in a chapter. Further studies on the role of women's economic empowerment and insecurity on domestic violence in the Chinese context are needed.

We are also aware of the weaknesses of CTS2. Even though CTS2 is commonly used in family violence surveys in many settings, the items in CTS2 cannot help to distinguish "common couple violence" and "patriarchal terrorism," which are two conceptually distinguished forms of violence as suggested by Johnson (1995). Johnson argues that the violent cases investigated in representative surveys mostly consist of common couple violence, which is more situational, less systemic, and a less severe form of abuse. With our data, we are unable to examine his argument and to distinguish the two forms of violence in the sample. Future studies with better measurements that can distinguish among types of violence may allow further investigation of the relationship between economic insecurity and the two forms of domestic violence.

Lastly, although Hong Kong is a good research site for family research in the Chinese context, generalizing the results from this study to other Chinese societies should be performed with extreme caution. Readers should note that Chinese societies such as Hong Kong, Taiwan, and mainland China share many cultural similarities but are also different in many aspects such as policy environment and social institutions. More studies, using samples from other Chinese societies, are called for to examine the relationship between economic insecurity and domestic violence in the Chinese context.

References

Anderson, K. L. (1997). Gender, status, and domestic violence: An integration of feminist and family violence approaches. *Journal of Marriage and the Family, 59*, 655–669.

Atkinson, M. P., Greenstein, T. N., & Lang, M. M. (2005). For women, breadwinning can be dangerous: Gendered resource theory and wife abuse. *Journal of Marriage and Family, 67*, 1137–1148.

Babcock, J. C., Waltz, J., Jacobson, N. S., & Gottman, J. M. (1993). Power and violence: The relation between communication patters, power discrepancies, and domestic violence. *Journal of Consulting and Clinical Psychology, 61*, 40–50.

Benson, M. L., Fox, G. L., DeMaris, A., & van Wyk, J. (2003). Neighborhood disadvantage, individual economic distress and violence against women in intimate relationships. *Journal of Quantitative Criminology, 19*, 207–235.

Blood, R., & Wolfe, D. (1960). *Husbands and wives: The dynamics of married living*. Glencoe: Free Press.

Campbell, J. C. (2002). Health consequences of intimate partner violence. *The Lancet, 359*, 1331–1336.

Chan, K. L. (2005). *Study on child abuse and spouse battering: Report on findings of household survey*. Hong Kong: Department of Social Work & Social Administration, The University of Hong Kong.

Cheung, F. M., Lai, B. L., Au, K. C., & Ngai, S. S. Y. (1997). Gender role identity, stereotypes, and attitudes in Hong Kong. In F. M. Cheung (Ed.), *Engendering Hong Kong society* (pp. 201–236). Hong Kong: The Chinese University Press.

Chiu, S. W. K., & Lui, T. L. (2004). Testing the global city-social polarization thesis: Hong Kong since 1990s. *Urban Studies, 41*, 1863–1888.

Choi, S. Y. P., & Ting, K. F. (2008). Wife beating in South Africa: An imbalance theory of resources and power. *Journal of Interpersonal Violence, 23*, 834–852.

Choi, S. Y. P., Au, W. T., Wong, W., Liong, C. C. M., Wong, F.Y., Lo, S. K. W., & Chao, K. C. (2012a). *Exploratory study on gender stereotyping and its impacts on male gender* (Research Report). Hong Kong: Equal Opportunities Commission.

Choi, S. Y. P., Cheung, Y. W., & Cheung, A. K. L. (2012b). Social isolation and spousal violence: Comparing female marriage migrants with local women. *Journal of Marriage and Family, 74*, 444–461.

Chow, N., & Lum, T. (2008). *Trends in family attitudes and values in Hong Kong*. Hong Kong: Department of Social Work and Social Administration, The University of Hong Kong.

Coleman, D. H., & Straus, M. A. (1986). Marital power, conflict and violence in a nationally representative sample of American couples. *Violence and Victims, 1*, 141–157.

Crossman, R. K., Stith, S. M., & Bender, M. M. (1990). Sex role egalitarianism and marital violence. *Sex Roles, 22*, 293–304.

Cubbins, L. A., & Vannoy, D. (2005). Socioeconomic resources, gender traditionalism, and wife abuse in urban Russian couples. *Journal of Marriage and Family, 67*, 37–52.

Cunradi, C. B., Caetano, R., Clark, C., & Schafer, J. (2000). Neighborhood poverty as a predictor of intimate partner violence among White, Black, and Hispanic couples in the United States: A multilevel analysis. *Annals of Epidemiology, 10*, 297–308.

Davis, S. N., & Greenstein, T. N. (2009). Gender ideology: Components, predictors, and consequences. *Annual Review of Sociology, 35*, 87–105.

DeMaris, A. (2000). Till discord do us part: The role of physical and verbal conflict in union disruption. *Journal of Marriage and Family, 62*, 683–692.

DeMaris, A., Benson, M. L., Fox, G. L., Hill, T., & van Wyk, J. (2003). Distal and proximal factors in domestic violence: A test of an integrated model. *Journal of Marriage and Family, 65*, 652–667.

Dobash, R. E., & Dobash, R. (1979). *Violence against wives: A case against the patriarchy*. New York: Free Press.

Dutton, D. G., & Strachan, C. E. (1987). Motivation needs for power and spouse-specific assertiveness in assaultive and nonassaultive men. *Violence and Victims, 2*, 145–156.

Ellsberg, M., Jansen, H., Heise, L., Watts, C. H., & Garcia-Moreno, C. (2008). Intimate partner violence and women's physical and mental health in the WHO multi-country study on women's health and domestic violence: An observational study. *The Lancet, 371*, 1165–1172.

Fergusson, D. M., Horwood, J., Kershaw, K. L., & Shannon, F. T. (1986). Factors associated with reports of wife assault in New Zealand. *Journal of Marriage and the Family, 48*, 407–412.

Fox, G. L., & Chancey, D. (1998). Sources of economic distress: Individual and family outcomes. *Journal of Family Issues, 19*, 725–749.

Fox, G. L., Benson, M. L., DeMaris, A., & van Wyk, J. (2002). Economic distress and intimate violence: Testing family stress and resources theories. *Journal of Marriage and the Family, 64*, 793–807.

Garcia-Moreno, C., Jansen, H., Ellsberg, M., Heise, L., & Watts, C. H. (2006). Prevalence of intimate partner violence: Findings from the WHO multi-country study on women's health and domestic violence. *The Lancet, 368*, 1260–1269.

Gelles, R. J. (1974). *The violent home*. Beverley Hills: Sage.

Goode, W. J. (1971). Force and violence in the family. *Journal of Marriage and Family, 33*, 624–636.

Haj-Yahia, M. (2000). The incidence of wife abuse and battering and some sociodemographic correlates as revealed by two national surveys in Palestinian society. *Journal of Family Violence, 15*, 347–374.

Harris, R. J., Firestone, J. M., & Vega, W. A. (2005). The interaction of country of origin, acculturation, and gender role ideology on wife abuse. *Social Science Quarterly, 86*, 463–483.

Hayes, A. F. (2009). Beyond Baron and Kenny: Statistical mediation analysis in the new millennium. *Communication Monographs, 76*, 408–420.

Hindin, M. J., & Adair, L. S. (2002). Who's at risk? Factors associated with intimate partner violence in the Philippines. *Social Science & Medicine, 55*, 1385–1399.

Hoffman, K. L., Demo, D. H., & Edwards, J. N. (1994). Physical wife abuse in a non-western society: An integrated theoretical approach. *Journal of Marriage and the Family, 56*, 131–146.

Hong Kong Census and Statistics Department. (2007). *Women and men in Hong Kong: Key statistics 2007*. Hong Kong: Census and Statistics Department.

Hornung, C. A., McCullough, B. C., & Sugimoto, T. (1981). Status relationship in marriage: Risk factors in spouse abuse. *Journal of Marriage and the Family, 43*, 675–692.

Hotaling, G. T., & Sugarman, D. B. (1986). An analysis of risk markers in husband to wife violence: The current state of knowledge. *Violence and Victims, 1*, 101–124.

Jewkes, R. (2002). Intimate partner violence: Causes and prevention. *The Lancet, 359*, 1423–1429.

Jewkes, R., Levin, J., & Penn-Kekana, L. (2002). Risk factors for domestic violence: Findings from a South African cross-sectional study. *Social Science & Medicine, 55*, 1603–1617.

Johnson, M. P. (1995). Patriarchal terrorism and common couple violence: Two forms of violence against women. *Journal of Marriage and the Family, 57*, 283–294.

Kaukinen, C. (2004). Status compatibility, physical violence, and emotional abuse in intimate relationships. *Journal of Marriage and Family, 66*, 452–471.

Lenton, R. L. (1995). Power versus feminist theories of wife abuse. *Canadian Journal of Criminology, 37*, 305–330.

Liu, M., & Chan, C. (1999). Enduring violence and staying in marriage: Stories of battered women in rural china. *Violence Against Women, 5*, 1469–1492.

MacKinnon, D. P., Lockwood, C. M., Hoffman, J. M., West, S. G., & Sheet, V. (2002). A comparison of methods to test mediation and other intervening variables effects. *Psychological Methods, 7*, 83–104.

Macmillan, R., & Gartner, R. (1999). When she brings home the bacon: Labor-force participation and the risk of spousal violence against women. *Journal of Marriage and Family, 61*, 947–958.

Mason, A., & Blankenship, V. (1987). Power and affiliation motivation, stress, and abuse in intimate relationships. *Journal of Personality and Social Psychology, 52*, 203–210.

McCloskey, L. A. (1996). Socioeconomic and coercive power within the family. *Gender & Society, 10*, 449–463.

Mood, C. (2009). Logistic regression: Why we cannot do what we think we can do, and what we can do about it. *European Sociological Review, 26*, 67–82.

Parish, W. L., Wang, T., Laumann, E. O., Pan, S., & Luo, Y. (2004). Intimate partner violence in China: National prevalence, risk factors and associated health problems. *International Family Planning Perspectives, 30*, 174–181.

Rodman, H. (1972). Marital power and the theory of resources in cultural context. *Journal of Comparative Family Studies, 3*, 50–69.
Sagrestano, L. M., Heavey, C. L., & Christensen, A. (1999). Perceived power and physical violence in marital conflict. *Journal of Social Issues, 55*, 65–79.
Salari, S. M., & Baldwin, B. M. (2002). Verbal, physical, and injurious aggression among intimate couples over time. *Journal of Family Issues, 23*, 523–550.
Schumacher, J. A., Feldbau-Kohn, S., Slep, A. M. S., & Heyman, R. E. (2001). Risk factors for male-to-female partner physical abuse. *Aggression and Violent Behavior, 6*, 281–352.
Smith, M. D. (1990). Patriarchal ideology and wife beating: A test of a feminist hypothesis. *Violence and Victims, 5*, 257–273.
Smith, M. D. (1994). Enhancing the quality of survey data on violence against women: A feminist approach. *Gender & Society, 8*, 109–127.
Stith, S. M., Smith, D. B., Penn, C. E., Ward, D. B., & Tritt, D. (2004). Intimate partner physical abuse perpetration and victimization risk factors: A meta-analytic review. *Aggression and Violent Behavior, 10*, 65–98.
Straus, M. A., & Gelles, R. J. (1995). *Physical violence in American families: Risk factors and adaptations to violence in 8,145 families*. New Brunswick: Transaction Publishers.
Straus, M. A., Gelles, R. J., & Steinmetz, S. K. (1980). *Behind closed door: Violence in the American family*. New York: Anchor.
Straus, M. A., Hamby, S. L., Boney-McCoy, S., & Sugarman, D. B. (1996). The revised Conflict Tactics Scale (CTS2): Development and preliminary psychometric data. *Journal of Family Issues, 17*, 283–316.
Sullivan, P. L. (2005). Culture, divorce, and family mediation in Hong Kong. *Family Court Review, 43*, 109–123.
Szinovacz, M. E., & Egley, L. C. (1995). Comparing one-partner and couple data on sensitive marital behaviors: The case of marital violence. *Journal of Marriage and the Family, 57*, 995–1010.
Tai, P. F. (2012). Gender matters in social polarization: Comparing Singapore, Hong Kong and Taipei. *Urban Studies*. http://usj.sagepub.com/content/early/2012/10/01/0042098012460734.abstract?rss=1. Accessed 5 Nov 2012. doi: 10.1177/0042098012460734
Tam, S. Y., & Tang, C. S. K. (2005). Comparing wife abuse perceptions between Chinese police officers and social workers. *Journal of Family Violence, 20*, 29–38.
Tang, C. S. K. (1999a). Wife abuse in Hong Kong Chinese families: A community survey. *Journal of Family Violence, 14*, 179–191.
Tang, C. S. K. (1999b). Marital power and aggression in a community sample of Hong Kong Chinese families. *Journal of Interpersonal Violence, 14*, 586–601.
Tang, C. S. K., & Lai, B. P. Y. (2008). A review of empirical literature on the prevalence and risk markers of male-on-female intimate partner violence in contemporary China, 1987–2006. *Aggression and Violent Behavior, 13*, 10–28.
Tang, C. S. K., Cheung, F. M. C., Chen, R., & Sun, X. (2002a). Definition of violence against women: A comparative study in Chinese societies of Hong Kong, Taiwan, and the People's Republic of China. *Journal of Interpersonal Violence, 17*, 671–688.
Tang, C. S. K., Wong, D., & Cheung, F. M. C. (2002b). Social construction of women as legitimate victims of violence in Chinese societies. *Violence Against Women, 8*, 968–996.
Websdale, N. (2010). *Familicidal hearts: The emotional styles for 211 killers*. New York: Oxford University Press.
World Bank. (2008). *World development indicator*. Washington, DC: World Bank.
World Health Organization. (2005). *WHO multi-country study on women's health and domestic violence against women: Full report*. Geneva: World Health Organization.
Xu, X., Zhu, F., O'Campo, P., Koenig, M. A., Mock, V., & Campbell, J. (2005). Prevalence of and risk factors for intimate partner violence in China. *American Journal of Public Health, 95*, 78–85.
Yllo, K. (1993). Through a feminist lens: Gender, power, and violence. In R. J. Gelles & D. R. Loseke (Eds.), *Current controversies on family violence* (pp. 47–62). Newbury Park: Sage.

Yount, K. M. (2005). Resources, family organization, and domestic violence against married women in Minya, Egypt. *Journal of Marriage and Family, 67*, 579–596.

Yount, K. M., & Carrera, J. S. (2006). Domestic violence against married women in Cambodia. *Social Forces, 85*, 355–387.

Yount, K. M., & Li, L. (2010). Domestic violence against married women in Egypt. *Sex Roles, 63*, 332–347.

Part III
Economic Stress and Health

Chapter 8
Economic Stress and Health Among Rural Chinese Elderly

Wei-Jun Jean Yeung and Zhenhua Xu

Economic Stress and Mortality Among the Oldest-Old in China

Two-thirds of Chinese elderly live in the rural areas where both public and private safety nets for the elderly have weakened in recent decades. Poverty rate for the oldest-old is the highest among all age groups in China. With China's oldest-old population projected to quadruple by 2050, there is a pressing need to understand the implications of economic stress for the oldest-olds' well-being. The impact of economic stress on health remains largely unexplored with the exception of several longitudinal studies conducted in European countries or in America (Stuckler et al. 2009). China, having undergone dramatic demographic and economic transformations since the 1950s, provides a unique context for understanding the link between economic stress and health under a different cultural and political regime.

Research has shown that economic stress can affect various indicators of physical and mental health. Evidence of the effect of economic stress on mortality is mixed, however. At an aggregate level, the Russian Federation suffered a major increase in male mortality in the early 1990s, and mortality increased in Thailand during the 1990s' Asian Economic Crisis, whereas on the other hand, short-term mortality effects of the South Korean economic crisis were relatively small (Khang et al. 2005; Khang and Lynch 2010). Studies have shown that poor macroeconomic conditions seem to induce a biological response in men and women (Catalano 2003; Catalano

W.-J.J. Yeung (✉)
Department of Sociology and Asia Research Institute, National University of Singapore, Singapore
e-mail: ariywj@nus.edu.sg

Z. Xu
Department of Sociology, University of North Carolina at Chapel Hill, NC, USA
e-mail: xuzhenhua521@gmail.com

W.J.J. Yeung and M.T. Yap (eds.), *Economic Stress, Human Capital, and Families in Asia: Research and Policy Challenges*, Quality of Life in Asia 4,
DOI 10.1007/978-94-007-7386-8_8, © Springer Science+Business Media Dordrecht 2013

et al. 2005). Ruhm (2000) and Van Den Berg et al. (2009) show the relationship between economic recession and individual health. A longitudinal study on women with breast cancer found that patients who reported worries about job security, medical costs, or financial stress at the baseline had significantly poorer functional, mental, and affective well-being over the subsequent 12 months (Ell et al. 2008). A body of research has shown that stress and depression tend to trigger inflammatory response, enhancing proinflammatory cytokine production (Goebel et al. 2000; Steptoe et al. 2007; Maes et al. 2000; Kendall-Tackett 2009; Miller et al. 2005).

Friedman and Thomas (2008) used data from the Indonesia Family Life Survey to examine the impact of the 1997 Asian financial crisis on individuals' psychological well-being. They found that the crisis had detrimental consequences on psychological well-being (depression, anxiety, and lowered aspirations) across the entire age group distribution over the crisis period. The impact was strongest on the low-education group, the rural landless, and residents in the hardest hit areas. Furthermore, the negative impact persisted after the financial crisis, suggesting that financial crisis has long-term deleterious effects on one's psychological well-being.

In view of the potential health consequences of economic stress, researchers such as Dooley and Catalano (1984) had long highlighted the epidemiology of economic stress, and others have argued that: "It, therefore, deserves to be seriously considered as a potential public health risk factor among families" (e.g., Olivius et al. 2004).

This chapter examines the relationship between economic stress and mortality among the oldest-old population in rural China. We start by describing the social-demographic contexts in China today that are crucial for understanding the relationships under investigation. We then move to describe a conceptual framework which integrates microeconomic and sociopsychological perspectives (Conger and Elder 1994). We examine the risk factors for economic stress and consider factors that may mediate and moderate the relationship between economic stress and mortality. Finally, we end with a discussion about the implications of our results for China's challenge in caring for the elderly.

Recent Social Contexts of the Elderly in China

China has experienced a dramatic decline in fertility due to the one-child policy and an unprecedented speed of socioeconomic development since the economic reform in the late 1970s. As a result, the Chinese population is aging at a rate faster than those in many developed countries. The proportion of those aged 65 and above has increased from 6.96 % in 2000 to 8.87 % in 2010 (National Bureau of Statistics of China 2010) and forecasted to be 17 % in 2030 and 27 % in 2050 (Chinese Ministry of Civil Affairs Report 2010). The proportion of the oldest-old (80 years and older) among the elderly (65 years and older) is expected to climb rapidly, from 14 % in 2000 to 34.4 % in 2050, amounting to 114 million (Zeng and George 2000). This demographic landscape presents a tremendous challenge for China to support and care for the elderly because both private and public assistance for the elderly have weakened in China since the past few decades.

The availability of family support for the Chinese elderly has dwindled as the number of children and kin, who can provide care, has declined and the old-age dependency ratio has increased drastically since the 1979 one-child policy. Many single children will shoulder the responsibility of caring for their parents, parents-in-law, and grandparents, resulting in the "4-2-1" problem. This problem is particularly salient in light of the combination of the nature of caregiving tasks and the increasingly skewed sex ratio in China since the initiation of the one-child policy. As the caregiving responsibility often falls on the shoulders of daughters and daughters-in-law, the "missing girls" problem makes the challenge of caring for the elderly even more formidable.

To address the challenge of elderly care, the Chinese government has explicitly written into the laws that require children to care for elderly parents in China. Marriage Law of People's Republic of China stipulates that children shall be under the obligation to support their parents; where any child fails to perform his or her obligations, the parents who are unable to work or who are living a difficult life shall be entitled to ask their child(ren) to provide aliments. The law of the Protection of Rights and Interests of the Aged also regulates the duty of children in supporting their elderly parents. Despite these laws, economic stress among the elderly remains pervasive, particularly among those who live in the rural areas, where many young adults migrate to the cities for work.

In the public domain, the social safety nets for the elderly in China have weakened since the economic reform, especially since the late 1990s. As the health care provision became increasingly privatized, the out-of-pocket medical costs have skyrocketed. Meanwhile, the health insurance and pension are not available to most rural elderly. China Health Services Report estimated that 85.8 % of elderly did not have medical insurance in rural areas in 2003, before the reform of the New Rural Cooperative Medical System (Center for Health Statistics and Information 2009). Between1998 and 2003, clinical and hospital expenses had increased by 14.7 % each year in rural areas, compared to a 2.4 % increase each year between 1993 and 1997(Center for Health Statistics and Information 2004). The out-of-pocket cost of health care had increased to 40 % by 1997, 49 % by 2006, and reached its peak of 59 % in 2000 (England 2005; You and Kobayashi 2011).

To appreciate the intricacy of China's public safety nets system, it is crucial to understand the *hukou* system initiated in the late 1950s, which has served as the predominant social stratification mechanism in China since then and has contributed to urban-rural economic and social inequality (Selden 1999; Wu and Treiman 2007). The system assigns people, according to an individual's birth place, to either agricultural or nonagricultural *hukou* status. Children inherit the *hukou* status of their parent (usually the mother). Since the late 1950s, this system was used by the Chinese government to officially differentiate between residential groups and to control population movement. The *hukou* system is also used to allocate socioeconomic benefits, such as income, housing, social security, medical care, education, and retirement benefits, according to one's residence (Cheng and Selden 1994). While the "urban aristocrats" are entitled to these benefits, those with rural *hukou* are left to fend for themselves with little social security or public health services.

Poverty Rate Among Chinese Elderly

Research by Wang and Zhang (2005) examined elderly poverty in China based on subjective assessment by the elderly of their own financial circumstances. The elderly were asked if they felt their financial resources were "more than sufficient," "have some surplus," "just sufficient to make ends meet," "somewhat insufficient," or "very insufficient." Those who felt that their financial situation was very insufficient were defined as "poor." This study found that there were 9.2–11.7 million elderly living in poverty in 2000, accounting for about 7.1–9.0 % of the elderly population. Moreover, the authors found poverty was twice as prevalent in rural as in urban areas, with 8.6–10.8 % rural elderly, as opposed to 4.2–5.5 % of urban elderly, living in poverty.

Research has shown that poverty rate in China is higher among the elderly than among other age groups. The Sampling Survey of the Aged Population in China conducted in 2000 showed that the proportion of the poor among those aged 60–64 was 11.3 %, and this proportion increased dramatically to 22.6 % for those aged 75–79, 27.7 % for those aged 80–84, and to 30.3 % for those aged 85–89 (Qiao et al. 2006).

Methods

We examine how economic stress affects the mortality hazard of the elderly based on the conceptual framework shown in Fig. 8.1.

This framework integrates two strains of thoughts: (1) microeconomic theories that see family members pooling resources and smoothing life course consumptions over time, and (2) the family stress theory that takes sociopsychological factors into account (Conger and Elder 1994). Objective economic stress, measured by indicators such as financial or material deprivation, often triggers a certain level of subjective economic strain or pressure among family members. The extent to which such economic pressure affects one's health status will likely depend on a set of moderators at individual, family, and community levels. These moderators include the psychological attributes of the individual and family members, stock of family wealth and human capital, and availability of social support networks that may buffer economic stress, as well as availability of community resources such as public assistance or favorable local labor market conditions.

We hypothesize that economic stress leads to poorer medical care and higher mental distress, which then raise the mortality hazard. Several factors may moderate the impact of economic stress on health including the human capital of the oldest-old, the availability of social support networks, and public assistance. Another potential moderator is the psychological resources of the elderly. A strong sense of control may help insulate the oldest-old from the harm of stressors and allow him or her to cope better in times of economic stress.

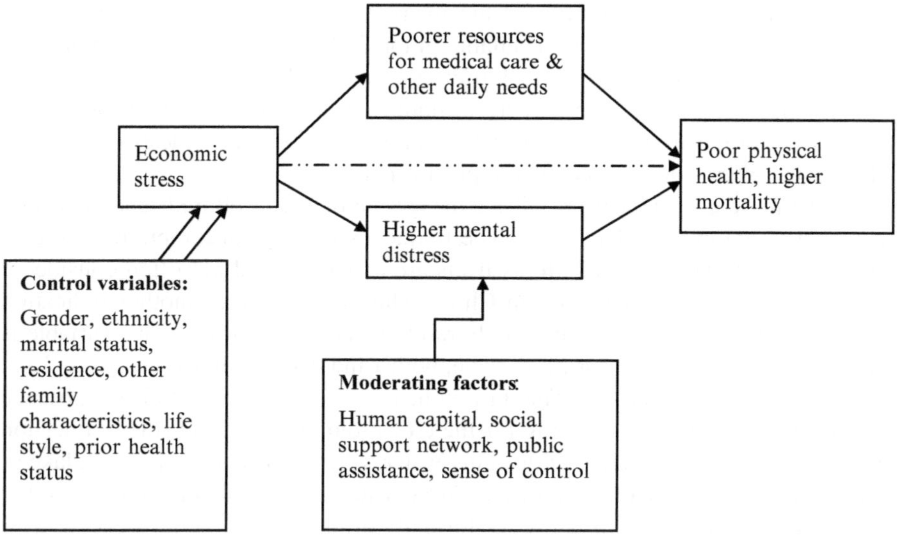

Fig. 8.1 Conceptual framework for the relationship between economic stress and health

The Data

We drew our data from the Chinese Longitudinal Healthy Longevity Survey (CLHLS) which was launched in 1998 in China. In 2000, 2002, 2005, and 2008, follow-up surveys were conducted. For details of the study, see documentations in the study Website (Center of the study of Aging and Human Development 2010). The sample was randomly collected from half of the counties and cities in 22 of China's 31 provinces, which constitutes about 85 % of the total population in China (Zeng 2008). We drew our data from the 2000, 2002, and 2005 panel surveys. Our sample included 7,398 men and women in rural areas between the ages of 80 and 105 in 2000.

Measures

Independent Variable

The main independent construct in our study is economic stress. We measure this construct with both objective indicators of economic hardships and a subjective indicator of the perceived economic strain for the elderly. It has been argued in previous research that data on family income collected from the elderly tend to be unreliable since they may not know or be confused about the amount (e.g., see Wang and Zhang 2005).

For the objective economic hardship measures, data for household income or earnings were unfortunately not available in the 2000 survey. We use several alternative indicators of economic hardship in this chapter. These measures include (1) whether the oldest-old were receiving welfare from the government or community assistance, (2) the frequency of fruit consumption among the oldest-old, and (3) whether the oldest-old had access to tapped water.

The Chinese government provides a meager amount of welfare to the very poor to support them in their daily lives. The frequency of fruit consumption is used as an indicator of the quality of life as fruits are expensive and not often considered as a basic necessity in daily life in China. Thus we take it as another indication of daily financial difficulty if an elderly rarely or never eats fruits. This variable is measured in the survey on a 4-point scale, with 1 indicating "almost every day" and 4 indicating "rarely or never." The third indicator of economic stress is the absence of tapped water for daily drinking for the oldest-old. The original survey question enquired regarding the source of drinking water, whether it was from a well, lake or river, spring, pond or pool, or tap water. We construct a variable indicating whether the oldest-old had access to tap water for daily drinking. Economic stress theories postulate that objective economic stress induces perceived (subjective) economic strain which then exerts a more direct impact on the well-being of the elderly. We measure subjective economic stress (economic strain) with an indicator that assesses whether the oldest-old perceived income from all sources as sufficient to support all of his or her daily expenditures at the time of the 2000 interview. These income sources include pension, spouse, child, grandchild, other relatives, local government or community, income from own work, and any other sources.

Dependent Variable

The dependent variable was the hazard rate of mortality – a time-variant variable, indicating whether the respondents in 2000 had or had not passed away by 2005 at different time points. The unit of time for the dependent variable is the number of days under risk.

Moderators

As depicted in the conceptual framework, several factors including one's human capital, social support network, public assistance, and sense of control can potentially moderate the impact of economic stress on health. We measure human capital with educational attainment and occupation of the oldest-old. As the Chinese oldest-old generally have low educational attainment, we divide the years of school into three categories: (1) none, (2) 1–5 years, and (3) 6 or more years. Occupational level is measured with the occupational status of one's job before the age of 60.

Occupational status is defined as high for professional and technical personnel and governmental, institutional, or managerial personnel and as low for all other occupations, including those in agriculture, forestry, animal husbandry, industry, service fishery work, military, housework, and others.

The social support network of the oldest-old is measured with (1) whether he or she had at least one living child, (2) whether the main financial support came from children in 2000, and (3) whether the oldest-old was receiving a pension.

Another potential mediator in this framework is the psychological attributes of the oldest-old, specifically the extent to which the elderly felt he or she was in control. We assess their sense of control by measuring the degree to which the elderly felt he or she had a say in matters concerning himself or herself in daily living. This scale ranges from 1 indicating "never" to 5 "always."

Mediators: Quality of Medical Care and Mental Distress

We hypothesize that the impact of economic stress on mortality was mediated by the quality of medical care and the psychological well-being of the oldest-old. The quality of medical care is measured in terms of whether the oldest-old was able to obtain immediate medical service when ill. We create a dichotomized variable for "poor medical care" from these data.

The mental well-being of the elderly was measured with four items in the 2000 and 2002 surveys: optimism ("I look at the bright side of things"), conscientiousness ("I like to keep my belongings neat and clean"), neuroticism ("I often feel fearful or anxious"), and loneliness ("I often feel lonely and isolated"). These items measure psychological resources for the well-being of the oldest-old (Smith et al. 2008; Wu and Schimmele 2006). Responses are recorded in a 5-point scale (0, always; 1, often; 2, sometimes; 3, seldom; and 4, never). The last items (neuroticism and loneliness) for the negative aspects of emotions are reverse coded. The overall index is derived from the average score on the four items with a range of "0" to "4" (Cronbach's alpha = 0.629), with a higher score indicating a higher level of mental distress. Both mediators are measured in two points of time – 2000 and 2002.

Other Control Variables

We control for basic demographic characteristics, the lifestyle, and diet consumption of the oldest-old. Basic demographic variables include age, gender, ethnicity, residence, and marital status. Ethnicity is measured by whether he or she was Han. We also control for three aspects of the life style – whether or not the oldest-old smoked, drank, or exercised in the past, all dichotomous variables. For diet, we create an index of protein consumption composed of the frequency of meat, fish, and egg consumption measured on a 3-point scale with 1 indicating "rarely or never" and 3 indicating "almost every day."

We also control for baseline health status, activities of daily living (ADL), and the cognitive functioning of the oldest-old. Self-reported health is measured on a 5-point scale, which we then collapse into 3 categories, with 1 indicating "very good and good," 2 indicating "so-so," and 3 indicating "poor and very poor." We create the cumulated activities of daily living index (ADL index) with six items – bathing, dressing, visiting the toilet, transferring, continence, and feeding (Katz et al. 1963). Each item ranges from 1 to 3, with 3 indicating the highest level of disability. Additionally, we measure the cognitive functioning of China's oldest-old using the Chinese version of mini-mental state examination (MMSE), which records four aspects of cognitive functioning – orientation, calculation, recall, and language (Folstein et al. 1975). MMSE has been widely used in measuring cognitive impairment (Nguyen et al. 2003; Schultz-Larsen et al. 2008). It covers 30 questions, and the respondents receive one point for answering each question correctly. Respondents who score less than 18 are considered cognitively impaired, based on previous studies (Zhang 2006).

In addition, about 36 % of the interviews were conducted with a proxy respondent at the time of the 2000 interview. This is often done when the respondents are too impaired to participate in the survey. We create a variable indicating whether a proxy respondent was used as a control for both the quality of the report and as an indicator of the disability status of the oldest-old.

Analytical Strategy

Sampling weights are applied to all analyses in this chapter to adjust for initial selection probability and attrition over time. First, we investigate potential risk factors for living under economic stress, including basic demographic characteristics, baseline health status, personal support network, and public assistance. Then we examine whether economic stress had an effect on mortality through (1) the quality of medical care and (2) emotional distress of the oldest-old.

Subsequently, we estimate the Kaplan-Meier survival curves (Kaplan and Meier 1958), comparing those who lived under economic stress in 2000 to those who did not. As shown in the formula below, n_j represents the number of respondents who had not died and were not censored at t_0 (the beginning of time period t), d_j represents the number of respondents who had died during this period, and $S(t)$ denotes the outcome of survival probabilities in t and the preceding periods:

$$S(t) = \prod_{j=t_0}^{t} \left\{ \frac{(n_j - d_j)}{n_j} \right\}$$

Finally, Cox's proportional hazard model is used to estimate the impact of economic stress on the hazard rates of mortality from 2000 to 2005. This model stipulates that the hazard rate for the nth subject is

$$h\left(t\middle|x_n\right) = h_0(t)\exp\left(x_n\beta_x\right)$$

where the regression coefficients β_x are to be estimated from the data (Cox 1972). The exponentiated individual coefficient $\exp(\beta_x)$ represents the ratio of the hazards for a one-unit change in the corresponding covariate.

Results

First, we examine the four indicators of the economic stress experienced by the oldest-old in 2000 in Fig. 8.2. About 17 % of the oldest-old felt they lived under economic stress. Sixty-seven percent did not have access to tap water, one-quarter rarely or never ate fruits, and about 16 % received welfare from government or community.

Figure 8.3 shows the living arrangements of the oldest-old in rural areas, indicating a majority of them lived with family members with 65 % living with children (with or without a spouse) and 13 % living only with a spouse. About 15 % of them lived alone and 6 % lived in an institution.

Figure 8.4 shows the distribution of the main source of income for the oldest-old. About three-quarters relied on their child(ren), and about 4 % on grandchild(ren), as his or her main source of income. Public assistance such as pension was not

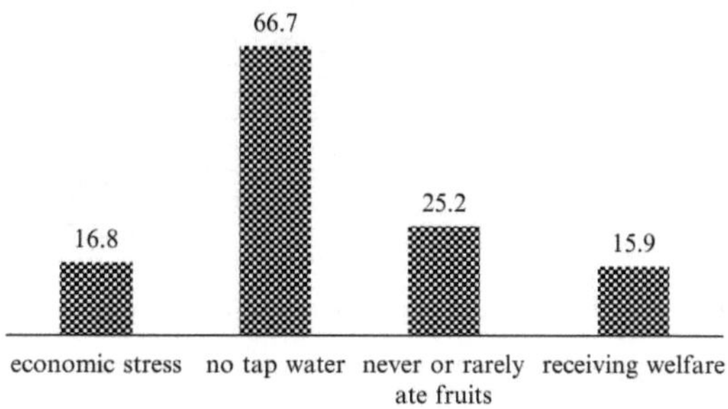

Fig. 8.2 Percent indicators of economic stress for oldest-old in rural areas

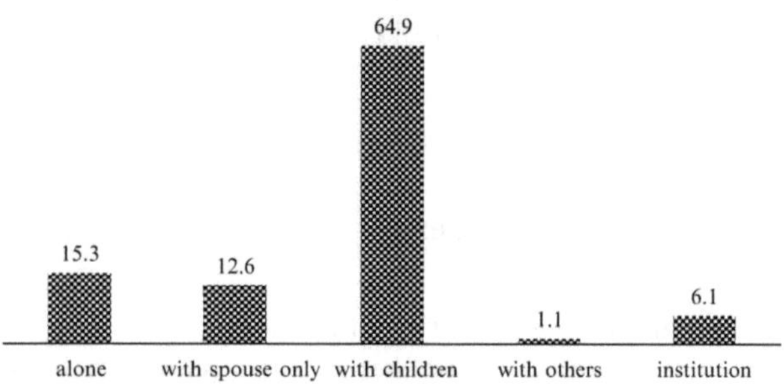

Fig. 8.3 Percent living arrangements for oldest-old in rural areas

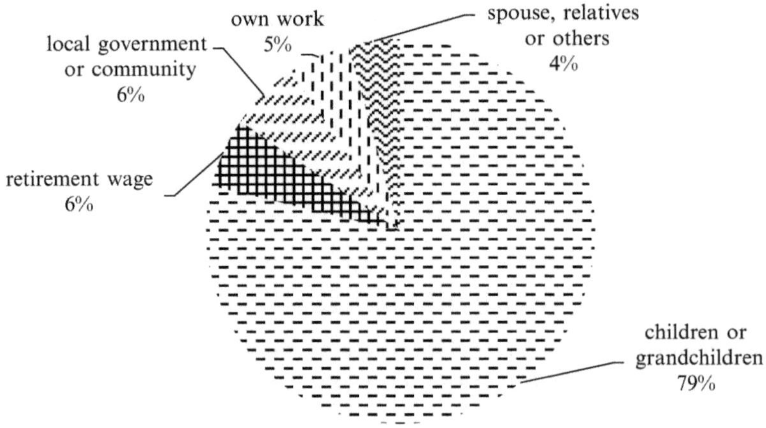

Fig. 8.4 Main financial source for the oldest-old in rural areas in 2000

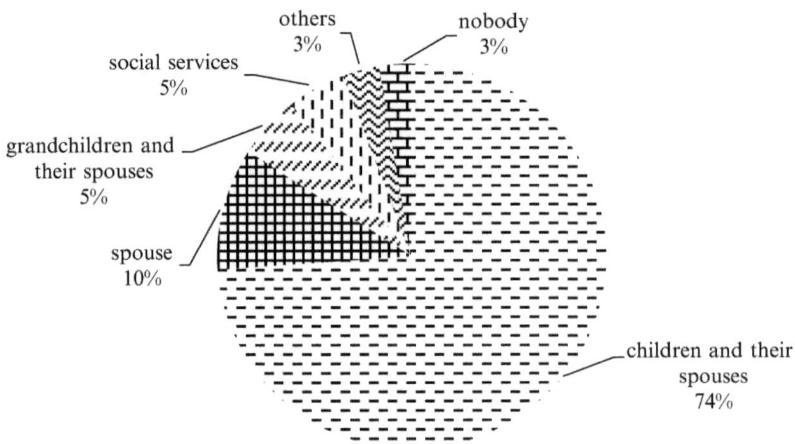

Fig. 8.5 Main caregiver of the oldest-old in rural areas in 2000

available to the majority of them; only 6 % received it. Figure 8.5 shows that the majority (three-quarters) of the oldest-old in rural areas rely on children as their main caregiver when they are ill.

Risk Factors of Economic Stress

What are the factors that increase the risk of economic stress in old age? Table 8.1 shows that these risk factors include being aged, being male, having low or no education, being widowed or never married, having no living children, no

Table 8.1 Logistic regression estimates for the risk factors for economic stress

	(1)	(2)
Variables	Receiving welfare (odds ratio)	Economic stress (odds ratio)
Age	1.034**	1.037***
	(0.011)	(0.011)
Female	0.758**	0.683***
	(0.069)	(0.061)
Minority	0.468***	2.837***
	(0.088)	(0.344)
Divorced	1.763	1.122
	(0.941)	(0.673)
Widowed	1.222*	1.006
	(0.107)	(0.084)
Never married	2.352**	0.341**
	(0.748)	(0.140)
Education (1–5 years)	0.950	1.061
	(0.093)	(0.100)
Education (>5 years)	0.662*	0.619**
	(0.115)	(0.110)
Good occupation	0.860	1.313
	(0.266)	(0.370)
Have living child	0.400***	0.638***
	(0.040)	(0.069)
Main financial source from children	0.279***	0.523***
	(0.023)	(0.045)
Pension	0.250***	0.372***
	(0.044)	(0.066)
Sense of control	0.994	0.784***
	(0.033)	(0.025)
Self-reported health	1.095	2.260***
	(0.058)	(0.110)
ADL index	1.743***	0.428***
	(0.244)	(0.071)
Cognitive impaired	0.585	8.011**
	(0.508)	(5.075)
Proxy	0.799**	0.682***
	(0.063)	(0.053)
Constant	0.065**	0.021***
	(0.057)	(0.018)
Observations	6607	6538
Log-likelihood	−2544.3381	−2594.5301

Standard errors in parentheses

***$p < 0.001$; ** $p < 0.01$; * $p < 0.05$

pension, and not having children as main source of financial support. Upon further investigation, we find that compared to females, more male oldest-old were never married (2.48 % vs. 0.24 %) and did not have children as their main source of income (32 % vs. 21 %). These factors partly explain why the male oldest-old was more likely to be under economic stress than his female counterpart. Previous studies did not control for many of these factors. Consistent with the descriptive data, a lower sense of control level, poor self-reported health status, and impaired cognitive conditions are all significantly related to subjective economic strain.

Mediating Mechanisms

We hypothesize that economic stress affects the health of the oldest-old through its negative effect on (1) the quality of medical care and (2) mental health.

Table 8.2 shows that the oldest-old who felt they were under economic strain were about seven times more likely to receive poor-quality medical care and were in greater emotional distress. Another indicator of economic stress, lack of fruit consumption (never or rarely ate fruits), was also associated with a higher likelihood of receiving poor-quality medical care in rural areas and a higher level of emotional distress. Having no access to tap water was significantly related to higher mental stress. Receiving welfare in fact reduced the likelihood of receiving poor-quality medical care but increased mental stress. This may be indicative of the general negative relationship between economic stress and one's mental health despite the benefit of some medical assistance from the government. However, when the oldest-old had his/her children as the main financial source, the negative impact of economic strain on emotional distress decreased by 0.16 %.

Economic Stress and Mortality Hazard

We now turn to the relationship between economic stress and mortality. First, we show the Kaplan-Meier survival curves of the probability of survival, against the number of elapsed days from 2000 to 2005 for those who were under economic strain in 2000 with those who were not (see Fig. 8.6). As can be seen, the probability of survival was higher for those who were not under economic strain and the gap seemed to increase as time advanced. At the end of 5 years, about 48 % who were not under economic strain, vs. 42 % of those who were, had survived. Log-rank test tells us that there is a statistically significant difference between the two survival curves, with $p = 0.000$.

Table 8.2 Estimates for the impact of economic stress on the quality of medical care and the emotional distress of the oldest-old in 2000

Variables	(1) Poor medicare (odds ratio)	(2) Emotional distress (coef.)
Receive welfare	0.532***	0.098***
	(0.093)	(0.018)
No tap water	1.228	0.061***
	(0.167)	(0.014)
Lack of fruit consumption	1.202*	0.047***
	(0.108)	(0.008)
Economic stresss	6.956***	0.291***
	(1.507)	(0.031)
Economic stress × main Financial source from children	0.797	−0.170***
	(0.205)	(0.036)
Age	0.973	−0.001
	(0.018)	(0.002)
Female	0.567***	−0.005
	(0.082)	(0.016)
Minority	0.506*	−0.076**
	(0.143)	(0.026)
Divorced	1.336	0.152
	(1.107)	(0.127)
Widowed	1.712***	0.030*
	(0.249)	(0.015)
Never married	0.872	−0.259***
	(0.510)	(0.071)
Education (1–5 years)	0.946	0.031
	(0.140)	(0.017)
Education (>5 years)	0.453*	−0.078**
	(0.150)	(0.027)
Good occupation	2.588*	−0.115*
	(1.016)	(0.046)
Have living child	0.401***	−0.028
	(0.069)	(0.022)
Main financial source from children	0.841	0.020
	(0.169)	(0.018)
Pension	0.589	0.029
	(0.175)	(0.027)
Sense of control	1.019	−0.098***
	(0.053)	(0.006)
Self-reported health	2.369***	0.205***
	(0.191)	(0.010)
ADL index	1.134	0.153***
	(0.222)	(0.028)

(continued)

Table 8.2 (continued)

	(1)	(2)
Variables	Poor medicare (odds ratio)	Emotional distress (coef.)
Proxy	1.171	−0.030*
	(0.144)	(0.013)
Constant	0.111	0.992***
	(0.175)	(0.160)
Observations	4940	6523
Log-likelihood	−1079.6553	–
R-squared	–	0.20

Standard errors in parentheses
***$p < 0.001$; **$p < 0.01$; *$p < 0.05$

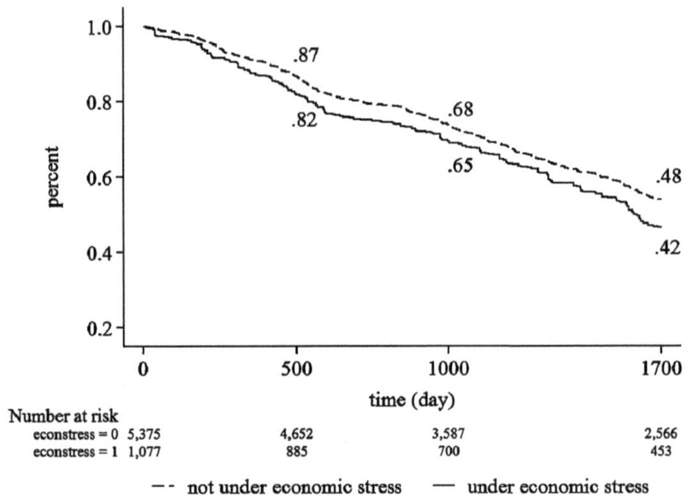

Fig. 8.6 Kaplan-Meier survival estimates by economic stress in rural areas

Hazard Models for Mortality

We turn now to examine the impact of economic stress on mortality hazard. Table 8.3 shows the Cox regression estimates. We show results of the model that includes the four indicators of economic stress; demographic controls; moderators including private social support network, public assistance, lifestyle, and sense of control; and indicators of prior health status. We also add two interaction terms to see if the impact of economic strain had changed when the oldest-old had children as his or her main source of income or had access to a pension. In the second model, we further add the two mediators – the quality of medical care and the mental well-being of the oldest-old.

Table 8.3 Cox regression estimates for mortality hazard

Variables	(1)	(2)	(3)	(4)
Receive welfare	1.037	0.984	1.075	1.151*
	(0.053)	(0.051)	(0.060)	(0.071)
No tap water	1.033	1.005	1.035	1.005
	(0.042)	(0.041)	(0.046)	(0.051)
Never or rarely eat fruits	1.111***	1.117***	1.107***	1.122***
	(0.028)	(0.028)	(0.030)	(0.036)
Economic stress	1.247***	1.179***	1.560***	1.397**
	(0.059)	(0.056)	(0.15)	(0.16)
Economic stress × main financial source from children			0.677***	0.773*
			(0.077)	(0.10)
Economic stress × pension			0.334***	0.337**
			(0.10)	(0.14)
Age		1.084***	1.067***	1.065***
		(0.0052)	(0.0057)	(0.0066)
Female		0.695***	0.693***	0.750***
		(0.032)	(0.039)	(0.048)
Minority		0.905	0.867	0.899
		(0.065)	(0.070)	(0.092)
Divorced		1.486	1.352	2.506**
		(0.48)	(0.44)	(0.84)
Widowed		1.137**	1.139**	1.126*
		(0.051)	(0.054)	(0.061)
Never married		0.975	1.093	1.025
		(0.18)	(0.24)	(0.26)
Education (1–5 years)		0.965	0.903	0.898
		(0.048)	(0.048)	(0.054)
Education (>5 years)		0.989	1.006	1.091
		(0.080)	(0.087)	(0.11)
Good occupation		1.060	1.036	1.168
		(0.13)	(0.14)	(0.17)
Have living child			0.985	0.837*
			(0.067)	(0.065)
Main financial source from children			1.325***	1.430***
			(0.084)	(0.10)
Pension			1.388***	1.536***
			(0.12)	(0.15)
Drank			1.120*	1.092
			(0.052)	(0.059)
Smoked			1.141**	1.254***
			(0.057)	(0.071)
Exercised			1.047	1.055
			(0.048)	(0.055)
Meat, fish, egg consumption			1.178***	1.213***
			(0.056)	(0.067)

(continued)

Table 8.3 (continued)

Variables	(1)	(2)	(3)	(4)
Sense of control			0.971	0.981
			(0.018)	(0.021)
Self-reported health			1.234***	1.239***
			(0.037)	(0.043)
ADL index			1.839***	1.769***
			(0.13)	(0.13)
Cognitive impaired			1.065	1.111
			(0.41)	(0.44)
Proxy			1.373***	1.381***
			(0.056)	(0.065)
Quality of medical care				1.047
				(0.088)
Mental health				1.056
				(0.048)
Observations	6263	6220	5803	4397
Log-likelihood	−24381.121	−24105.795	−21681.665	−15980.741

Standard errors in parentheses
$^{***}p < 0.001$; $^{**}p < 0.01$; $^{*}p < 0.05$

Two of the indicators – lack of fruit consumption and perceived economic strain – contributed significantly to a higher mortality hazard. These effects remain rather stable as we add the moderators and mediators. Economic strain and the lack of fruit consumption are associated with an increase in mortality hazard by 40 % and 12 %, respectively, in the final model. Having children as a main financial source reduced the mortality hazard by about 23 % and receiving pension reduced the mortality hazard by 66 %. In the final model, the two mediators reduce the effects of economic strain although only mental distress has a direct impact on the mortality hazard. The control variables are related to mortality rates in expected directions.

Summary and Discussions

Despite the limitation that we do not have direct measures of family income but only crude measures of economic stress, our findings lend some support to the concern that economic stress is a potentially serious public health issue. The Chinese oldest-old in rural areas relies heavily on children and has almost no access to public assistance. The financial hardships increase emotional distress and the probability of the elderly not receiving adequate medical care when needed. The negative impact of economic strain is ameliorated by the presence of private (children) and public (pension) support networks. For most of the upcoming generation of elderly in China, relying heavily on children for care is not a viable option because those who grew up under the one-child policy would have fewer children (and many have no sons) to rely on than their predecessors who were the respondents in this study. In addition, the unusually high sex ratio in China as a result of the one-child policy means that there will be fewer daughters and daughters-in-law to perform caregiving tasks which have traditionally been the responsibility of females. The shrinking private and public support will pose a great challenge to China's ability to care for its elderly. Although pension reform is under way, a majority of the elderly population still do not have access to these government resources.

Several factors exacerbate the problem of elderly care in China's rural areas: (1) the large number of young people migrating from rural to urban areas, (2) the substantially higher sex ratio in the rural than urban areas, and (3) the absence of a social security system in the rural areas. Currently, the medical system in China is effectively only serving those who can afford the high cost. For the elderly who have the highest poverty rates, adequate medical care remains largely inaccessible. The New Corporative Medical Scheme (NCMS) in rural China is a step in a positive direction. Whether the government can set up adequate public safety nets in time to alleviate the pension crisis and whether social security can extend coverage to rural elderly are critical to the well-being of the elderly in China.

References

Catalano, R. (2003). Sex ratios in the two Germanies: A test of the economic stress hypothesis. *Human Reproduction, 9*, 1972–1975.

Catalano, R., Bruckner, T., Anderson, B., & Gould, J. (2005). Fetal death sex ratios: A test of the economic stress hypothesis. *International Journal of Epidemiology, 34*, 944–948.

Center for Health Statistics and Information. (2004). Medical expenses for residents. In *Analysis report of national health services survey in China, 2003* (pp. 93–95). Beijing: Peking Union Medical College Press.

Center for Health Statistics and Information. (2009). Demands and utilization of health services for elderly. In *Analysis report of national health services survey in China, 2008* (pp. 93–95). Beijing: Peking Union Medical College Press.

Center of the Study of Aging and Human Development. (2010). *Chinese longitudinal healthy longevity survey (2010)*. Duke University. http://centerforaging.duke.edu/index.php?option=com_content&view=article&id=115&Itemid=152

Cheng, T., & Selden, M. (1994). The origins and social consequences of China's Hukou System. *The China Quarterly, 139*, 644–668.

Chinese Ministry of Civil Affairs Report. (2010). http://cws.mca.gov.cn/article/tjbg/201006/20100600081422.shtml

Conger, R. D., & Elder, G. H., Jr. (1994). *Families in troubled times: Adapting to change in rural America*. Hillsdale: Aldine.

Cox, D. C. (1972). Regression models and life-tables. *Journal of the Royal Statistical Society. Series B (Methodological), 34*(2), 178–220.

Dooley, D., & Catlano, R. (1984). The epidemiology of economic stress. *American Journal of Community Psychology, 12*(4), 387–409.

Ell, K., Xie, B., Wells, A., Nedjat-Haiem, F., Lee, P.-J., & Vourlekis, B. (2008). Economic stress among low-income women with cancer: Effects on quality of life. *Cancer, 112*, 616–625.

England, R. S. (2005). China's social service programs. In *Aging China: The demographic challenge to China's economic prospects* (pp. 99–108). Washington, DC: Praeger Press.

Folstein, M. F., Folstein, S. E., & McHugh, P. R. (1975). Mini-mental state: A practical method for grading the cognitive state of patients for the clinician. *Journal of Psychiatric Research, 12*, 189–198.

Friedman, J., & Thomas, D. (2008). Psychological health before, during, and after an economic crisis: Results from Indonesia, 1993–2000. *World Bank Economic Review, 23*, 57–76.

Goebel, M. U., Mills, P. J., Irwin, M. R., & Ziegler, M. G. (2000). Interleukin-6 and tumor necrosis factor-alpha production after acute psychological stress, exercise, and infused isoproterenol: Differential effects and pathways. *Psychosomatic Research, 62*, 591–598.

Kaplan, E. L., & Meier, P. (1958). Nonparametric estimation from incomplete observations. *Journal of the American Statistical Association, 53*, 457–481.

Katz, S., Ford, A. B., Moskowitz, R. W., Jackson, B. A., & Jaffe, M. W. (1963). Studies of illness in the aged. The index of ADL: A standardized measure of biological and psychosocial function. *Journal of the American Medical Association, 185*(12), 914–919.

Kendall-Tackett, K. (2009). Psychological trauma and physical health: A psychoneuroimmunology approach to etiology of negative health effects and possible interventions. *Psychological Trauma: Theory, Research, Practice, and Policy, 1*, 35–48.

Khang, Y.-H., & Lynch, J. (2010). Asian economic crises and health: Population health impacts and policy responses. *Journal of Epidemiology and Community Health, 64*(4), 282–283.

Khang, Y.-H., Lynch, J. W., & Kaplan, G. A. (2005). Impact of economic crisis on cause-specific mortality in South Korea. *International Journal of Epidemiology, 34*(6), 1291–1301.

Maes, M., Christophe, A., Bosmans, E., Lin, A., & Neels, H. (2000). In humans, serum polyunsaturated fatty acid levels predict the response of proinflammatory cytokines to psychologic stress. *Biological Psychiatry, 47*, 910–920.

Miller, G. E., Rohleder, N., Stetler, C., & Kirschbaum, C. (2005). Clinical depression and regulation of the inflammatory response during acute stress. *Psychosomatic Medicine, 67*, 679–687.

National Bureau of Statistics of China. (2010). *Communique of the National Bureau of Statistics of People's Republic of China on major figures of the 2010 Population Census (No.1).*http://www.stats.gov.cn/english/newsandcomingevents/t20110428_402722244.htm

Nguyen, H. T., Black, S. A., Ray, L. A., Espino, D. V., & Markides, K. S. (2003). Cognitive impairment and mortality in older Mexican Americans. *Journal of the American Geriatrics Society, 51*, 178–183.

Olivius, G., Ostergren, P. O., Hanson, B. S., & Lyttkens, C. H. (2004). Parental economic stress: Evidence of an overlooked public health risk among Swedish families. *European Journal of Public Health, 14*(4), 354–360.

Qiao, X., Zhang, K., & Sun, L. (2006). Analysis on population characteristic of the aged poor in China. *Population Journal, 4*, 3–8 (in Chinese).

Ruhm, C. J. (2000). Are recession good for your health? *Quarterly Journal of Economics, 115*(2), 617–650.

Schultz-Larsen, K., Rahmanfard, N., Kreiner, S., Avlund, K., & Holst, C. (2008). Cognitive impairment as assessed by a short form of MMSE was predictive of mortality. *Journal of Clinical Epidemiology, 61*, 1227–1233.

Selden, M. (1999). Poverty alleviation, inequality and welfare in rural China. *Economic and Political Weekly, 34*(45), 3183–3190.

Smith, J., Gerstorf, D., & Li, Q. (2008). Psychological resources for well-being among octogenarians, nonagenarians, and centenarians: Differential effects of age and selective mortality. In Y. Zeng, J. D. L. Poston, D. A. Vlosky, & D. Gu (Eds.), *Healthy longevity in China* (pp. 329–345). Dordrecht: The Netherlands Springer Press.

Steptoe, A., Hamer, M., & Chida, Y. (2007). The effect of acute psychological stress on circulating inflammatory factors in humans: A review and meta-analysis. *Brain, Behavior, and Immunity, 21*(7), 901–912.

Stuckler, D., King, L., & McKee, M. (2009). Mass privatisation and the post-communist mortality crisis. *Lancet, 373*, 399–407.

Van Den Berg, G. J., Lindeboom, M., & Lopez, M. (2009). Inequality in individual mortality and economic conditions earlier in life. *Social Science and Medicine, 69*(9), 1360–1367.

Wang, D., & Zhang, K. (2005). The Chinese elderly: How they live and how many of them are in poverty. *Chinese Journal of Population Science, 1*, 58–66 (in Chinese).

Wu, Z., & Schimmele, M. (2006). Psychological disposition and self-reported health among the oldest-old in China. *Ageing and Society, 26*, 135–151.

Wu, X., & Treiman, D. J. (2007). Inequality and equality under Chinese socialism: The hukou system and intergenerational occupational mobility. *American Journal of Sociology, 113*(2), 415–445.

You, X., & Kobayashi, Y. (2011). Determinants of out-of-pocket health expenditure in China: Analysis using China health and nutrition survey data. *Applied Health Economics & Health Policy, 9*(1), 39–49.

Zeng, Y. (2008). Introduction to the Chinese longitudinal health longevity survey (CLHLS). In Y. Zeng, J. D. L. Poston, D. A. Vlosky, & D. Gu (Eds.), *Healthy longevity in China* (pp. 23–37). Dordrecht: The Netherlands Springer Press.

Zeng, Y., & George, L. (2000). *Extremely rapid ageing and the living arrangements of older persons: The case of China*. United Nations technical meeting on population ageing and living arrangements of older person: Critical issues and policy responses. New York: Population Division, Department of Economic and Social Affairs, United Nations Secretariat.

Zhang, Z. (2006). Gender differentials in cognitive impairment and decline of the oldest-old in China. *Journal of Gerontology: Social Sciences, 61B*(2), S107–S115.

Chapter 9
Poverty, Perceived Economic Strain, and Psychological Distress Among Thai Older Adults

Kattika Thanakwang

Introduction

Indeed, poverty among older persons is still a major problem in many developing countries as well as several developed ones (Glasgow 1993; Smeeding and Weaver 2002). It has been widely documented that poverty is negatively associated with health and well-being (Chan et al. 2002; Zimmer 2008). Hence, older persons living in poverty may be vulnerable to economic hardships and health problems. Prior studies conducted in the United States have found that the rates of transition into poverty in old age are higher for women, ethnic minorities, those with lower educational attainments, the disabled, widows and widowers, those living alone, and those living in rural areas (Angel et al. 2003; Glasgow 1993; Smeeding and Weaver 2002). However, there have been only a few studies which explored the impacts of poverty on health and well-being in older persons, particularly in poor countries (Zimmer 2008).

Poverty is significantly related to subjective measures of economic conditions such as perceptions of income adequacy or economic strain (Malmgren et al. 1996). Much evidence has shown that financial strain influences the psychological health and well-being of the elderly (Chou and Chi 2000; Cheng et al. 2002; Krause et al. 2008). Cheng and colleague (Cheng et al. 2002) indicate that perceived financial sufficiency is the strongest predictor of elderly mental health. The 3-year longitudinal study of Chou and Chi (2002) also found that financial strain was the strongest predictor of life satisfaction among the Chinese elderly in Hong Kong. In an 18-month longitudinal study of American elders, Krause (1987) reported that financial strain at the baseline brought to bear a significant impact on depression at follow-up. Chi and Chou (1999) similarly found that financial strain caused depression in both older men and women.

K. Thanakwang (✉)
Institute of Nursing, Suranaree University of Technology, Nakhon Ratchasima, Thailand
e-mail: kattika@sut.ac.th

W.J.J. Yeung and M.T. Yap (eds.), *Economic Stress, Human Capital, and Families in Asia: Research and Policy Challenges*, Quality of Life in Asia 4,
DOI 10.1007/978-94-007-7386-8_9,

In Thai society, family members, particularly children, play a major role in providing resources and assistance to older parents. At present, the family structure has become predominantly nuclear; co-residence with children has declined and living alone or only with a spouse has increased (Knodel and Chayovan 2009a, b). However, children are still the most common source of income for older Thais (Zimmer and Amornsirisomboon 2001). Knodel and Chayovan (2009a) reported that 52.3 % of elderly's income came from their children and 28.9 % from paid work. Financial dependence on children increases for older persons aged 70 years and over and for elderly females, whereas income from work decreases with age because labor force participation and income generating activities decline with increasing age.

Amid social changes and economic constraints, intergenerational relationships may be impacted. Given the projected demographic changes, the old-age economic dependence ratio will increase and this trend is expected to continue into the foreseeable future. The potential support ratio (PSR), which denotes the ratio of working-age people aged 15–59 years per person aged 60 years and over, is shrinking from 10.3 in 1980 to 5.7 in 2010 and 2.4 in 2030 (Knodel and Chayovan 2009a). This means that the elderly will be supported by fewer working-age people and the burden on family members caring for their elderly parents will increase significantly in the near future.

While numerous studies in Western countries have focused on the social and economic constraints facing older persons, especially older women, few studies have focused on those facing older Thai people (Thanakwang and Soonthorndhada 2007). There is also a lack of research on socioeconomic status and its impacts on the health and well-being among older adults in a non-Western society, particularly in Thailand (Zimmer and Amornsirisomboon 2001). Although it is well established that more than one-fourth of Thai elders have an annual income below the poverty line and that children are their main income source, little research has focused on whether poverty and family support influence economic strain and psychological well-being. To date, there are still significant gaps in our understanding of the intervening mechanisms of objective poverty and family support on perceived economic strain and psychological distress. Therefore, the present study attempts to explore the relationships between poverty, measured by having an income below the poverty line, perceived economic strain, and psychological distress among Thai older adults. The mediating role of perceived economic strain in the relationship between poverty and psychological distress is examined, and the moderating effects of sources of income and family support in the links between poverty and perceived economic strain and psychological distress are assessed. The following hypotheses are examined:

1. Poverty is associated with perceived economic strain and psychological distress in Thai older adults.
2. Perceived economic strain mediates the linkage between poverty and psychological distress.
3. Sources of income and family support moderate the effects of poverty on perceived economic strain.
4. Family support moderates the effect of poverty on psychological distress.

Poverty and Economic Security of Thai Older Adults

Recently, the problems of poverty and economic security in Thai older adults have become a challenge for policy makers (Suwanrada 2009). In prior studies on economics of Thai elders, Chayovan (2005) found that one-fourth (25 %) of them had an average income of less than 10,000 baht per year (USD332), considered as lower than the poverty line, and approximately 14 % of them faced poverty or possessed insufficient income. Similarly, the Thailand Population Health Examination Survey III found that 13 and 19 % of elderly males and females, respectively, had no income and experienced economic hardships in their daily lives, and a substantial proportion (71 % of men and 58 % of women) reported that they had insufficient income and suffered economic hardships (Porrapakkam and Punyaratabandhu 2006).

Thanakwang and Soonthorndhada (2007) found that nearly one-third (32 %) of Thai elders could be considered as poor. Most poverty-stricken older adults were mainly found in the following groups: women, the oldest old, rural inhabitants, the disabled, those with low levels of education, those engaged in low-status occupations, and those unprepared financially for old age.

In addition, most impoverished older persons lack crucial knowledge that would allow them to prepare for their old age, especially with regard to financial security. Only one out of five makes any kind of preparation for their economic well-being before old age (Chayovan 2005). Consistent with the study by Choolert (2008) in Kanchanaburi province of Thailand, only 24.3 % of the elderly farmers had prepared themselves economically for old age. The National Economic and Social Development Board (NESDB) (2008) also reported that, among all Thai elders, 31.3 % did not have savings or any financial assets. Therefore, a financial arrangement to ensure economic security in later life is needed for Thai people. This is due to current demographic and socioeconomic changes. First, life expectancy is increasing. Secondly, the number of children per couple has declined due to a low fertility rate, potentially resulting in dramatic decline in future support ratio. Thirdly, co-residence with children is decreasing, and more elderly live alone or live only with a spouse because of the increased migration of adult children.

Economic Strain and Psychological Distress

Malmgren et al. (1996) state that low-income and older adults below the poverty line are likely to suffer from greater financial hardships, poorer medical care, and a higher number of health problems. Poverty is significantly related to subjective economic strain (Angel et al. 2003). However, their relationship may somewhat be weak (Chan et al. 2002) as individuals in similar economic circumstances may have different perceptions of their circumstances (Szanton et al. 2008), or some may possess mediating or moderating factors while others may not.

A growing body of research has begun to catalogue the relationship between economic constraints and psychological distress in older adults. Szanton and colleagues (Szanton et al. 2008) state that economic strain is the subjective measure of perceived financial sufficiency based on resources and needs of individuals. It has been widely documented that a subjective measure of income is an important indicator for measuring the economic situation among older persons. Therefore, many studies have used subjective measures of income, such as self-perceived financial adequacy, self-rated economic condition, financial strain, or financial satisfaction to predict psychological health, particularly depression and psychological distress (Cheng et al. 2002; Ferraro and Su 1999; Chou and Chi 2001; Chou et al. 2004; Krause 1987; Litwin and Sapir 2009).

Psychological sense of economic hardship could have an impact on emotional distress and result in discouragement, loss of hope, low self-esteem, or demoralization (Angel et al. 2003; Barrera et al. 2001). Krause and colleagues (Krause et al. 1991) report that the more financial strain the older adults perceive, the lesser their sense of psychological well-being, indicated as lower personal control and self-worth. In a cross-cultural research, Ferraro and Su (1999) found that financial strain was the strongest predictor of psychological distress among older people in four countries: Korea, Malaysia, Fiji, and the Philippines. Similarly, Krause et al. (1991) also found a positive association between economic strain and depressive symptoms among older people in the United States of America and Japan. Consistent with the cross-sectional study findings, several longitudinal studies found that a higher financial strain at the baseline significantly impacted levels of depression during the follow-up (Chi and Chou 1999; Krause 1987).

Sources of Income and Family Support as Moderators

The major source of income of older Thai persons come from adult children (Knodel and Chayovan 2009b; Zimmer and Amornsirisomboon 2001), followed by income from work. There are limited sources of income that come from retirement pensions or savings and government welfare (Suwanrada 2009). However, some older adults may receive income from several sources. Therefore, it is expected that sources of income may moderate the impact of poverty on economic strain. Income from pension or savings may lead older persons to financial independence (Chou et al. 2004). This may be the case for older persons who receive government welfare too.

Family support may be tangible or intangible and it leads the older parents to believe that he/she is cared for, loved and valued, and belongs to a network of members with mutual obligation, subsequently improving the well-being of the elderly. It has been noted that family support in relation to older parents in the Thai context is a part of the cultural tradition of filial obligations based on Buddhist values (Caffrey 1992; Kespichayawattana 1999). Family support has been mostly examined as the moderator on the links between economic stress and health outcomes. Krause (1987) found that social support reduces the impact of financial strain on the sense of psychological distress. Specifically, Krause (2005) indicated that emotional support from family and friends significantly acts as a buffer against the deleterious effects of financial strain on life satisfaction.

Conceptual Framework

The Stress Process Model proposed by Pearlin and colleagues (Pearlin et al. 1990; Pearlin and Skaff 1996) is used to explain the effects of poverty on psychological distress via perceived economic strain, sources of income, and family support. The Stress Process Model includes five major conceptual domains: (a) contextual characteristics; (b) sources of stress, both objective and subjective stressors; (c) role and intrapsychic strains; (d) internal and external mediators; and (e) outcomes of health and well-being. Therefore, the impact of stress on psychological distress is subject to external social resources available and the internal resources of individuals. Specifically in the Thai context, the cultural aspect of filial support is believed to be an important intrinsic mediator.

This present study contributes to the knowledge of objective poverty on psychological distress and examines the effect of mediators. The analysis uses nationally representative data from Thailand and the conceptual model for this study is shown in Fig. 9.1.

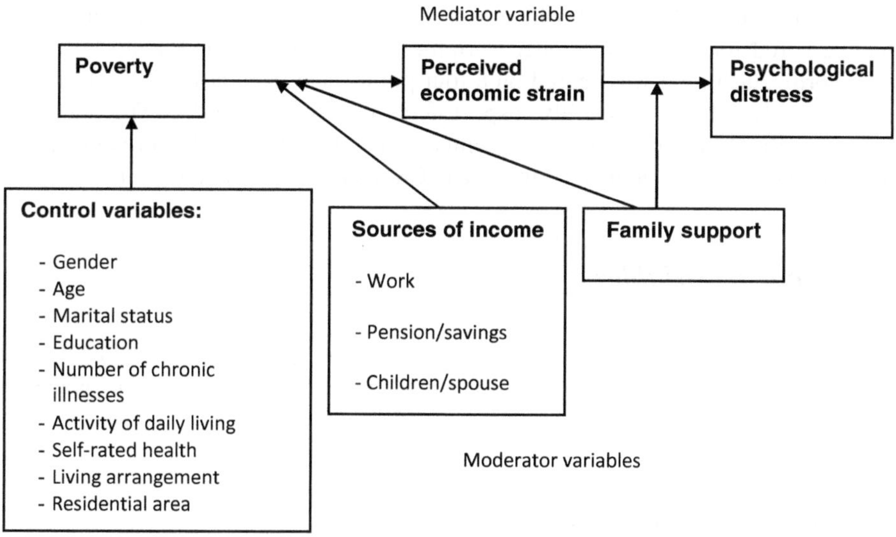

Fig. 9.1 A conceptual model of psychological distress of Thai older adults

Material and Method

Data Source

The source of data was the 2002 Survey of the Elderly in Thailand conducted by the National Statistical Office (2002). Stratified two-stage sampling was employed to produce nationally and regionally representative samples. Seventy-six provinces in five regions (North, Northeast, Central, and South, including Bangkok) of Thailand in the year 2002 were surveyed. All persons aged 50 years and older in selected households were eligible to be interviewed. Data were collected from April to June 2002, yielding 43,447 completed interviews. In this study, the analysis was restricted to the older population aged 60 years and older, which reduced the sample to 21,417 persons. Sampling weights were applied in order to make the sample nationally representative.

Measurement of Variables

Dependent Variable

Psychological distress. Psychological distress was measured using ten items from the subjective sense of well-being for living with other persons (Knodel et al. 2005). Negative aspects included (1) feeling discontented about the dwelling, (2) feeling family members considered them fussy, (3) feeling uneasy, (4) feeling lonely, and (5) feeling a lack of peace. Positive aspects included (1) feeling comfortable, (2) feeling cared for, (3) feeling inner warmth, (4) feeling respected, and (5) feeling self-worth. Each item was scored on a four-point scale from never (0), a little (1), moderate (2) to high (3). Positive aspect items were reverse coded. The scale was the unweighted sum of the ten items, with a range of 0–30. A high score indicated a greater level of psychological distress. The Cronbach's alpha coefficient was 0.73.

Independent Variables

Poverty. According to Chayovan (2005), an older person who averaged less than 10,000 baht per year as income was categorized as "poor" (1), others as "nonpoor" (0).

Mediating and Moderating Variables

Perceived economic strain. The measure was based on self-rated economic condition from a single question: "Do you think you have sufficient money to cover your daily expenses?" The respondents rated their income adequacy on a three-point scale ranging from insufficient (1), enough money (2), to more than enough (3). For the present analysis, this variable was reverse coded.

Family support. Family support was defined by the receipt of social support from family members including spouse, children, grandchildren, son-in-law and daughter-in-law, or relatives. Types of support included financial assistance; material goods including food, clothes, and groceries; and daily living support, with 1 indicating receiving support and 0 indicating no support. A sum of the scores of these five items was computed, with a range of 0–5, a high score indicated a greater level of receiving family support.

Sources of income. Four sources of income were considered, income from work, pension/savings or interest, support from children, and government welfare, 1 indicating support, 0 indicating no support.

Control Variables

Sociodemographic variables. The analysis adjusted for sociodemographic and health-related indicators. The sociodemographic variables included gender (1 = female, 0 = male), age (in years at the time the survey was conducted.), marital status (1 = currently married, 0 = not married.), education (none, primary school or less, secondary school, diploma, and bachelor degree or above), and residential area (1 = rural, 0 = urban). Living arrangement was coded as 1 or 0, depending on whether the older person (a) co-resided with a spouse only, (b) co-resided with children, and (c) co-resided with relatives. The reference group was those co-residing with others were.

Health status: Activity of Daily Living (ADL) limitations, number of chronic illnesses, and self-rated health were included as measures of health status. Respondents were coded as having physical limitations if they indicated having one or more ADL limitations in eating, dressing, and bathing. The number of chronic illnesses was treated as a continuous variable. Self-rated health was coded as very poor (1), poor (2), fair (3), good (4), and very good (5).

Data Analysis

Descriptive statistic and bivariate analysis were used to describe correlations among the study variables. Secondly, the mediating effect of economic strain on the linkage between poverty and psychological distress was examined after controlling for sociodemographic and health status variables. The analytic method suggested by Baron and Kenny (1986) that three conditions must hold was used. The first condition is that the independent variable must significantly affect the mediator variable. The second condition is that the independent variable must significantly affect the dependent variable. The third condition is that the mediator must significantly affect the dependent variable. A mediating effect exists if the following conditions are met: (a) Variations in the independent variable (poverty) significantly predict variations in the mediator (perceived economic strain), (b) variations in the mediator variable significantly predict variations in the dependent variable (psychological distress), and (c) when the association in (a) and (b) are controlled in the model, the direct relationship between the independent variable (poverty) and the dependent variable (psychological distress) becomes nonsignificant. If the direct relationship between the independent variable (poverty) and the dependent variable (psychological distress) is significantly reduced, this indicates the presence of a partial mediating effect.

Lastly, the moderating effects of sources of income and family support were tested using a hierarchical multiple regression analysis. Nine control variables of sociodemographic and health status variables were entered in the first step, followed by main effect variables (second step), and interaction terms (third step). If the interaction terms explain a statistically significant amount of variance in the dependent variable, a moderator effect is present (Bennett 2000). Centered variables were used for poverty, four sources of income, and family support to reduce multicollinearity problems that could be augmented between the direct effects and interaction terms (Aiken and West 1991).

Results

Characteristics of the Sample

The descriptive information which includes all study variables is provided in Table 9.1. In this nationally representative sample, elderly women were higher in number than elderly men (53.3 % vs. 46.7 %). The respondent majorities were currently married (66.7 %), co-resided with children (74 %), and lived in rural areas (68.6 %). Most achieved an educational attainment of primary school (72.4 %). The mean age of this sample was 68.54 years. Most respondents had no ADL limitation (93.5 %) and reported that their health was rather good (mean = 3.22). The mean number of chronic illnesses was 2.27. Specifically, about one-third of the sample (31.9 %) was poor. More than one-third of the respondents (36.1 %) reported perceived income inadequacy. Children were the main source of income (82.9 %). The majority of the respondents received social support from family members (mean = 3.55). The mean score of psychological distress was 7.83 with a standard deviation of 4.53.

Table 9.1 Study variable distributions ($N = 21{,}417$)

Variables	Number	Percentage
Gender: female	11,408	53.3
Marital status: married	14,292	66.7
Education		
None	4,414	20.6
Primary school or less	15,515	72.4
Secondary school	959	4.5
Diploma	176	0.8
Bachelor degree or above	353	1.6
ADL limitation: none	20,015	93.5
Living arrangement		
Live with only spouse	3,731	17.4
Live with children	15,848	74.0
Live with relatives	848	4.0
Live with others	990	4.6
Residential area: rural	14,700	68.6
Poverty: poor	6,838	31.9
Sources of income		
Working	8,033	37.5
Pension/savings/interest	4,434	20.7
Children support	17.760	82.9
Government welfare	599	2.8
Economic strain		
Enough money	13,534	63.2
Insufficient	7,731	36.1
More than enough	153	0.7
Variables	Mean	SD
Age (60–98)	68.54	7.22
Self-rated health (1–5)	3.22	0.98
Number of chronic illnesses (0–6)	2.27	1.51
Family support (0–5)	3.55	1.55
Psychological distress (0–26)	7.83	4.53

Correlations of the Study Variables

The correlations between the study variables were analyzed using Pearson's correlation coefficient. Most variables showed significant relationships at a mild to moderate level. Bivariate results indicated that education and self-rated health negatively correlated with perceived economic strain ($r = -0.15$, $p < 0.001$) and psychological distress ($r = -0.13$, $p < 0.001$). High levels of psychological distress were associated with a high economic strain ($r = 0.12$, $p < 0.001$) and poverty ($r = 0.06$, $p < 0.001$). Likewise, poverty was positively related to a high level of perceived economic strain ($r = 0.21$, $p < 0.001$), which meant that those who had greater poverty were more likely to suffer from perceived economic strain.

A source of income from a pension or savings/interest, which denotes that the respondents may have financial independence, was negatively associated with perceived economic strain ($r = -0.23$, $p < 0.001$). Family support was positively associated with poverty ($r = 0.14$, $p < 0.001$), indicating that the poor were more likely than the nonpoor to receive support from family members. Moreover, family support negatively correlated with perceived economic strain ($r = -0.03$, $p < 0.01$).

Mediating Effect of Perceived Economic Strain

The results of the multiple regression models for testing the mediating effect of perceived economic strain in the linkage between poverty and psychological distress among Thai older adults are presented in Table 9.2. Poverty was significantly and positively associated with the mediator, namely, perceived economic strain ($\beta = 0.18$, $p < 0.001$). Poverty was also significantly and positively associated with the dependent variable, namely, psychological distress ($\beta = 0.02$, $p < 0.01$), as shown in the second regression model. Lastly, perceived economic strain was significantly associated with psychological distress ($\beta = 0.09$, $p < 0.001$), as shown in the third regression model. The beta coefficient for poverty became statistically

Table 9.2 Perceived economic strain as a mediator in the relationship between poverty and psychological distress

	Perceived economic strain		Psychological distress		Psychological distress	
Predictor variables	*b*	Beta	*b*	Beta	*b*	Beta
Gender: female	−0.05	−0.05***	−0.12	−0.02	−0.07	−0.01
Age	−0.01	−0.13***	−0.02	−0.04***	−0.02	−0.02**
Marital status: married	0.02	0.02**	−0.46	−0.05***	−0.48	−0.05***
Education	−0.06	−0.08***	−0.54	−0.08***	−0.49	−0.07***
ADL limitations: none	−0.02	−0.01	−1.52	−0.08***	−1.50	−0.08***
Number of chronic illnesses	0.01	0.04***	−0.06	−0.02**	−0.07	−0.03**
Self-rated health	−0.06	−0.11***	−0.47	−0.10***	−0.42	−0.09***
Live with only spouse[a]	0.02	0.01	−1.93	−0.16***	−1.95	−0.16***
Live with children[a]	0.06	0.06***	−2.94	−0.29***	−2.99	−0.29***
Live with relatives[a]	0.03	0.01	−2.66	−0.11***	−2.68	−0.12***
Residential area: rural	0.11	0.10***	0.30	0.03***	0.21	0.02**
Poverty	0.19	0.18***	0.22	0.02**	0.06	0.01
Perceived economic strain					0.85	0.09***
F	179.232***		106.655***		112.821***	
R^2	0.091		0.056		0.065	

Note:
*$p < .05$; **$p < .01$; ***$p < .001$
[a]Live with others is the reference

insignificant ($\beta = 0.01, p > 0.05$) when both poverty and perceived economic strain were included, indicating that perceived economic strain is a complete mediator in the relationship between poverty and elderly psychological distress.

Moderating Effects of Sources of Income and Family Support

Table 9.3 shows the four regression models that were separately regressed to examine the moderating effects of various sources of income from work, pension or savings/interest, children, and government welfare in the relationship between poverty and perceived economic strain. To test the moderating effect of a source of income from work in the relationship between poverty and perceived economic strain, a hierarchical regression model was constructed, and the predictive variables including sociodemographic variables and health status variables, poverty, and the source of income from work were added in the first block where the dependent variable was perceived economic strain. In the second block, an interaction effect between poverty and source of income from working was added. The moderating effects of a source of income from a pension or savings/interest, children, and government welfare in the relationships between poverty and perceived economic strain were examined in models 2, 3, and 4, respectively.

The findings reveal that the interaction effects between poverty and sources of income in all four regression models were statistically significant. In the moderating effect of a source of income from work, the sign of multiplicative term was positive, indicating that the impact of poverty on perceived economic strain was higher among elderly respondents who had a source of income from work than those who did not. The sign of multiplicative term of poverty and a source of income from government welfare was positive, indicating that the impact of poverty on perceived economic strain was higher among the respondents who had a source of income from government welfare than those who did not. In case of the moderating effect of a source of income from a pension or savings/interest, the sign of multiplicative term was negative, indicating that the impact of poverty on perceived economic strain was lower among the respondents who had a source of income from a pension or savings/interest than those who did not. Similarly, the sign of multiplicative term between poverty and source of income from children was negative, indicating that the impact of poverty on perceived economic strain was lower among the respondents who had a source of income from children than those who did not. Thus, sources of income from a pension or savings/interest and from children significantly moderated the harmful impact of elderly poverty on perceived economic strain.

Table 9.4 shows that the impact of poverty on perceived economic strain was lower among the respondents who had a higher level of family support than those with a lower level of family support. Similarly, the impact of poverty on psychological distress was lower among the respondents who had a higher level of family support than those with a lower level of family support. This suggests that family support significantly moderated the harmful impact of both elderly poverty on perceived economic strain and elderly poverty on psychological distress.

Table 9.3 Sources of income as a moderator in the relationship between poverty and perceived economic strain

	Model 1		Model 2		Model 3		Model 4	
	b	Beta	*b*	Beta	*b*	Beta	*b*	Beta
Predictor variables								
Gender: female	−0.03	−0.04***	−0.05	−0.05***	−0.05	−0.05***	−0.05	−0.05***
Age	−0.01	−0.10***	−0.01	−0.12***	−0.01	−0.13***	−0.01	−0.13***
Marital status: married	0.01	0.01	0.03	0.03**	0.02	0.02**	0.02	0.02**
Education	−0.05	−0.07***	−0.03	−0.04***	−0.06	−0.08***	−0.06	−0.08***
ADL limitations: none	−0.02	−0.01	−0.01	−0.01	−0.02	−0.01	−0.02	−0.01
Number of chronic illnesses	0.02	0.04***	0.01	0.04***	0.01	0.04***	0.01	0.04***
Self-rated health	−0.06	−0.12***	−0.05	−0.10***	−0.06	−0.11***	−0.06	−0.11***
Live with only spouse[a]	0.02	0.01	0.02	0.01	0.02	0.01	0.02	0.01
Live with children[a]	0.07	0.06***	0.06	0.05***	0.06	0.06***	0.06	0.06***
Live with relatives[a]	0.03	0.01	0.04	0.02*	0.02	0.01	0.03	0.01
Residential area: rural	0.09	0.09***	0.09	0.08***	0.11	0.10***	0.11	0.10***
Poverty	0.20	0.19***	0.16	0.15***	0.18	0.17***	0.18	0.17***
Sources of income from work	0.11	0.10***						
Sources of income from pension/savings/ interest			−0.19	−0.16***				
Sources of income from children					−0.02	−0.02*		
Sources of income from government welfare							0.04	0.02*
R^2	0.099		0.113		0.091		0.091	

Interaction effect								
Poverty × sources of income from work	0.07	0.03***						
Poverty × sources of income from pension/saving/interest			−0.06	−0.02*				
Poverty × sources of income from children					−0.09	−0.03***		
Poverty × sources of income from government welfare							0.11	0.02**
F	170.262***		195.272***		155.671***		154.565***	
Total R^2	0.100		0.114		0.092		0.092	

Note:
*$p < .05$; **$p < .01$; ***$p < .001$
[a]Live with others is the reference

Table 9.4 Family support as a moderator in the relationships between poverty and perceived economic strain and between poverty and psychological distress

	Perceived economic strain		Psychological distress	
	b	Beta	*b*	Beta
Predictor variables				
Gender: female	−0.05	−0.05***	−0.13	−0.01
Age	−0.01	−0.12***	−0.02	−0.03***
Marital status: married	−0.02	−0.02*	−0.47	−0.05***
Education	−0.07	−0.09***	−0.56	−0.08***
ADL limitations: none	−0.02	−0.01	−1.52	−0.08***
Number of chronic illnesses	−0.02	−0.05***	−0.05	−0.02*
Self-rated health	−0.06	−0.11***	−0.48	−0.10***
Live with only spouse[a]	0.02	0.01	−1.94	−0.16***
Live with children[a]	0.07	0.06***	−2.92	−0.28***
Live with relatives[a]	0.02	0.01	−2.69	−0.12***
Residential area: rural	0.12	0.11***	0.33	0.03**
Poverty	0.19	0.18***	0.24	0.03**
Family support	−0.03	−0.08***	−0.09	−0.03***
R^2 change	0.097		0.057	
Interaction effect				
Poverty × family support	−0.03	−0.04***	−0.22	−0.03***
F	167.592***		94.716***	
R^2 change	0.002		0.001	
Total R^2	0.099		0.058	

Note:
*$p < .05$; **$p < .01$; ***$p < .001$
[a]Live with others is the reference

Discussion

The findings indicate that perceived economic strain fully mediates the relationship between poverty and psychological distress. This explains the possible mechanisms of poverty that indirectly influence psychological distress through perceived financial strain. This also indicates that perceived economic strain is a crucial factor influencing psychological health. As noted in several studies, economic strain is significantly detrimental on the older adults' psychological health with respect to depressive symptoms (Chi and Chou 1999; Chou and Chi 2000; Krause et al. 1991) and psychological distress (Ferrraro and Su 1999; Tran and Dhooper 1997).

Sources of income moderate the effects of poverty on economic strain. The findings suggest that sources of income from a pension, savings, or interest and from children buffer the deleterious effects of poverty on perceived economic strain. Older adults who have sources of income from a pension, savings, or interest may be considered financially independent (Chou et al. 2004). Typically, it is well known that children are the main source of economic support to elderly parents in Thai society due to the traditional culture of filial piety related to Buddhism. Financial assistance from adult children is very important in meeting the financial needs of the elderly; a large majority of older parents report receiving income from their children (Knodel and Chayovan 2009b; Suwanrada 2009; Zimmer and Amornsirisomboon 2001). In particular, adult children who leave the parental household often provide more financial support than co-residential children to elderly parents (Knodel and Saengtienchai 2007).

The findings also indicate that sources of income from work and government welfare enhance the impact of poverty on perceived economic strain. It has been documented that Thai older persons who receive government welfare are somewhat poor and the allowance is quite low and limited (Suwanrada 2009). Thus, a financial source from welfare may not help to alleviate the effect of poverty on perceived economic strain. At present, the Thai government is developing the old-age allowance system and has increased its allowance to 500 baht per head per month as well as expanded the pool of recipients covering about 2.3 million older Thais (Suwanrada 2009). As the government welfare system is changing, future research could examine how government welfare policies affect the poverty level and the perceived economic strain. More importantly, the moderating effect of sources of income from work reveals that the impact of poverty on perceived economic strain is higher among older persons who have a higher level of income from work. The findings also indicate that older adults who are still working are more likely to suffer from economic strain and psychological distress than those who do not. This could be possibly so because they have to work for a living due to various reasons such as lack of familial support, unavoidable responsibilities to care for their significant others, and the lack of a retirement pension or financial savings. Moreover, their income may be inadequate. This finding is congruent with the study on older adults in Hong Kong done by Chou and colleagues (Chou et al. 2004).

Specifically, the findings of this present study show that family support acts as the moderator on the links between both poverty on perceived economic strain and poverty on psychological distress. This finding is consistent with numerous studies that have indicated that support from children or family members significantly moderate the harmful psychological impact of economic stress (Chou and Chi 2001; Ferraro and Su 1999; Krause 1987). This is also supported by the social stress theory on the stress-buffering effect of social support on the impact of stressors on psychological health (Cobb 1976; Pearlin et al. 1990). The moderating function of family support involves a protective effect against the deleterious influence of poverty and economic strain. The older adults who receive higher levels of family support experience less negative psychological effects of economic hardships. There are several plausible explanations why family support is the most important factor influencing the older persons' economic and psychological well-being. First, nearly one-third of Thai elders lack financial preparation before entering later life (Chayovan 2005; Choolert 2008; NESDB 2008). Second, based on the social norms of filial obligations and reciprocal exchanges, the culture of repaying elderly parents for their care and nurture continues to be cultivated (Caffrey 1992; Kespichayawattana 1999); thus, the elders' expectation of support from family members may be deeply ingrained. Thirdly, most of the Thai elderly had suffered from limited opportunities for educational attainment, literacy, and employment, which could have made them financially independent in old age (Knodel and Chayovan 2009a). Lastly, because of the limitations of social welfare programs for the aged population, the older parents are therefore dependent on their younger family members for financial assistance (Ingersoll-Dayton et al. 2001; Suwanrada 2009).

Policy makers should explore how to strengthen the social support systems and welfare among the poor older people, particularly the poor and those who have limited support from family members. Given the changes in the population structure, financial support from adult children is expected to gradually decrease in future and the financial security of Thai older persons will be heavily challenged (Knodel and Chayovan 2009a; Thanakwang and Soonthorndhada 2007). To combat poverty and enhance the economic security of the Thai elderly, Suwanrada (2009) suggests three important policy options which should (1) promote the establishment of a community-based social welfare fund, (2) expand the coverage of the old-age allowance system, and (3) establish a national pension system, which covers employed persons who do not currently receive coverage.

Taken together, the findings of the present study can contribute to the planning and instatement of practical measures to alleviate poverty, economic strain, and psychological distress among Thai older adults. Projected demographic changes show that the rate of the aging population is dramatically increasing whereas the rate of fertility is declining, which will result in a diminished potential support ratio (Knodel and Chayovan 2009b; Suwanrada 2009). Undoubtedly, there are fewer family members available to care for and assist older parents in the near future. Intergenerational solidarity within the family and filial obligations should be continuously promoted, and economic preparation before aging among the working population to ensure economic security in later life should be also encouraged.

Although this present study extends previous research in several significant ways in a national sample of older adults, some limitations must be addressed when reviewing the results. First, the respondents in this study did not include older adults who lived alone. Therefore, the pattern of relationships described here may be not absolutely generalized to all elderly Thais. A second limitation is that its analysis is based on cross-sectional data and is restricted by the information made available. The data set did not provide enough details to employ poverty as a multidimensional concept. Perhaps annual income and the poverty line may not completely reflect the state of actual poverty among Thai older adults. Lastly, the cross-sectional nature of this present study may decrease the robustness of the causal influences between poverty, perceived economic strain, family support, and psychological distress. Further longitudinal research is needed to trace the comprehensible mechanisms of this model on Thai older adults.

Acknowledgements The author would like to express appreciation to the National Statistical Office, Thailand, for providing data from the 2002 National Survey of the Elderly in Thailand and to Professor W. Jean Yeung and Angelique Chan who provided useful comments on several drafts of this chapter.

References

Aiken, I. S., & West, S. G. (1991). *Multiple regressions: Testing and interpreting interactions*. Newbury Park: Sage.

Angel, R. J., Frisco, M., Angel, J. L., & Chiriboga, D. A. (2003). Financial strain and health among elderly Mexican-origin individuals. *Journal of Health and Social Behavior, 44*, 536–551.

Baron, R. M., & Kenny, D. A. (1986). The moderator-mediator variable distinction in social psychological research: Conceptual, strategic, and statistical considerations. *Journal of Personality and Social Psychology, 51*, 1173–1182.

Barrera, M., Caples, H., & Tein, J.-Y. (2001). The psychological sense of economic hardship: Measurement models, validity, and cross-ethnic equivalence or urban families. *American Journal of Community Psychology, 29*, 493–517.

Bennett, J. A. (2000). Mediator and moderator variables in nursing research: Conceptual and statistical differences. *Research in Nursing & Health, 23*, 415–420.

Caffrey, R. A. (1992). Caregiving to the elderly in Northeast Thailand. *Journal of Cross-Cultural Gerontology, 7*, 117–134.

Chan, A., Ofstedal, M. B., & Hermalin, A. I. (2002). Changes in subjective and objective measures of economic well-being and their interrelationship among the elderly in Singapore and Taiwan. *Social Indicators Research, 57*, 263–300.

Chayovan, N. (2005). Vulnerable elderly groups in Thailand. *Journal of Demography, 21*(1), 1–24.

Cheng, Y. H., Chi, I., Boey, K. W., Ko, L. S. F., & Chou, K. L. (2002). Self-rated economic condition and the health of elderly persons in Hong Kong. *Social Science & Medicine, 55*, 1415–1424.

Chi, I., & Chou, K. L. (1999). Financial strain and depressive symptoms among Hong Kong Chinese elderly: A longitudinal study. *Journal of Gerontological Social Work, 32*(4), 41–60.

Choolert, P. (2008). *The economic preparation of becoming elderly among farmers in Kanchanaburi, Thailand, using the Kanchanaburi Demographic Surveillance System*. Master thesis of Population and Social Research, Graduate Studies, Mahidol University, Nakhon Pathom.

Chou, K. L., & Chi, I. (2000). Financial strain and depressive symptoms in Hong Kong elderly Chinese: The moderating or mediating effect of sense of control. *Aging & Mental Health, 5*(1), 23–30.

Chou, K. L., & Chi, I. (2001). Stressful life events and depressive symptoms: Social support and sense of control as mediators or moderators? *International Journal of Aging & Human Development, 52*(2), 155–171.

Chou, K. L., & Chi, I. (2002). Financial strain and life satisfaction in Hong Kong elderly Chinese: Moderating effect of life management strategies including selection, optimization, and compensation. *Aging & Mental Health, 6*(2), 172–177.

Chou, K. L., Chi, I., & Chow, N. W. S. (2004). Sources of income and depression in elderly Hong Kong Chinese: Mediating and moderating effects of social support and financial strain. *Aging & Mental Health, 8*(3), 212–221.

Cobb, S. (1976). Social support as moderator of life stress. *Psychosomatic Medicine, 38*, 300–314.

Ferraro, K. F., & Su, Y.-P. (1999). Financial strain, social relations, and psychological distress among older people: A cross-cultural analysis. *Journals of Gerontology Series B: Psychological Sciences and Social Sciences, 54B*(1), S3–S15.

Glasgow, N. (1993). Poverty among rural elders: Trends, context, and directions for policy. *Journal of Applied Gerontology, 12*(3), 302–319.

Ingersoll-Dayton, B., Saengtienchai, C., Kespichayawattana, J., & Aungsuroch, Y. (2001). Psychological well-being Asian style: The perspective of Thai elders. *Journal of Cross-Cultural Gerontology, 16*(3), 283–302.

Kespichayawattana, J. (1999). Katanyu Katavedi and caregiving for frail elderly parents: A perspective of Thai families in metropolitan Bangkok. *Journal of Nursing Science Chulalongkorn University, 11*(3), 51–64.

Knodel, J., & Chayovan, N. (2009a). Older persons in Thailand: A demographic, social and economic profile. *Ageing International, 33*, 3–14.

Knodel, J., & Chayovan, N. (2009b). Intergenerational relationships and family care and support for Thai elderly. *Ageing International, 33*, 15–27.

Knodel, J., & Saengtienchai, C. (2007). Rural parents with urban children: Social and economic implications of migration on the rural elderly in Thailand. *Population, Space and Place, 13*(3), 193–210.

Knodel, J., Chayovan, N., Mithranon, P., Amornsirisomboon, P., & Arunsombat, S. (2005). *Thailand's older population: Social and economic support as assessed in 2002*. Bangkok: National Statistical Office.

Krause, N. (1987). Chronic financial strain, social support, and depressive symptoms among older adults. *Psychology and Aging, 2*, 185–192.

Krause, N. (2005). Exploring age differences in the stress-buffering function of social support. *Psychology and Aging, 20*(4), 714–717.

Krause, N., Jay, G., & Liang, J. (1991). Financial strain and psychological well-being among the American and Japanese elderly. *Psychology and Aging, 6*(2), 170–181.

Krause, N., Newsom, J. T., & Rook, K. S. (2008). Financial strain, negative interaction, and self-rated health: Evidence from the two United States nationwide longitudinal surveys. *Ageing and Society, 28*, 1001–1023.

Litwin, H., & Sapir, E. V. (2009). Perceived income adequacy among older adults in 12 countries: Findings from the survey of health, ageing and retirement in Europe. *The Gerontologist, 49*(3), 397–406.

Malmgren, J. A., Martin, M. L., & Nicola, R. M. (1996). Health care access of poverty-level older adults in Subsidized Public Housing. *Public Health Reports, 3*, 260–263.

National Economic and Social Development Board. (2008, June). *Data and index on poverty and income distribution 1988–2007*. Office of the National Economic and Social Development Board, Bangkok.

Office, N. S. (2002). *Report on the 2002 survey of elderly in Thailand*. Bangkok: National Statistical Office.

Pearlin, L. I., & Skaff, M. M. (1996). Stress and the life course: A paradigmatic alliance. *The Gerontologist, 36*, 229–247.

Pearlin, L. I., Mullan, J. T., Semple, S. L., & Skaff, M. M. (1990). Caregiving and the stress process: An overview of concepts and measures. *The Gerontologist, 30*, 583–594.

Porrapakkam, Y., & Punyaratabandhu, P. (2006). *The report of Thailand Population Health Examination Survey III*. Nonthaburi: Health System Research Institute.

Smeeding, T. M., & Weaver, R. K. (2002). *The senior income guarantee (SIG): A new proposal to reduce poverty among the elderly*. Chestnut Hill: Center for Retirement Research at Boston College.

Suwanrada, W. (2009). Poverty and financial security of the elderly in Thailand. *Ageing International, 33*, 50–61.

Szanton, S. L., Allen, J. K., Thorpe, R. J., Seeman, T., Bandeen-Roche, K., & Fried, L. P. (2008). Effect of financial strain on mortality in community-dwelling older women. *Journals of Gerontology Series B: Psychological Sciences and Social Sciences, 63*(6), S369–S374.

Thanakwang, K., & Soonthorndhada, K. (2007). Determinants of economic security among Thai elderly: Evidence from a cross-sectional national survey. *Asia Journal of Global Studies, 1*(2), 35–49.

Tran, T. V., & Dhooper, S. S. (1997). Poverty, chronic stress, ethnicity and psychological stress among elderly Hispanics. *Journal of Gerontological Social Work, 27*(4), 3–19.

Zimmer, Z. (2008). Poverty, wealth inequality and health among older adults in rural Cambodia. *Social Science & Medicine, 66*(1), 57–71.

Zimmer, Z., & Amornsirisomboon, P. (2001). Socioeconomic status and health among older adults in Thailand: An examination using multiple indicators. *Social Science & Medicine, 52*, 1297–1311.

Part IV
Social Support During Economic Hardships

Chapter 10
Social Networks and Reduction of Risk in Disasters: An Example of the Wenchuan Earthquake

Zhao Yandong

Disaster, Risk, and Social Networks

Social Aspects of Disaster and Risk

Disaster is a natural hazard with complex social impacts. When disaster strikes, normal social order is interrupted. This might lead to serious aftermath such as social disorder and social conflicts. Kreps (1984: 312) defined disaster as "events, observable in time and space, in which societies or their larger subunits (e.g. communities, regions) incur physical damages and losses and/or disruption of their routine functioning" and argued that both the cause and consequences of the disaster are related to social structure. Thus, the social science of disasters is of great value for the better understanding of disaster and for devising better management policies.

Sociologists are extremely interested in disasters not only because they hope to answer practical questions like "how to mitigate the social impact of disasters" but also because disasters provide a "natural laboratory" for understanding social structure and social process. In recent years, sociologists have started to focus on the importance of "social networks" and "social capital" in disaster studies.

Social Networks

"Social networks" form the basis for a set of theories and methods to study social structure. The basic idea is to view actors (that could be persons or organizations) as "nodes" and the relationship between actors as "ties." These nodes and ties add

Zhao Y. (✉)
Institute of Science, Technology and Society, Chinese Academy of Science and Technology for Development, Beijing, China
e-mail: zhaoyd@casted.org.cn

W.J.J. Yeung and M.T. Yap (eds.), *Economic Stress, Human Capital, and Families in Asia: Research and Policy Challenges*, Quality of Life in Asia 4,
DOI 10.1007/978-94-007-7386-8_10,

up to construct a network-like structure. In social network analysis, the structure of the society is exactly this network-like structure (Scott 1991; Wasserman and Faust 1994).

While the methods of network analysis are becoming more advanced and more complex, the theoretical development of social network was not advancing very quickly until the emergence of the concept of "social capital." The concept of social capital has transcended the traditional definition of "visible" capital. It implies that social relationships and interaction among social members and the social norms and structure based on these network relationships are all important types of "capital," which is beneficial both for individuals and for the society. Originating in sociological studies, this concept has rapidly gained popularity in economics, political studies, management, and social science generally in recent years (Portes 1998; Putnam et al. 1993).

Early disaster researchers had already noticed the role of social networks and social capital in disasters. Drabek et al. (1981) argues that social networks and social associations are the basic social units that respond in a disaster. Dynes (2005) holds that disaster destroys all types of capital, including economic, human, and social ones. However, compared to economic and human capital, social capital is the least damaged in disaster. Thus, social capital and social networks may be the most dependable resources in the aftermath of disaster.

Several empirical studies have considered the importance of social networks and social capital in disasters (e.g., Haines et al. 1996; Hurlbert et al. 2000). Nevertheless, few studies have given a comprehensive overview of how social networks reduce risks during and after disasters. Based on the survey data of the Wenchuan earthquake in 2008, this chapter will describe and discuss the role of social networks in reducing risk after disaster.

In May 12, 2008, an earthquake measuring 8.0 on the Richter scale hit Wenchuan County of Sichuan province, China. The seriously damaged area included more than 100,000 km^2 covering four provinces. According to statistics up to September 8, 2008, 69,226 people were confirmed to have been killed in this earthquake, 17,923 were reported missing, and 374,643 were injured. The total direct economic loss amounted to 845.1 billion yuan. As one of the most catastrophic disasters in the history of China, the Wenchuan earthquake has put great economic and social stress on the affected population. During the earthquake, around 6.9 million houses collapsed and 23.4 million houses were damaged. Around 15 million people were displaced. Food, water, shelter, and health care became the urgent needs of the affected population. According to a representative survey in the earthquake-hit area conducted in July 2008,[1] 32 % of the interviewed households had their houses totally destroyed in the earthquake. When asked about their most urgent needs, almost half (49 %) of the affected people declared that "new houses or improved housing" was their most urgent need, around 8 % selected "new jobs," and around 5 % selected "medical care." With the help from the government and society, the

[1]More details of the survey follow in this paper.

people in the disaster area are actively reconstructing their homeland. This disaster also provides researchers with an opportunity to observe how social network reduces risks in disasters.

Data and Measurement of Social Networks

Data

The data came from the Post-Wenchuan Earthquake Rapid Needs Assessment. In July 2008, the Chinese Academy of Science and Technology for Development conducted a rapid needs assessment survey in the Sichuan earthquake area, which was the first large-scale study of post-disaster rapid needs assessment in China.[2] As many as 174 clusters (villages, residential committees, or camps) and 5,000 households in the affected area were randomly sampled, and trained interviewers were sent to conduct face-to-face questionnaire interviews. The questionnaire mainly focused on the living conditions of residents, including their losses in the disaster, housing and infrastructure, education, health, employment, social networks and social participation, attitude, and evaluation. The field work was conducted from July 7 to July 19. Finally, 144 clusters and 4,526 households were interviewed, and 3,652 questionnaires were successfully collected. The response rate was 80.7 %.

Measurement of Social Networks

To measure the social networks of the respondents, we used "spring festival network" indicators. Developed as a revised version of "position generator" in Chinese context by Bian and Li (2000), the spring festival network has proven to be a good indicator for measuring the core social networks in the Chinese society (Bian and Li 2000; Zhao 2002, 2007). We asked the respondents, "In the spring festival of 2008, how many relatives, friends and other acquaintances did you contact?" With this question, we could arrive at two basic indicators of the network. One is the size of the network (total number of contacts). The other is the composition/structure of the network (the proportion of the relatives in the network).

We also measured the change in the network due to the disaster. First, we asked if any of the network members had died in the earthquake. This is considered as the "deterioration of networks." Second, we asked if the respondents had any new network members after the earthquake. This represented the reconstruction of networks.

Table 10.1 showed the basic characteristics of networks in our survey. The mean size of spring festival networks is 17.8 members. Among network members, the

[2]The survey is funded by the Norwegian Ministry of Foreign Affairs and supported by Fafo Institute of Applied International Studies, Norway.

Table 10.1 Statistics of social networks of residents in the earthquake area

	Mean	Std. deviation
Size of networks	17.80	17.68
Composition of networks (proportion of relatives)	0.68	0.41
Death of network members (yes = 1)	0.10	0.30
Have new network members (yes = 1)	0.04	0.20

Table 10.2 Statistics of control variables

	Mean	Std. deviation
Years of education	5.03	3.98
Household income per capital (logged)	4.98	2.08
Self-assessed economic status before the earthquake (1 = lowest , 5 = highest)	2.31	0.85
Loss in the disaster (1 = yes)	0.69	0.46
Live in temporary house (yes = 1)	0.40	0.49
Got governmental economic aid (1 = yes)	0.70	0.46
Self-reported health status in last 2 weeks (1 = very bad , 4 = very good)	2.83	0.82
Party membership (1 = no)	0.87	0.32
Gender (1 = female)	0.23	0.41
Age	59.77	14.19

average proportion of relatives is 68 %. Around 10 % of local residents lost some of their network members in the earthquake. Only 4 % of the people obtained new network members through the earthquake.

Control Variables

To better measure the impact of social networks, some control variables were also included in the analysis. We measured the "years of education" of the respondents as the indicator of their human capital and the "household income per capita" and "self-estimated economic status" as indicators of their economic capital. We also measured the respondents' loss in the earthquake with two variables. One is "the type of house currently living in." Those who were living in temporary housing were considered as more severely affected by the disaster, compared to those who had their own homes. The other variable is "self-estimated loss" in the earthquake. If the respondents reported that their lives became worse after the earthquake, they were considered as have losses in the disaster. We measured whether the respondents "received governmental economic aid" after the earthquake to see the impact of governmental support. To control for the health status before the earthquake, "self-reported health before the earthquake" was measured. Moreover, we also measured some individual characteristic variables, such as sex, age, and hukou registration status.

The statistics of control variables are listed in Table 10.2.

How Social Network Reduces Risks in the Wenchuan Earthquake?

Search and Rescue

During the initial period after a disaster, the normal workings of the social system is temporarily suspended, which leaves an "institutional vacuum" in which informal social institutions like social networks could play a prominent role. One example is search and rescue efforts.

Aguirre et al. (1995) found that search and rescue efforts after disaster are conducted primarily by other victims belonging to the social network of trapped ones. When external rescue personnel do arrive, they also need to locate remaining victims with the help of their neighbors. Based on a study of the 1980 Italy earthquake, Lechat (1989) also reported that 97 % of the injured victims who were successfully evacuated and transported to medical care were rescued by other people who used their bare hands and shovels, not heavy equipment.

The Wenchuan data shows similar patterns. In the survey we found some 130 respondents had been trapped in debris. Among them, around 95 % were rescued by relatives, neighbors, and other members of the public. Only a very small percentage of trapped victims were rescued by external rescue personnel, including PLA (People's Liberation Army) soldiers, professional rescue teams, or volunteers (see Fig. 10.1).

Information

Knowledge and information are of great importance in reducing risks before and after the disaster. A varied literature has shown that one of the main functions of social networks is to facilitate information flow (Granovetter 1973; Lin 1982). Disaster researchers also found that social networks are an important channel for transmitting warning messages before a disaster (Aguirre 1988; Fitzpatrick and Mileti 1994).

Our survey showed that social networks played an indispensable role in facilitating information flows in the disaster affected area. After the earthquake, around 16 % of residents had acquired information about the government's disaster relief efforts through the channel of "relatives, friends, and other social ties." Among all the information channels, social networks were the third most frequently used channel, only less than "television" and "local cadres" (see Fig. 10.2).

Further analysis was conducted to see who were more likely to use social networks as their main information channel. The result of logistic regression shows that those with lower proportion of relatives in their networks were more likely to use the social network to get information. This finding is consistent with that

Fig. 10.1 Rescuers in the Wenchuan earthquake

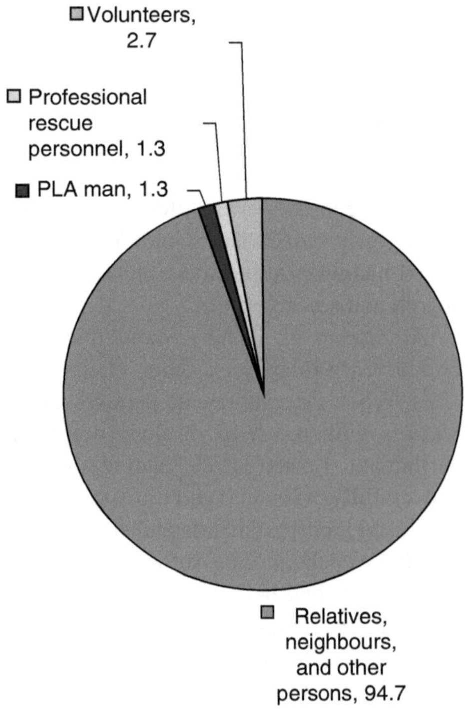

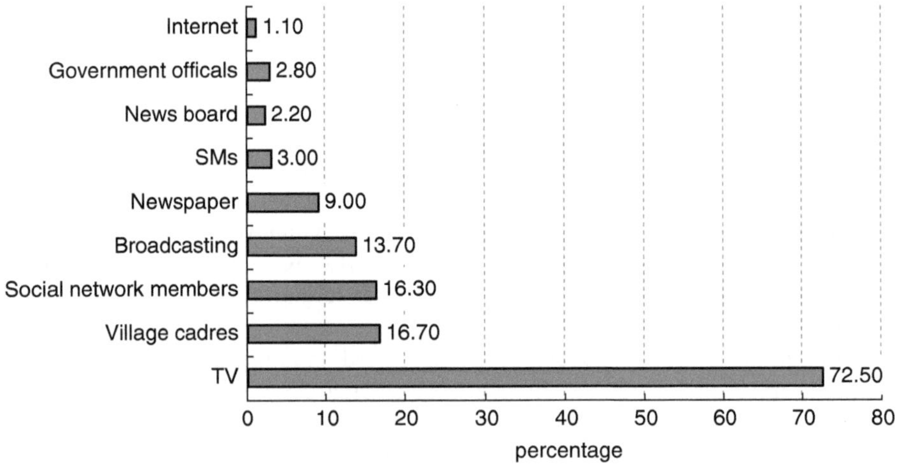

Fig. 10.2 Main channels of policy-related information after the earthquake

of existing literature. Granovetter (1973) argues that weak ties in one's social networks, such as acquaintances, are usually more different or heterogeneous than the strong ties such as relatives and close friends. As a result, weak ties have a higher probability of bringing in new information and knowledge than strong ties.

Table 10.3 Logistic regression of likelihood of using social networks to get information after the earthquake

	B		Std. error
Network size	0.00		0.01
Network composition	−0.32	#	0.20
Death of Network members (1 = yes)	−0.34		0.31
Have new network member (1 = yes)	0.00		0.01
Education years	−0.04	#	0.03
Household income per capital (logged)	0.00		0.04
Self-assessed economic status before the disaster	−0.08		0.10
Loss in the earthquake (1 = yes)	0.20	*	0.20
Living in temporary house (1 = yes)	0.61		
Self-reported health in last 2 weeks	−0.03		0.09
Sex (female = 1)	−0.11		0.20
Age	0.01		0.01
Party membership (yes = 1)	0.72	*	0.34
Hukou (urban = 1)	0.05		0.22
Constant	−4.71		1.02
−2 Log-likelihood	1355.10		
Chi square	36.15	**	
df	14		
N	3, 404		

Note: #, $p < 0.10$; *$p < 0.05$; **$p < 0.01$

Our finding also suggests that after disaster, the more heterogeneous network, i.e., the networks with more non-relatives, is better for getting new information (Table 10.3).

Social Support

After the disaster, the victims are in urgent need of various types of assistance and support. Researchers of the effects of disasters have found that the degree of loss in disaster is strongly related to the support/assistance received (Rossi et al. 1982; Kaniasty and Norris 1995a, b). Among the external support, social support is one of the most important.

Social support is defined as social interactions that provide individuals with actual assistance or embed them into a web of social relationships perceived to be loving, caring, and readily available in times of need (Hobfoll 1988). The source of social support can be divided into formal and informal ones. The formal source of social support may be viewed as coming from the people outside of an individual's social network, while the informal source is within the social network (Vaux 1988).

Our data showed that after the Wenchuan earthquake, the victims obtained various types of support. Though the government was the main support provider,

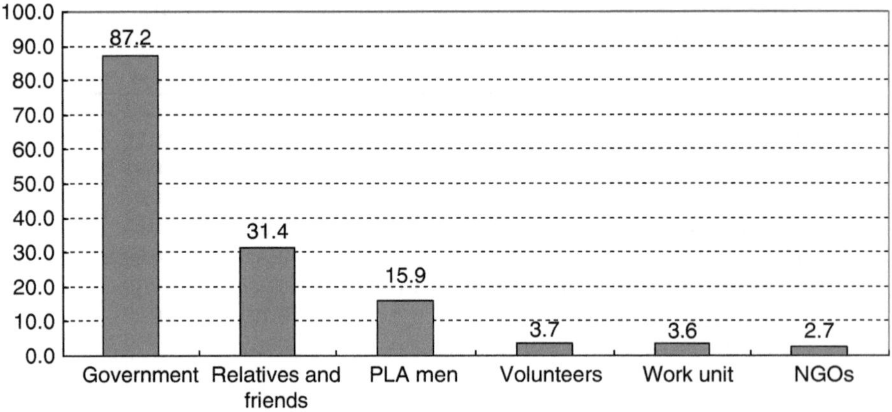

Fig. 10.3 The most important support providers

social networks played an important supplementary role in providing support to the victims. When asked "among those who provide support to you, who is the most important?" the majority of respondents (87.2 %) selected "government," while "relatives and friends" was the second most frequently option selected. More than 30 % of respondents thought social networks were their most important support providers (Fig. 10.3).[3]

An important issue in the wake of a disaster is the distribution of support resources among the victims. Some believe there is a "rule of relative needs," i.e., those in need of more support will be provided with more (Hobfoll and Lerman 1989; Kaniasty and Norris 1995a). Others insist on the "rule of relative advantages," which holds that some social groups are more likely to receive support than others regardless of their needs (Drabek and Key 1984; Kaniasty and Norris 1995a).

To test these two conflicting theories and to see if social networks also played a role in providing support, we further analyzed what kind of households was more likely to get more support than others after the earthquake. We set "the amount of support received" as the dependent variable. In addition to social network variables, we also included control variables such as highest education of household members, household income per capital (loggEd.), self-assessed social status of the household before the earthquake, any loss in the earthquake, type of houses, and the type of residence of the household.

In Table 10.4, the result of an ordinary least squares regression is shown. The network size has a significant influence on the amount of support received, which means that a bigger network will bring more social support. The number of new network members is also a significant variable. If the household has more newly obtained network members, it will receive more support. The results indicate

[3]Please note that since this question is a multi-choice one, the percentage adds up to more than 100.

Table 10.4 Ordinary least squares regression of the factors influencing the amount of support received

	B		Std. error
Network size	0.01	***	0.00
Network composition	0.01		0.06
Death of Network members (1 = yes)	0.24	***	0.08
Have new network member (1 = yes)	0.02	***	0.00
Highest completed education years in household	−0.08	***	0.03
Household income per capital (logged)	0.02	*	0.01
Self-assessed economic status before the disaster	−0.01		0.03
Loss in the earthquake (1 = yes)	0.47	***	0.05
Living in temporary house (1 = yes)	0.88	***	0.05
Residence (1 = urban)	0.05		0.06
(Constant)	0.92	***	0.15
R^2	0.20		
F	80.77	***	
N	3,260		

Note: $*p < 0.05$; $***p < 0.001$

that social network is a very important channel of various types of support after the disaster. Having a bigger social network size, i.e., knowing more people, is apparently one of the "relative advantages" one has in the distribution of support.

Mental Health

The impact of disaster is not only confined to the loss of lives and properties but also affects the mental health of survivors. During the disaster, the victims may experience the loss of relatives, neighbors and friends, the damage to property, and other losses. The great stress brought by these losses may create short-term and long-term psychological distress.

Several studies have found that social networks reduce the negative impact of trauma induced by disasters. After the disaster, social networks can provide the victims with emotional support, help them to release their stress and trauma, and help them to recover from psychological distress (Bolin and Klenow 1983; Kaniasty and Norris 1995a).

The impact of social networks on victims' mental health is quite significant in our survey. The mental health score of the residents in the earthquake area is measured by the CHQ-12 scale. CHQ (Chinese Health Questionnaire) is a revised Chinese version of GHQ (General Health Questionnaire), which aims at measuring the mental health status of the respondents. CHQ was developed in Taiwan and has been tested in several Chinese cities (Yang et al. 2003). We set the mental health score as the dependent variable (the higher the score, the better mental health status) and social network indicators as independent variables in addition to a number of control variables.

Table 10.5 Ordinary least squares regression of the factors influencing mental health status of survivors

	B		Std. error
Network size	0.02	**	0.01
Network composition	0.49		0.26
Death of Network members (1 = yes)	−0.82		0.36
Number of new network member after earthquake	0.03		0.05
Education years	0.10	*	0.03
Household income per capita (logged)	0.15	*	0.05
Self-assessed economic status before the disaster	0.66	**	0.13
Loss in the earthquake (1 = yes)	−1.40	**	0.25
Living in temporary house (1 = yes)	−0.25	**	0.24
Got governmental economic aid (1 = yes)	0.08		9.26
Self-reported health status in last 2 weeks	3.07	**	0.12
Sex (1 = female)	0.05		0.29
Age	−0.02		0.01
Party membership (1 = yes)	−0.21		0.33
Hukou (1 = urban)	0.42		0.28
(Constant)	45.23	**	1.29
R^2	0.23		
F	61.82	***	
N	3,391		

Note: #, $p < 0.10$; *$p < 0.05$; **$p < 0.01$; ***$p < 0.001$

The results of regression are shown in Table 10.5.

From the results we could clearly see that social network is very important in maintaining the mental health of disaster victims. A bigger network will bring better psychological outcomes. Secondly, the higher proportion of relatives in the network, the better mental health status one is in. A high proportion of relatives provides higher density and lower heterogeneity to the network than one with a low proportion of relatives. This result is consistent with existing arguments that a dense and homogenous network is good for providing emotional support (Lin 1982). Finally, death of network members is negatively related with mental health. Apart from the obvious conclusion that people are affected when those they are close to die, the result also supports the argument that the damage to networks will have significant negative impact on individuals' psychological health (Kreps 1984). It is also interesting to note that obtaining governmental aid after the earthquake has no significant impact on respondents' mental health. This finding further implies that after the disaster, informal resources like social networks play a more important role in social lives of survivors than formal/institutional resources.

Other control variables like level of education and economic status have impact on the mental health. Those with relatively high education and better economic status tend to report better mental health. Experiencing loss in earthquake and living in temporary houses lead to decreased mental health. In terms of self-reported health status, the B coefficient shows that when the self-rated health status increases by one level, mental health will also increase by around three points.

Conclusion

The study has shown that social networks play an important role in reducing risks during and after disaster. In the early phase of disaster, most of the search and rescue endeavors come from social network members. In the aftermath of disaster, social networks can facilitate the flow of information, provide various types of support, and help in maintaining the mental health of the victims.

The study also indicates that changes in the social network in disaster is an important topic that needs further study. In the disaster, part of people's social networks will be damaged, and they actively reconstruct their networks after the disaster. These dynamics and their social impact deserve further study.

Some policy implications can also be drawn from the study. Firstly, as mentioned above, the social network members are the most dependable rescuers during the initial phase of the disaster. Therefore, the government should put more emphasis on improving the preparedness of local people in disaster-prone areas, including providing training for basic rescue skills to local dwellers. Secondly, since social networks are indispensable in disaster, it is necessary to take them into consideration when designing disaster management and mitigation policies. For example, after disaster hits, the government should assist the survivors in keeping their social networks intact during rescue and displacement and tap existing social networks in the reconstruction processes. Finally, the government should understand that social networks and social capital require long-term accumulation. Helping people to freely communicate and associate with each other is the best way to help them build up social networks and social capital that build resilience to disaster.

References

Aguirre, E. (1988). The lack of warning before the Saragosa Tornado. *International Journal of Mass Emergencies and Disasters, 6*, 65–74.

Aguirre, E., Wenger, D., Glass, T., Diaz-Murillo, M., & Vigo, G. (1995). The social organization of search and rescue: Evidence from the Guadalajara Gasoline Explosion. *International Journal of Mass Emergencies and Disasters, 13*, 93–106.

Bian, Y., & Li, Y. (2000). Social network capital of Chinese urban families. *Tsinghua Sociological Review, 2*, 1–18.

Bolin, R., & Klenow, D. (1983). Response of elderly to disaster: An age-stratified analysis. *International Journal of Aging and Human Development, 16*, 283–296.

Drabek, T., & Key, W. (1984). *Conquering disaster: Family recovery and long-term consequences*. New York: Irvington.

Drabek, T., Taminga, J., Kilijanek, T., & Adams, C. (1981). *Managing multiorganizational emergency responses: Emergent search and rescue networks in natural disasters and remote area settings*. Boulder: Institute of Behavior Science, University of Colombia.

Dynes, R. (2005). *Community social capital as the primary basis for resilience* (Preliminary Paper No. 344). Newark DE: University of Delaware, Disaster Research Center.

Fitzpatrick, C., & Mileti, D. (1994). Public risk communication. In R. Dynes & K. Tierney (Eds.), *Disasters, collective behavior, and social organizations* (pp. 71–84). Newark: University of Delaware Press.

Granovetter, M. (1973). The strength of weak tie. *American Journal of Sociology, 78*, 1360–1380.
Haines, V., Hurlbert, J., & Beggs, J. (1996). Exploring the determinants of support provision: Provider characteristics, personal networks, community contexts, and support following life events. *Journal of Health and Social Behavior, 37*(3), 252–264.
Hobfoll, S. (1988). *The ecology of stress*. New York: Hemisphere.
Hobfoll, S., & Lerman, M. (1989). Predicting receipt of social support: A longitudinal study of parents' reactions to their child's illness. *Health Psychology, 8*, 61–77.
Hurlbert, J., Haines, V., & Beggs, J. (2000). Core networks and tie activation: What kinds of routine networks allocate resources in nonroutine situations? *American Sociological Review, 65*(4), 598–618.
Kaniasty, K., & Norris, F. (1995a). In search of altruistic community: Patterns of social support mobilization following Hurricane Hugo. *American Journal of Community Psychology, 23*, 447–477.
Kaniasty, K., & Norris, F. (1995b). Mobilization and deterioration of social support following natural disasters. *Current Directions in Psychological Science, 4*(3), 94–98.
Kreps, G. (1984). Sociological inquiry and disaster research. *Annual Review of Sociology, 10*, 309–330.
Lechat, M. (1989). *Corporal damage as related to building structure and design*. Lovain: Center for Research on the Epidemiology of Disaster, Catholic University.
Lin, N. (1982). Social resources and instrumental action. In P. Marsden & N. Lin (Eds.), *Social structure and network analysis* (pp. 131–147). Beverly Hills: Sage Publications.
Portes, A. (1998). Social capital: Its origins and applications in modern sociology. *Annual Review of Sociology, 24*, 1–24.
Putnam, R., Leonardi, R., & Raffaella, Y. N. (1993). *Making democracy work: Civic traditions in modern Italy*. Princeton: Princeton University Press.
Rossi, P. H., Wright, J. D., & Weber-Burdin, E. (1982). *Natural hazards and public choice: The state and local politics of hazards mitigation*. New York: Academic.
Scott, J. (1991). *Social network analysis: A handbook*. London: Sage Publications Ltd.
Vaux, A. (1988). *Social support: Theory, research, and intervention*. New York: Praeger.
Wasserman, S., & Faust, K. (1994). *Social network analysis*. Cambridge: Cambridge University Press.
Yang, T., Huang, L., & Wu, Z. (2003). The validity of Chinese health questionnaire in the mental disorder studies in mainland China. *Chinese Journal of Epidemiology, 24*, 769–773.
Zhao, Y. (2002). Social capital in re-employment: Its efficacy and limit. *Sociological Research, 100*(4), 43–54. Retrieved online at: http://en.cnki.com.cn/CJFD_en_New/Detail.ashx?t=e&url=/Article_en/CJFDTOTAL-SHXJ200204006.htm.
Zhao, Y. (2007). Social capital and post-disaster recovery: A sociological study on disaster. *Sociological Research, 131*(5), 164–187. Retreived online at: http://en.cnki.com.cn/Article_en/CJFDTOTAL-SHXJ200705009.htm.

Chapter 11
Human and Social Capital Dynamics in Economic Crises: The Impact on Poor Chinese Migrant Children in Hong Kong During the Far East Economic Crisis

Sam Wong

Introduction

Human capital and social capital both play a significant role in economic development and social well-being. The Organisation for Economic Co-operation and Development (OECD) defines human capital as "the knowledge, skills and health embodied in individuals," whereas social capital is defined as "the norms and networks facilitating co-operation either within or between groups" (OECD 1998: 12). In its World Development Reports, the World Bank recommends building both capitals to alleviate global poverty (World Bank 1990, 2000). During times of economic crisis, human capital and social capital come under tremendous pressure (Bhutta et al. 2009; Knowles et al. 1999). In response to the "capital deficit," policy makers are often inclined to implement various social policies. The effectiveness of their interventions, however, depends, to a great extent, on how human capital and social capital interact. Is human capital complementary or substitutive to social capital? Does one facilitate, or hinder, the development of the other?

Interrogating the relationship between human and social capital is not new in literature. In his influential study, Coleman (1988) asserts that parents' social capital has a significant impact on children's school attainments. Putnam (2000) makes a similar finding and argues that families with higher human capital may have led to the decline of social capital in the USA, since dual earners are so preoccupied with their jobs that they reduce social interactions with other community members. This idea of the causal relationship between human and social capital has, however, sparked fierce debate. According to Schuller and Field (1998), social capital is "internally differentiated and constantly changing" in nature (p. 234). Any simplistic

S. Wong (✉)
Department of Geography and Planning, University of Liverpool, Merseyside, L69 7ZT, UK
e-mail: s.wong@liv.ac.uk

W.J.J. Yeung and M.T. Yap (eds.), *Economic Stress, Human Capital, and Families in Asia: Research and Policy Challenges*, Quality of Life in Asia 4,
DOI 10.1007/978-94-007-7386-8_11,

public policies, which do not take into account the "dynamic context which captures the interactions between policies and institutions and the differing time scales," Schuller warns (2001: 19), are highly undesirable.

This chapter revisits the old debate and underlines human and social capital interactions in the contexts of economic crises. Unlike the quantitative studies that aim to offer correlations between human and social capital (see Felicio et al. 2009; Goldin and Katz 1999), this chapter explores these complex relationships with an ethnographic, qualitative approach. It draws on Mainland Chinese migrant children in Hong Kong whose families received less than half of the median monthly household incomes of the general population in Hong Kong, i.e., below HK$8,250.00, during the Far East Economic Crisis (1998–2002) as a case study (Hong Kong Government 2002a). It makes two observations. Firstly, the rising unemployment rate and reduction in salaries, caused by the economic crisis, had forced the migrant parents to reduce the family budget for activities and social involvement. This led to a reduction in the social capital, but not the human capital, of the migrant children. Secondly, the economic crisis changed gendered relations within the affected families. Unemployed men found they could not cope with their new social role as family carer. They felt embarrassed to take their children to attend private tuition and computer classes intended to provide Mainland students with extra support for homework and examination. The human capital building of the Mainland Chinese children was affected when they were unable to receive the support they need given in these classes.

This chapter begins by offering a contextual understanding of the lives of poor Mainland Chinese migrant children in Hong Kong. After discussing the research methodology, it will explore how the process of migration had shaped the social and human capital building of migrant families. The next section will explore the impact of the Far East Economic Crisis in Hong Kong in the early 2000s and examine how it had affected the migrant families trying to cope with diminishing human and social capital.

Mainland Chinese Migrant Children in Hong Kong

Schuller (2001) compares and contrasts human capital and social capital and points out that the former is individually owned while the latter is socially shared. He also mentions that the former is measured by the duration of schooling and the number of qualifications, while the latter is measured by levels of trust and associational membership.

Before the handover of Hong Kong back to China, the British and Chinese governments reached an agreement in 1995 to grant a daily quota of 150 legitimate Chinese immigrants a one-way permit to Hong Kong. Among these 150 migrants, two-thirds were children aged below 15 (Lui and Wong 1995). These children came from cross-border marriages, and the motivations for these marriages were complex. Middle-aged men failed to find partners in Hong Kong because of their working class background and low social status. Economic disparities between Hong Kong and the Mainland in the 1980s, however, made these men highly desirable in the eyes of Mainland women because they earned relatively more and held Hong Kong citizenship (Wong 2007). Another reason for cross-border marriage relates to the process of deindustrialization of Hong Kong in the 1980s. Many factories were relocated to the Mainland in order to capitalize on the low production costs there. Hong Kong workers were considered more skilled in staff management and quality control and were recruited as supervisors of Chinese workers. Once settled in Mainland China, a few of them met their partners and decided to start a family in the Mainland while retaining Hong Kong citizenship. For the sake of the long-term well-being of their children, most of these fathers would move back to Hong Kong and apply for their families to settle in Hong Kong.

The quota system was, however, criticized for failing to consider the family as a whole migration unit (Lui and Wong 1995). In many cases, parents and their children were granted the right of abode at different times, which led to the "split-family phenomenon" (Kuah 1999). Fathers in Hong Kong often took up the childcare responsibilities while simultaneously managing their full-time jobs and waiting for the reunion with their Mainland wives, which meant that many of them became pseudo-single families.

The Mainland Chinese children faced numerous adjustment difficulties in Hong Kong. Not all of them could speak Cantonese, the local dialect in Hong Kong. Owing to the different education systems in Hong Kong and the Mainland, academic qualifications attained from the Mainland were not recognized. Ng and Liu (1999) found that 50 % of migrant children in primary and 80 % in secondary school had to repeat their grades. As a result, most of them were older than their fellow students. Compared to their Hong Kong counterparts, they were also slow in learning English, and the same research showed that 55 % of the migrants felt they lagged behind at the secondary school level. A study by the Boys' and Girls' Clubs Association of Hong Kong (1999) also suggested that the split-family phenomenon was to blame for poor family relationships. Low self-esteem among the migrant children was also identified as being due to poor academic performance, especially in English language (Wong 2008: 237).

Research Methodology

Within these social contexts, how did the Far East Economic Crisis exert extra pressure on the Mainland Chinese migrant families? How did these families draw on their human and social capital to cope with the changes? What was the short- and long-term impact of their coping strategies on the well-being of their children? Cleaver (2005) suggests that human beings do not always make strategic choices in their lives; instead, they let social institutions think on their behalf. To explore the migrants' complex "investment patterns," I have adopted an ethnographic approach to examine the complex decision-making process among the Mainland Chinese migrant families in Hong Kong. I was particularly interested in exploring the changes in the social and human capital of the migrant children during the economic crisis in the period between 1998 and 2002 in Hong Kong.

I spent 12 months in Hong Kong during 2001 and 2002 to investigate the lives of 15 migrant families and their children, who had already been living in Hong Kong for more than a year. This qualitative study did not aim to make any generalized claims; instead, it intended to demonstrate the multiple realities facing the migrants and to expose the institutional constraints that prohibited them from maximizing their social and human capital. I approached migrant families through nongovernmental organizations (NGOs) and snowball networking. Initially, I approached 20 NGOs which were providing services for Mainland migrants. After a long period of negotiation, I obtained support from three of these NGOs. They were a community currency project in Wanchai, a support group for abused women in Tsuen Wan, and a female migrants' mutual-help group in Mongkok. They were from different locations in Hong Kong and had different objectives and activities. While the first and the second groups were explicit about their intention to foster mutual understanding between migrants and local people, the third NGO was exclusively for migrants and its purpose was to strengthen in-group solidarity by highlighting the member's migrant identity. The abused women's support group was run by feminist social workers who were in favor of public demonstrations to fight for battered women's interests. I worked as volunteers with all three NGOs, participating in their committee meetings and daily activities, in an attempt to develop interpersonal relationships with the group members. Apart from informal conversations and observations, I also conducted in-depth interviews with the migrant parents and their children.

Since many of the participants in these three NGO groups were female, I asked social workers and the migrants themselves to introduce to us some of their female and male migrant friends who did not participate in NGOs. The 15 migrant families were chosen according to their diverse social backgrounds and experiences. My intention was to explore their diverse motivations and strategies for building human and social capital (Brewer 2000). I took notes during the interviews and made my analysis by coding.

Perceptions of the Education System in Hong Kong

The female migrants who were married to Hong Kong men had, at best, only received primary education. Most of them worked as factory workers before their marriage. However, they considered their children's education as a top priority. They agreed, in interviews, that they would try to ensure that their children received the best education possible and also wanted them to achieve the highest academic achievements.

When asked why education played such an important role, they mentioned that good education and high qualifications would pave the way to a good life with decent salaries. Having once lived in poverty, this mattered most to the female migrants. Investing in their children's human capital, they believed, was the best way to avoid falling back into poverty. Apart from this economic motive, my study also showed that the migrants had been strongly influenced by Confucian values. They considered education as a way to teach their children to become good people. Not only would this mean that their children would take up filial responsibilities in due course but that they would also cherish social harmony. Confucian values also helped to shape the discourse of "good parenthood." The idea of being good parents meant that they would sacrifice anything in return for good education for their children. When asked who should emigrate to Hong Kong first, they or their children, the parents did not hesitate to let their children go first, since their children could "learn English earlier in Hong Kong" (interview, 08/06/02). However, if they, themselves, were granted the right of abode in Hong Kong before their children were, they would regularly send remittances in order to help raise their children's living standards. In a nutshell, the Confucian values provided the migrant parents with an inspiration to maximize their children's education opportunities. Yet, these values also created strong social pressure on them as they did not want to be seen as "bad" parents.

The female migrants learned of the different educational systems in Hong Kong and the Mainland from relatives and friends. The Hong Kong system of education used both Chinese and English as the medium of instruction in primary and secondary schools. In Hong Kong, children started learning English vocabulary and simple sentences as early as in kindergarten. Although English as the medium of instruction posed a dilemma to the migrant parents, they welcomed it because English was considered an elite language. As one migrant put it, "I want my daughter to be a lawyer, and it would be nice if she can start learning English as young as possible" (interview with a female migrant, 07/05/02). On the other hand, they were worried that their children might encounter difficulties in learning English and that this would adversely affect their academic performance in school. Another learning obstacle came from the use of Chinese characters. Hong Kong uses complex Chinese characters, while Mainland China has adopted a simplified version. The migrant parents were concerned that this would affect their children's motivation in learning.

To facilitate their children's adjustment to the new educational system, the female migrants would ask their husbands to gather information about schools around their neighborhood in Hong Kong. They then submitted applications to their chosen schools to reserve a place, long before their applications of resettlement were accepted. The parents also provided English and Chinese textbooks to their children to read. Migrants who could afford leaving their hometowns in rural areas would move to the towns near the border. These towns had a large cluster of primary and secondary schools which provided programs to prepare children for an English medium education. These schools claimed that their English tutors were experienced teachers from Hong Kong. The courses were expensive, yet they were very popular since many well-off parents wanted to ensure a smooth transition in their children's education. In my particular study, however, there were only two families out of 15 who actually moved to the towns near the border.

Coping Strategies After Migration

My study noted that the children of the female migrants played a significant role in helping their mothers make the necessary social adjustments in the host society. Their parents met other migrants in local parks and playgrounds as well as at school entrances before and after school. Many migrants with children in the same schools or classes formed a close bond among themselves. They built informal social networks via telephone conversations and by having social gatherings during which they could share their common concerns about adjustment to their new way of life as well as concerns about their children's studies.

Many migrant children encountered difficulties in learning, not only in subjects taught in English but also in computer skills. This was exacerbated by the Hong Kong government's move to develop the city as a "knowledge society" in the mid-1990s. From then on many primary school students were encouraged to engage in online learning and to complete their assignments by computer. Yet, many poor migrant families could not afford a family computer. Recognizing the chief concerns of migrant parents about their children's education, some NGOs in Hong Kong initiated remedial programs that catered to the children's educational needs. All three NGOs in my study provided the migrant children with free, private tuition services and computer classes after school. Migrant parents waiting for their children in school were approached by social workers who invited them to join their social programs. After the migrants had developed interpersonal relationships, the social workers organized capacity-building workshops for them with the intention of empowering them to build their human capital and to promote community cohesion by bridging the gap between migrants and local people. The social workers also formalized group participation and arranged for the migrants to join organizing committees in order to train them in leadership skills. I also volunteered at the NGOs to conduct English language and computer classes, so that I could approach suitable migrants for observations and interviews.

Apart from group participation in the host society, the female migrants built and maintained their cross-border social capital by making regular trips to their hometowns in the Mainland. Many female migrants in my study returned to Mainland China with their children at least once a year. Some of them sought emotional support from their families and friends, whereas others wanted to show off their success after becoming a "Hong Kong bride." No matter what their motivation, they often made their decisions about when to make these visits based on their children's school calendars, in order not to interrupt their children's education. Therefore, many migrants made their trips during the Chinese Lunar New Year and the summer holidays.

Migrant Children's Lives During the Far East Economic Crisis

The Far East Economic Crisis started in Thailand in 1997 when the baht was drastically devalued over a very short period of time. Many other Asian countries then followed suit and devalued their currencies in order to maintain the competitiveness of their economies. The currency crisis turned into a large-scale economic crisis, and Hong Kong was hit hard. Unemployment in 1998 reached a record high of 8 %. Low-skilled and lowly educated labor, including many Mainland Chinese families in Hong Kong, faced redundancy (Fung and Hung 1999). Some were lucky enough to keep their jobs but faced salary reductions and longer working hours (Weisbrot 2007).

In Hong Kong, the economic crisis forced the migrants to rethink their economic priorities and social commitments. A quantitative, longitudinal survey by the Hong Kong government in 2002 highlighted the changing sources of income for migrant families between 1998 and 2002 (Hong Kong Government 2002a). The findings, shown in Table 11.1, showed that wages from the formal labor sector remained the most significant source of migrant incomes, but employment in this sector declined drastically from 76.5 % in 1998 to 56.2 % in 2000. Simultaneously, the numbers of migrants receiving financial support from their relatives and from public assistance rose significantly – from 13.2 to 23.9 % and from 10.5 to 15.5 %, respectively. This survey offers us a glimpse of the changing self-help pattern among the migrants during the economic crisis.

Unlike Thailand or Indonesia, where parents were forced to disinvest in human capital by withdrawing their children from school in order to cope with the economic hardship (Bhutta et al. 2009; Knowles et al. 1999), Hong Kong's robust education system which offered 9 years of free education to every child in the city-state was not affected by the crisis. For those who progressed to the upper secondary schools, the fees were low and bursaries were available. The economic crisis, however, affected the human and social capital development of the migrants and their children. During the economic crisis, the construction industry was hit particularly hard. Many female migrants' husbands who were working in this industry lost their jobs. To compensate for the reduction in family income, the female migrants had no choice but to

Table 11.1 Major sources of family incomes of new arrivals from 1998 to 2002

	1998 (Q3) (%)	1999 (Q2) (%)	2000 (Q3) (%)	2002 (Q2) (%)
Wages	76.5	71.8	56.2	69.4
Financial assistance from relatives	13.2	12.4	23.9	12.8
Public assistance	10.5	6.6	15.5	12.5
Others	0	8.6	4.4	5.3

Source: Hong Kong Government (2002a: 12)

start looking for jobs. Facing a very competitive employment market, many of them ended up working as cleaners in restaurants – employment characterized by low pay, low status, and long working hours. Other migrants who had very low qualifications and limited work experience had to find work in the informal sector, such as in rubbish collection and recycling companies. Owing to the heavy workload as working mothers and due to exhaustion, many of the female migrants in my study stopped taking their children for recreation in local parks and playgrounds. A few of them mentioned in interviews that they were too exhausted even to maintain contact with their friends. To offer some assistance to their parents, some older migrant children withdrew from extracurricular activities to look after their siblings after school.

During my ethnographic study, I met a 10-year-old girl, Siu Ying (not her real name), in my English class. When we met, she had already settled in Hong Kong for 3 years. She was smart, industrious, and always eager to improve her English. She performed very well in the first semester. However, in the second semester, she was a different person. She was often late for class, did not submit assignments punctually, and even dozed off in class. I went to see her mother who was embarrassed to tell me that since her husband was made redundant a year ago, she had no choice but to start collecting rubbish from the streets. Siu Ying was eager to help, and they both worked until midnight. Without proper sleep, Siu Ying found it difficult to concentrate in school, and this was affecting her academic performance (interview, 15/07/02).

Although education itself in Hong Kong is free, many essential items such as textbooks, transport, meals, school uniform, school trips, and extracurricular activities are payable. During the economic crisis, many migrant couples had considered enrolling their children in full-day schools. The benefit of such schools was that both parents were then free to work. Yet, the drawback was that this would involve higher costs than half-day school. Another tough decision that the migrant parents had to make was to limit their children's engagement in after-school activities. This was especially if the private tuition and computer skills training centers were some distance from home. Many of these classes targeted poor families, including Mainland migrant children. They intended to provide them with extra support, not only in English and computer skills but also in building their self-confidence. However, high transport costs meant that the children had to withdraw from these activities. Some migrants felt that this would affect the long-term development of their children and affect their psychological development. Some of them felt inferior when they could not afford the video games and expensive toys that their friends and classmates had.

A few migrant parents felt tempted to send their children to Mainland China and ask their own parents to look after them. However, under pressure from the discourse of "good parenthood," they feared that they would be accused of being "failed parents" and would be condemned for not acting in their children's best interests by discontinuing their education in Hong Kong.

The NGOs considered the financial crisis as a golden opportunity for them to further develop their services in a wider migrant community. The community currency project, for instance, initiated the setting up of a secondhand goods bazaar. The social workers encouraged poor migrants to exchange goods and to provide childcare services to one another. Migrants were also encouraged to set up their own food stalls in the bazaar to generate income. The group for abused women, in my case study, adopted a different strategy. Social workers encouraged their members to exercise their civil rights and apply for public assistance. Both approaches tried to foster mutual support and to build migrants' confidence during the economic downturn.

The Hong Kong Catholic Commission for Labour Affairs (1999) suggested that the economic crisis had soured the relationship between Hong Kongers and the "outsiders" and triggered social discrimination. When the economy was good, the influx of Mainland migrants was appreciated for they helped to maintain a steady population growth and, with it, economic growth. Yet, during the economic crisis, hostility toward the Mainlanders increased. A survey by the Hong Kong Psychological Society (1999) found that local residents believed that Chinese migrants were "bad" by nature. Some 54 % of respondents thought migrants brought bad influences to Hong Kong and 55 % believed that migrants had only themselves to blame for their own poverty. These negative attitudes made the social integration of the migrant children even harder (Wong 2007). The rising levels of discrimination against migrants also caused deep concern among the Hong Kong authorities, and the government launched an investigation into discrimination against Chinese migrants (Home Affairs Branch 1997).

Gender Impact

The economic crisis affected different industries differently and changed the structure of the employment market. Men and women were also hit differently, and that had some impact on the gendered relations of the migrant families. The service industry of Hong Kong was more suited to women because they were more open to taking up low-skilled and low-paying jobs than the men. These changes transformed the traditional gender norms of men as breadwinners and women as carers. Some men could not come to terms with this change as they felt that their economic superiority was threatened by the rising economic power of their migrant wives. The large age gap between the spouses also made men feel vulnerable as they were afraid that their wives would look for younger men.

Although unemployment could provide men with an opportunity to spend more time with their children, the stigma of being stay-at-home fathers undermined men's confidence in handling their new social role. They disliked the feeling of being "idle" at home and felt too embarrassed to take their children to school. They were also reluctant to take their children to private tuition and computer classes provided by the NGOs. Students' loss of opportunity to patronize support programs not only affected their human capital building, but it further reduced their limited social capital.

Driven by the notion of "good motherhood," many women could not bear to see their children suffer in this way. To address these problems, they took their children to schools or NGOs themselves, rather than wait for the assistance of their husbands. This became another burden added to their full-time employment and heavy domestic workloads. These multiple demands on their time and energy explain their struggle to maintain social capital within Hong Kong and across the border in Mainland China.

Conclusion

This chapter has drawn on the experiences of Mainland Chinese migrant children in Hong Kong as a case study to demonstrate the complex social and human capital interactions resulting from the Far East Economic Crisis in Hong Kong between 1998 and 2002. Despite Hong Kong's sound and resilient education system, the economic crisis may have increased poverty and led to a disinvestment in human capital, such as withdrawal from after-school tuition, and in social capital, such as reduced participation in extracurricular activities, among poor migrant children. The changing gendered relations, arising from high levels of unemployment among men, also had some negative impact on the human and social capital formation of the migrant children. This was particularly the case when the migrant fathers were unable to adapt to their new role as carer, and their children suffered as a result when they lost access to free private tuition and computer lessons provided by the schools and NGOs.

I am aware of the limitations of my research. My study lasted for only 12 months in Hong Kong, with no subsequent follow-up. The negative impact on the human and social capital building among the migrant children could be a short-term effect while the Hong Kong economy was gradually recovering from the crisis. The Hong Kong government was also proactive in 2002, initiating the setting up of a HK$300 million Community Investment and Inclusion Fund. Its main goal was to "enable us to move forward during this difficult time and work toward building a strong, caring and harmonious community" (Hong Kong Government 2002b: 2). Wong (2006) states that the Fund has been successful in encouraging more social welfare organizations to "formulate the sustainability plan for bringing longer and continued impact on both individual and community levels with social capital" (p. 87). However, Kwok (2004) argues that social workers need to critically reflect their own power relations and work practices with the marginalized groups in Hong Kong in order to "become effective social capital builders" (p. 23). Thus far, there are not many studies focusing on the impact of the Fund on Chinese migrants in Hong Kong. The Fund might be useful in helping the migrant children rebuild their bond, as well as bridge social capital (Wong 2009). It might also be useful in developing the social resilience of the migrant community in facing another crisis in the near future.

References

Bhutta, Z., Bawany, F., Feroze, A., & Rizvi, A. (2009). *The impact of the food and economic crisis on child health and nutrition*. Draft working paper for UNICEF Conference East Asia and the Pacific Islands, 6–7 January, Singapore.

Boys' and Girls' Clubs Association of Hong Kong. (1999). *Coping strategies of poor Mainland Chinese children in Hong Kong*. Hong Kong [in Chinese].

Brewer, J. (2000). *Ethnography*. Buckingham: Open University Press.

Cleaver, F. (2005). The inequality of social capital and the reproduction of chronic poverty. *World Development, 33*(6), 893–906.

Coleman, J. (1988). Social capital in the creation of human capital. *American Journal of Sociology, 94*, S95–S120.

Felicio, A., Couto, E., & Caiado, J. (2009). Interrelationshipsbetweenhumancapitalandsocialcapital insmallandmediumsizedfirms:Theeffectofageandsectorofactivity (CEMAPRE Working Papers). Lisbon: Centre for Applied Mathematics and Economics, Portugal.

Fung, K. K., & Hung, X. L. (1999). Re-examining the Working Female New Arrivals. In The Hong Kong Council of Social Services (Ed.), *Convention and innovation: Community development in the 21st century* (pp. 53–72). Hong Kong [in Chinese].

Goldin, G., & Katz, L. (1999). Human capital and social capital: The rise of secondary schooling in America, 1910–1940. *Journal of Interdisciplinary History, 29*, 683–723.

Home Affairs Branch. (1997). *Equal opportunity: A study of discrimination on the ground of race. A consultation paper*. Hong Kong: Hong Kong Government.

Hong Kong Catholic Commission for Labour Affairs. (1999). *Co-operation and mutual understanding: A report on the newly arrived Chinese migrant "problems"*. Hong Kong [in Chinese].

Hong Kong Government. (2002a). *Surveys on new arrivals from the mainland*. Hong Kong: Home Affairs Department.

Hong Kong Government. (2002b). *Community investment and inclusion fund. Application guide and form*. Hong Kong SAR Government.

Hong Kong Psychological Society. (1999). *Study on attitudes towards newly-arrived Chinese migrants in Hong Kong*. Hong Kong: HKPS [in Chinese].

Knowles, J., Pernia, E., & Racelis, M. (1999). *Social consequences of the financial crisis in Asia* (Economic Staff Paper 60). Manila: ADB.

Kuah, K. E. (1999). The split-family phenomenon: A new immigrant family structure. In G. Wang & J. Wong (Eds.), *Hong Kong in China: The challenges of transition* (pp. 203–230). Singapore: Time Academic Press.

Kwok, J. (2004). Social welfare, social capital and social work: Personal reflection of a Hong Kong social worker. *Journal of Social Policy and Social Work, 8*, 23–32.

Lui, T. L., & Wong, H. (1995). *Disempowerment and empowerment – An exploratory study of low-income households in Hong Kong*. Hong Kong: Oxford University Press.

Ng, C., & Liu, C. (1999). Teaching English to Chinese immigrants in Hong Kong secondary schools. *Language, Culture and Curriculum, 12*, 229–237.

OECD. (1998). *The well-being of nations. The role of human and social capital*. Paris: Centre for Educational Research and Innovation.

Putnam, R. (2000). *Bowling alone: The collapse and revival of American community*. London: Simon and Schuster.

Schuller, T. (2001). The complementary roles of human and social capital. *ISUMA, 2*(1), 18–24.

Schuller, T., & Field, J. (1998). Social capital, human capital and the learning society. *International Journal of Lifelong Education, 17*(4), 226–235.

Weisbrot, M. (2007). *Ten years after: The lasting impact of the Asian Financial Crisis*. Washington, DC: Center for Economic and Policy Research.

Wong, C. K. (2006). *The role of the community investment and inclusion fund (CIIF) in building social capital in Hong Kong*. Unpublished M.A. dissertation of Public Administration. Hong Kong: University of Hong Kong.

Wong, S. (2007). *Exploring unseen social capital in community development*. Amsterdam: Amsterdam University Press.
Wong, F. K. (2008). Differential impacts of stressful life events and social support on the mental health of Mainland Chinese immigrants and local youth in Hong Kong: A resilience perspective. *British Journal of Social Work, 38*(2), 236–252.
Wong, S. (2009). Is identity clash inevitable? Identity and network building amongst Mainland Chinese migrants in Hong Kong. In E. Kolig, V. Angeles, & S. Wong (Eds.), *Identity in crossroad civilizations: Ethnicity, nationalism and globalism in Asia* (pp. 85–96). Amsterdam: Amsterdam University Press.
World Bank. (1990). *World Bank world development report 1990: Attacking poverty*. Washington, DC: World Bank.
World Bank. (2000). *World Bank world development report 2000/2001: Attacking poverty*. Washington, DC: World Bank.

Part V
Economic Stress and Public Policy

Chapter 12
Conditional Cash Transfers (CCTs): A Child Policy Strategy in Asia

Shirley Gatenio Gabel and Sheila B. Kamerman

Conditional Cash Transfers (CCTs): A Child Policy Strategy in Asia

More than one billion children – or more than half the children in the world – are deprived of at least one of their basic human needs, and 30 % (650 million) are deprived of two or more severe basic needs (Gordon et al. 2003). Children suffering from one or more forms of severe deprivation of basic human need are defined as severely deprived. Two regions, South Asia and sub-Saharan Africa, have severe deprivation rates of over 80 % (Gordon et al. 2003). About half the poor in developing countries (with incomes less than $1.25USD a day) are children, and poor children constitute 40 % of the children in developing countries.

Children deprived of their basic needs experience severely limited opportunities to develop in a way that lets them reach their full potential as adults. Limiting human well-being is a violation of children's rights. Having a large proportion of a population growing up in poverty is a major constraint on human capital development and often exposes children to hazardous and exploitative conditions that may lead to physical and mental damage. Children who are deprived of their basic needs often find themselves taking on adult roles while they are children themselves, such as the orphans and street children who frequently have to fend not only for themselves but for the welfare of younger siblings. We know too that

S. Gatenio Gabel (✉)
Graduate School of Social Service, Fordham University, NY, USA
e-mail: gateniogabe@fordham.edu

S.B. Kamerman
School of Social Work, Columbia University, NY, USA
e-mail: sbk2@columbia.edu

W.J.J. Yeung and M.T. Yap (eds.), *Economic Stress, Human Capital, and Families in Asia: Research and Policy Challenges*, Quality of Life in Asia 4,
DOI 10.1007/978-94-007-7386-8_12, © Springer Science+Business Media Dordrecht 2013

children with little or no education are more likely to live in poverty as adults because their prospects for escaping poverty are slim and are much more unlikely to be able to provide their own children with adequate opportunities to reach their full potential.

As is well established by now, cash income transfer policies are a key to reducing child poverty in the European Union (EU) and Organization of Economic Cooperation and Development (OECD) countries and enhancing the economic situation of children and their families (Kamerman et al. 2003; Vleminckx and Smeeding 2001). There is growing evidence as well that cash transfers are an effective strategy for reducing child poverty in developing countries (Barrientos and De Jong 2006). Thus, cash benefits are instrumental in promoting the well-being of children. *No one factor alone may be key to eliminating child poverty; and reducing deprivation requires more than cash benefits.* Nonetheless, the evidence is clear that income transfers play an essential role in child well-being (Fiszbein and Schady 2009; Kamerman et al. 2003).

Frustrated by the persistence of poverty in the region, Latin America became a laboratory for economic and social policy experiments aimed at eliminating or reducing poverty since the mid-1970s (Saracostti 2008). A new income transfer, conditional cash transfers (CCTs) initiated in Latin America and in Bangladesh in the late 1990s, has expanded exponentially and globally since then. Today, conditional cash transfers are being used as an incentive in both developing and industrialized countries to reduce poverty, enhance child health and nutrition, and improve students' performance in schools. Its application to South and Southeast Asian countries is being seriously tested. At a meeting in Manila in July 2009, the vice-president of the Asian Development Bank urged Asian-Pacific governments to consider the use of CCTs to help vulnerable families affected by the 2008 global financial crisis, but several Asian countries had already taken note of CCTs following the 1997 Asian financial crisis.

The purpose of this paper is to explore the use of CCTs as a policy tool in several Asian countries. The political and economic conditions that ushered in CCTs in Latin America are compared to those in Asia. The effectiveness of CCTs in Asia has received less attention than in Latin American countries. To date the evaluations of CCTs in Asia are generally positive, but more research is needed on which conditions lead the CCTs to achieve their goals of reducing child poverty, increasing school enrollment, and improving health and nutrition. Higher levels of school attainment, better childhood health, and not living in deprived conditions during childhood are all conditions that are linked with improved levels of well-being both during childhood and adulthood. We discuss the effectiveness of CCTs in modifying individual behavior in these countries, provide highlights of the CCT programs in several countries, compare the effectiveness of CCTs to other types of income benefits such as unconditioned cash transfers, and conclude with lessons learned.

Overview of Conditional Cash Transfers

To date, over 30 countries have implemented about 40 conditional cash transfer programs, some of which are pilot programs (see Table 12.1). Although the majority are in Latin America and the Caribbean, CCTs have also spread to several countries in Africa and to Southeast and East Asia. CCTs are seen as going beyond traditional social assistance policies because they seek not only to reduce income poverty but also to create incentives for behavioral change and to increase investment in human capital. In particular, we will explore the effectiveness of the experience in the Southeast and East Asian countries.

Table 12.1 Countries with conditional cash transfer programs, 2011

Africa	**Latin America and Caribbean**
Burkina Faso: conditional cash transfers for poor families	*Argentina*: Plan Familias
Kenya: Cash Transfer Program for Orphans and Vulnerable Children	*Brazil*: Bolsa Familia
Malawi: Malawi Social Action Fund	*Chile*: Chile Solidario
Morocco: Tayssir Program	*Colombia*: Familias en Accion
South Africa: Conditional Cash Transfers to Support Vulnerable Children and Households in the Context of HIV/AIDS and Poverty	*Costa Rica*: Superemonos
Egypt: pilot program, Ain el-Sira in Cairo	*Dominican Republic*: Programa Solidaridad
Ghana: LEAP – Empowerment Against Poverty Social Grants Program	*Ecuador*: Bono de Desarrollo Humano/Programa de Protecccion Social
Nigeria: pilot program	*El Salvador*: Red Solidaria
Yemen: education conditional cash transfer	*Honduras*: Programa de Asignacion Familiar (PRAF)
Asia and Pacific	*Jamaica*: Program of Advancement through Health and Education (PATH)
Bangladesh: Income Generation for Vulnerable Group Development program. A focus on girls. Food for Education (later, Cash for Education). Female Secondary School Assistance	*Mexico*: Oportunidades
Cambodia: Cambodia Education Sector Support Program (CESSP)	*Nicaragua*: Red de Proteccion Social
India: several CCT program for families of girls in 5 areas, conditioned on school attendance, birth registration, immunizations, and others	*Paraguay*: Programa Tekopora
Indonesia: Program Keluarga Harapan (PKH), PNPM Generasi	*Peru*: Programa Nacional de Apoyo Directo a los Mas Pobres-Juntos
Mongolia: Child Money Program, a CCT supported mainly by the Asian Development Bank. A universal program	*Trinidad y Tobago*: Targeted Conditional Cash Transfer Program (TCCTP)
Pakistan: Bait-ul-Mal Child Support Program. A focus on girls	*Uruguay*: Ingreso Ciudadano
Philippines: the 4Ps, enhancing the role of parents	

CCTs are particularly attractive in countries with high levels of income inequality where the extreme poor are characterized by very low levels of income, consumption, human capital, and ties to formal employment (Kakawani et al. 2006). In Latin America, the appeal of CCTs had to do with its ability to address a key determinant of chronic poverty – low educational attainment (de Britto 2008). Unlike traditional social assistance, CCTs are not viewed as creating work disincentives, rather they are seen as investments in human capital and opportunities to increase citizenship (Saracostti 2008; Farrington and Slater 2006). This focus on beneficiaries and their roles and responsibilities in long-term investments in human capital acknowledges demand-side barriers to such investment including lack of information, the additional costs of access to health and education services, and the opportunity costs of schooling because of reliance on child labor (de Janvry and Sadoulet 2006; Handa and Davis 2006; Soares et al. 2006; Attanasio et al. 2005). According to Bastagali (2007), CCTs can be used to increase citizenship by including populations that would otherwise have been excluded from education and by providing a minimal income.

While the goals of CCTs may be laudable, CCTs have been criticized by some scholars as "redolent of the 'conditionalities' imposed by the IMF, World Bank and other donors when making loans or implementing budget support programs, a perpetuation of the mind-set that imposed 'structural-adjustment' and enforced poverty reduction strategies" earlier (Freeland 2007: 75). From this perspective, CCTs are contractual arrangements between beneficiaries and society that beneficiaries generally do not participate in formulating the contract, and as such, CCTs may be viewed as paternalistic. In the United States, using cash as incentives for student performance has been negatively characterized as bribery (Miller 2008).

Freeland (2007) and Hanlon et al. (2010), among others, argue that there are many times when conditionalities are not necessary and unconditional cash transfers would be as or more effective to achieve the human investment goals of CCTs. Numerous studies demonstrate that poor families want to send their children to school and to receive health-care services, but their limited incomes prevent them from doing so (Hanlon et al. 2010). Imposing conditions on what are human rights to adequate standards of living, education and health is exclusionary. Conditionalities suggest that certain populations are less deserving of their rights and that by modifying their behaviors through the use of conditionalities, they will become "deserving." The implication of conditionalities is that poor people, especially poor parents, are incapable of knowing what is in their and their children's best interest.

Although conditionalities are characteristic of all CCTs, experience suggests some programs are stricter than others in imposing the meeting of conditionalities on the receipt of cash benefits (Hanlon et al. 2010). For example, Mexico's *Progresa*, now *Opportunitades*, initially required voluntary labor that it later relaxed. In Brazil, families who fall short of meeting required conditions are given additional social support services.

Philosophically, the draw to imposing conditions on cash transfers to the poor is that it captures northern, especially US, notions of a social contract. The public and policy makers generally support conditioning social benefits on recipient behaviors. According to one conservative American scholar (Mead 1997), the public supports a social contract that requires welfare recipients to satisfy behavioral requirements, such as working or staying in school, as well as income rules in order to receive aid, because it stresses traditional values of work and personal responsibility. Fiszbein and Schady (2009) argue that globally the two broad justifications for attaching conditions to cash transfers are that it requires parent's investment in the human capital of their children where it is often low and that it is easier to garner public support for conditioned benefits because they are seen as helping those who are trying to improve their lots not just perpetuating handouts.

Elements of CCT Programs

There is considerable variation in the design, target groups, conditionalities, benefits, and administration of CCTS. The two conditionalities most often associated with CCTs are education and health care/nutrition. The education component is usually a cash grant targeted to school-aged children, sometimes specifically for groups who are least likely to attend school, such as girls in grades 4–9 in Yemen and girls who have dropped out of school in Pakistan. In some countries, conditionality extends to adolescents' participation in secondary education. Students are often required to attend school 80–85 % of school days to be eligible for the cash grant, which is usually paid to the mother. The grant may cover direct educational costs (school fees and supplies, transportation) as well as the opportunity costs of the income a child would have earned if they were working rather than attending school.

The health and nutrition component is a cash grant most often targeted to preschool-age children and pregnant or lactating women. Women may be required to attend health-care centers during pregnancy and thereafter, and children may be required to obtain vaccinations and regular health checkups. The cash grants received may cover the cost of food to bring a family out of extreme poverty, reduce consumption costs of improving a family's diet, or reduce the opportunity costs of travel and waiting times for parents to health-care centers.

All CCT programs are means-tested[1] and categorical. They may target specific households or geographic locations, and some focus on population subgroups. Targeting is generally used to reach the poorest of the poor (Coady et al. 2004). In some countries, CCT programs are gender-targeted to address intra-household disparities in human capital investments. For example, in Pakistan, India, and Bangladesh, girls receive school stipends to increase female enrollment in public schools (Chaudhury and Parajuli 2006). And in many countries, the grants are targeted on mothers as a strategy for ensuring that children benefit.

---

[1]Means-tested programs are those that consider income and assets in establishing eligibility. They are most often targeted to the poor and sometimes known as social assistance cash benefits.

Effectiveness

The rapid popularity of CCTs is making them a central policy instrument for fighting poverty and enhancing child well-being. On the economic side, research has shown that the elasticity of poverty to growth is much lower in countries with higher inequality. Growth is seen as necessary but insufficient by itself to reduce poverty; redistribution also plays an important role (Perry et al. 2006; Soares et al. 2006). On the social side, these longer-term investments in health and education are expected to contribute to breaking intergenerational poverty by helping today's children become productive members and full citizens of society tomorrow (Skoufias and Parker 2001). Another study suggests that CCTs can go beyond benefiting recipients. Angelucci and De Giorgi (2009) used the unique design of the experimental data for the evaluation of Mexico's *Progresa* to show that food consumption in villages where *Progresa* was implemented increased by over 10 % for non-beneficiary households, about half the size of the increase in food consumption for eligible households. The increased income of beneficiary households fueled higher consumption in the community by increasing loans and transfers from family and friends and reducing savings. These results show how positive program benefits can extend beyond an eligible group to benefit a community.

A growing body of evidence now exists on the effects of CCTs on meeting policy and program objectives. In general, CCTs have been successful in meeting the basic consumption needs of beneficiaries by increasing total and food expenditures, decreasing malnutrition and its effects on young children, raising educational levels and lowering dropout rates, and reducing child labor. Evaluations of CCT programs show that household consumption for CCT beneficiaries increased and stunting of children under age 6 decreased (Attanasio et al. 2005; Skoufias 2005; Hoddinott and Skoufias 2005; Maluccio and Flores 2004).

Several research studies have reported an increase in the use of health services, greater for disadvantaged children and generally for 1–5 year olds compared to infants (Gertler 2000; Maluccio and Flores 2004). Studies report mixed effects of CCTs on immunization coverage and mixed effects on other health outcomes such as anemia and childhood illness (Lagarde et al. 2007). The literature indicates that while CCTs increase the use of health services, their overall effect on health status is less clear than the increased demand generated by CCTs (Lagarde et al. 2007).

With regard to education objectives, primary school attendance and student learning were mixed. CCTs had the largest effects on older, preschool children who were the most delayed along various dimensions, including language acquisition, memory, and social skills, and for whom the delays were related to household consumption levels. Favorable education outcomes were drawn mostly from the experience of Mexico's *Progresa* (now *Opportunitades*) indicating that there was a significant increase in the enrollment of boys and girls, particularly the latter. The program also increased enrollment in secondary schools by 6 and 9 percentage points for boys and girls, respectively. For girls, who often dropped out before secondary school, the transition rate to secondary school rose by 15 percentage points.

The impact of CCT programs on enrollment rates is greater in countries where preprogram enrollment rates are extremely low. In countries such as Colombia, Mexico, and Turkey, CCT programs hardly increased enrollment rates at the primary level because these countries already had high primary enrollment rates before the program. In countries where school enrollment rates were above 90 %, CCTs had little, if any, effect. Relatively little impact was demonstrated on school attendance rate, on school achievement, or in attracting dropouts to schools. CCTs showed greater effects in countries where school enrollment rates were between 60 and 80 % (Attanasio et al. 2005; Skoufias 2005; Maluccio and Flores 2004). CCT programs in Bangladesh and Nicaragua significantly raised primary school enrollment by 9 and 13 percentage points, respectively. In these cases, the programs were particularly effective because both countries had a large proportion of children who were not enrolled in primary school.

The effects of CCTs on child labor have been assessed positively in Bangladesh where child labor rates decreased by 4–14 % (Patrinos 2007). In Cambodia, the CESSP program, which gives transfers to children in transition from primary to lower-secondary school, was found to reduce child labor by 11 percentage points (Fiszbein and Schady 2009). Others note that CCTs may not reduce child labor but may affect the frequency, duration (hours per day), and work conditions (hazardous) or child being sent away for work (Barrera-Osario et al. 2008; Attanasio et al. 2005; Glewwe and Olinto 2004).

CCTs have been found to be efficient in reaching the poorest of the poor and are believed to be more efficient than unconditional cash transfers in changing parental decisions regarding school, labor, and health; but this efficiency may not fully recognize the costs of implementing targeted programs in many areas (de Janvry and Sadoulet 2006). In addition to the demand-side effects of cash transfers, supply-side improvements may also account for some of the positive health and education effects. There is little direct evidence supporting whether the demand-side interventions were more effective than the supply-side interventions.

Conditionality

A key question is whether conditionality is needed to achieve observable improvements in school attendance and health, especially in areas where the social infrastructure is only just being developed. The issue is complicated because it not only reflects child outcomes (e.g., improvement in health and education indicators) but also considers the effectiveness of programs to redirect behavior, household and individual goals, and societal capacity to implement change. Among advanced industrialized countries, the evidence is inconclusive with regard to the value of conditionality. For example, Europe makes far less use of conditionality and has far higher indicators of child well-being. A UNICEF Innocenti Report Card comprehensively assessing the lives and well-being of children and young people in 21 industrialized nations on six dimensions – material well-being, health and safety, education, peer and family relationships, behaviors and risks, and young people's own subjective sense of well-being – found that European countries dominate the top half of the overall table, with Northern European countries claiming the top four rankings (2007). The European countries, particularly the Northern European countries, are most likely to provide universal, unconditional cash benefits to children and their families (Gatenio and Kamerman 2006). The countries that traditionally have been more likely to offer assistance in the form of means-tested cash benefits sometimes linked to a conditionality, the United States and the United Kingdom, scored the lowest on the UNICEF Innocenti Report Card (2007).

There is a long history of imposing conditionalities on the poor in the United States particularly for poor families with children. Despite the generally positive outcomes attributed to welfare reform in the United States, when the effects of behavior-conditioned initiatives are studied separately, the outcomes are less positive (Gatenio and Kamerman 2009). The effects of conditionality in the United States suggest no or limited impact on behavior: no success in reducing nonmarital births, no positive impact from efforts at promoting marriage, minimal increases in school attendance, and some positive impact from workfare. Behavioral changes were more often achieved by positive reinforcements. Thus far, researchers have been reticent to attribute causality because of the difficulty in disentangling the effects of the policy and the effects of a strong economy and relative ease of obtaining employment at the time of the studies. Furthermore, no one policy alone appears able to modify behavior although the cumulative impacts of multiple interventions can make a difference.

Can these evaluations be translated to the developing world? Are the limited effects of conditionalities consistent or in contrast to research findings on conditionality imposed on benefits in developing countries? It is only recently that researchers have explored contrasting the value of conditioned vs. unconditioned transfers. As Schubert and Slater have noted, banks are "spending millions of dollars on administering conditionality without ever having analyzed how much the conditions contribute to the impact of the social cash transfer programmes and whether this contributions is worth the costs involved" (2006).

Untangling the effects of conditionality is challenging. Schady, a proponent of CCTs, among others, undertook several studies in Latin American countries to capture conditionality effects – none of which yielded robust evidence.[2] In reviewing this research, Hanlon et al. (2010) have argued that the positive results reported may be due to mediating factors such as mothers who have higher educational levels in the benefit group, increased benefit levels as girls go onto secondary education levels, or rewarding accomplishments rather than behavioral change.

The largest unconditional cash transfer program among developing countries is South Africa's Child Support Grant (CSG). The program was introduced to address the social exclusion and growing poverty and inequalities experienced, and

[2]See Paxson and Schady (2007) and Schady and Araujo (2008).

benefits were initially available to children from birth to their seventh birthday and then extended in three phases to include children up to their fourteenth birthday. The CSG has increased student enrollment and attendance and increased household consumption (Lund et al. 2008). And while the CSG does not condition benefits, Lund et al. (2008) observe that over time some formal conditionalities have been incorporated (e.g., birth registration) and how some administrative requirements have become de facto conditionalities. Like CCTs, CSG links to health- and nutrition-related programs but stops short of officially requiring these linkages due to supply-side constraints. Conditionality is administratively complex and requires adequate quantity and quality of services. This raises the question whether conditionality should be implemented where access (either due to supply shortfalls or exclusionary practices) is an obstacle to participation and how to guard against conditionalities creating further disadvantages among those who may be in most need.

Other researchers have looked at how imposing conditionalities affects women since women often bear the burden of seeking assistance, attending meetings as required, and ensuring compliance. A quantitative and qualitative assessment of the effect of *Progresa* on women's status and intra-household relations found that the program increased women's empowerment but that it also placed extra demands on women's time (Adato et al. 2000). On the other hand, Molyneux (2006) found that Progresa placed additional burdens on women's already scarce time without offering them further remuneration.

Factors Influencing the Launching of CCTs

The Latin American debt crisis of the 1980s left long-term political and economic effects on countries, especially those that had been hit the hardest, notably Brazil, Argentina, and Mexico. The severe economic crisis in the region contributed to the collapse of authoritarian regimes and the rethinking about poverty and the role of government. By the late 1990s, the economic situation was nowhere as devastating as it had been in the 1980s, yet limited economic recoveries followed by downturns were characteristic of the 1990s throughout Latin America.

Popular opinion in the postcrisis period was that poverty was caused by societal injustice and that government needed to help provide opportunities for people to escape poverty. Policy debates during this period focused on how the state could fulfill its obligations and at the same time what policy instruments could tackle the causes of poverty. Education was seen as crucial for breaking the intergenerational cycle of poverty, but mere enrollment was not sufficient: poor students also needed support to maintain a minimum level of attendance.

From this, the concept of conditional cash transfers (CCTs) was born and promulgated by the then Brazilian President Fernando Henrique Cardoso into a national program. Facing similar challenges and struggling to hold onto his presidency in a time of political and economic turmoil, Mexico's President Ernesto Zedillo led the implementations of conditional cash transfers in Mexico. Interestingly, it was subsequent administrations in both Brazil and Mexico that expanded CCTs and used CCTs to garner political support. In both countries, CCTs were important in stabilizing popular support for incoming governments in the aftermath of fallen authoritarian regimes and economic crises. Political leaders in both countries played on growing public understanding of the causes of poverty to be multidimensional and for solutions necessitating co-responsibility and cross-sectoral approaches (de Britto 2008).

The financial crisis that swept through South East Asia between June 1997 and January 1998 was a shock to previously prospering countries. In the decades leading up to the crisis, the "tiger economies" of Thailand, Malaysia, Singapore, Indonesia, Hong Kong, and South Korea had economies whose GDP was growing by 6–9 % each year. This Asian miracle, however, came to an abrupt end in the late 1997 when in one country after another, local stock markets and currency markets imploded, their currencies rapidly depreciated, and country economies were threatened by bankruptcy. Although there were and remain important differences between the individual countries, a number of elements were common to most. A combination of inexpensive and relatively well-educated labor, export-oriented economies, falling barriers to international trade, and heavy foreign investment left the domestic economies exposed to external factors with little in the way of social protection measures to provide cushioning and smooth consumption during periods of crises.

Triggered by economic crises, countries in both Latin America and Southeast Asia were challenged to find new ways to rapidly respond to widespread poverty and its consequences. In both regions, a reconceptualization of poverty, its causes, and responsibilities of the state and individual took place before new policy responses took place. Although CCTs were implemented in a relatively short period in Latin America in the late 1990s, public debates on poverty and co-responsibility had begun following the economic crises in the 1980s. At first, immediate cash and in-kind transfers were made available that showed signs of failing, and in response, systemic approaches to chronic and intergenerational poverty were conceived and implemented. The pattern is similar in Southeast Asia. The financial crises of 1997–1998 caused a rethinking of the relationship between the state and individuals. Initially, widespread cash and in-kind transfers were introduced to respond to the immediate suffering such as in Indonesia, but by the mid- 2000s, longer-term and comprehensive solutions were sought as strategies for improving living standards and breaking intergenerational poverty.

The situation in other parts of Asia differed. Reliance on family-based social protection was typical throughout the region. In the more developed countries of Korea, Taiwan, Malaysia, Thailand, and Singapore, social risk was somewhat mitigated by access to health and education institutions, higher school enrollment rates, higher proportions of formal labor, and their coverage by social insurance schemes. The 1997 crisis was a call to expand social insurance in several of these countries, such as Thailand's subsequent introduction of a universal health-care scheme and Korea's Minimum Living Standards Guarantee Scheme.

In South Asia, long colonial histories had previously introduced programs of conditioned transfers such as food for work and other social assistance programs for the poor. Added to this was a myriad of different kinds of programs that relatively new independent governments and international NGOs introduced. Social assistance was also used to garner political support, and new social programs were often promised and added to expand political allegiance. The result is a patchwork of different approaches and programs to address poverty. The challenge in this region is to improve administrative capacity and to develop evaluative measures to improve the effectiveness of efforts.

The Experience in Asia

Nearly half of Asia's 1.27 billion children live in poverty – deprived of food, safe drinking water, health care, adequate income, or shelter. Almost half of these lack access to a basic human need, and in South Asia, over 80 % of children lack access to a basic need (Gordon et al. 2003).

In the last decade, evidence that CCTS can be an effective policy strategy to address children's basic needs has grown. CCTs are a means of addressing the low educational achievement in the region, especially of secondary school children in rural areas (sharp increase in dropout rates between elementary and secondary school is a major issue); high maternal and infant mortality rates; and high malnutrition rates, particularly in rural areas.

Increasingly, CCTS are viewed as a means of meeting immediate basic needs and simultaneously as an investment in human capital and economic development because of the contingencies placed on social assistance.

A World Bank report (Fiszbein and Schady 2009) describes the experiences of six Asian countries having at least one CCT, Cambodia, Indonesia, Philippines in East Asia and Bangladesh, India, and Pakistan in South Asia. We briefly highlight these below and include Mongolia as well.

Bangladesh. In Bangladesh, children account for about 45 % of the total population that approaches 150 million. Almost half of all children in Bangladesh live below the national poverty line with one-quarter living in extreme poverty. About half of the child population are poor children deprived of basic social needs – shelter, food, heath, education, water, sanitation, and information – and currently live below the international poverty threshold of US $1.25 per person per day (UNICEF Bangladesh 2010). And almost two-thirds of children aged 3–17 are deprived of sanitation, one-third are deprived of food, 16 % health care, and 8 % education. The extent of child poverty, deprivation, undernutrition, and vulnerability is directly connected to the presence of child labor and the level of their parents' education. "Social polarization, increasing food prices, income inequality, rapid urbanization, lack of land ownership, and the devastating effects of natural disasters ... all contribute to the high levels of poverty" (IRIN Asia Humanitarian News and Analysis December 28, 2009).

Primary net education enrollment rates increased over the course of the last 20 years, and although coverage is still not universal, the gender gap in enrollment has all but disappeared. The primary school completion rate (i.e., the proportion of pupils starting grade one that reach grade five) rose from 43 to 55 % over the same time period but remains far below the MDG target of 100 % completion, and repetition rates also remain high (39 %), resulting in an average of 6.6 years needed to complete a 5-year primary education cycle. CCTs have contributed to improved educational levels and the closing of the gender gap in education in Bangladesh and are being expanded.

Bangladesh embarked on a program of macroeconomic stabilization during the early to mid-1980s along the conditionality arrangements of the IMF and the World Bank. These reforms took priority in the 1990s and were primarily aimed at reducing agricultural and food subsidies. The government was also directed to implement cost-effective, safety nets for the poor to reduce poverty. The floods of 1998, which were the most devastating floods suffered in the region, reinforced already ongoing efforts to prevent the anticipated famine, disease, and suffering. As a result of these factors, government spending priorities shifted in Bangladesh in the 1980s and 1990s with a substantially greater proportion of public expenditures that continue to go toward social welfare, education, and health. Social assistance was further developed after the end of military authoritarian regimes in Bangladesh in the 1990s, yet these efforts were scattered and not well targeted.

Bangladesh actually has a history of conditional transfer programs preceding the current popularity of CCTs. One of its oldest is the Food for Work (FFW) program. It was introduced in 1974 in response to the famine in Bangladesh. During the lean season, beneficiaries are employed in the construction and maintenance of rural infrastructure (repair of roads and digging and re-excavation of small irrigation channels) in return for food. An offshoot of the FFW program is the Rural Infrastructure Maintenance-Test Relief (TR) program. The TR program sought to aid the development of educational and benevolent organizations and aid the unemployed, rural poor during the monsoon season by undertaking smaller-scale projects such as the maintenance of embankments and roads; the development/maintenance of schools, colleges, madrasas, mosques, orphanages, and public places; tree plantings; and the construction of bridges. Another employment-related conditioned transfer is the Vulnerable Group Development (VGD) program originated as part of the Vulnerable Group Feeding (VGF) program of 1975. In 1986 VGD became a separate food aid-supported development program targeted to very poor rural women who receive food in return for participating in training and work efforts. Many of these women are at risk of social exclusion due to family circumstances. An outgrowth of the VGD program is the Vulnerable Group Development for Ultra-Poor (VGD-UP) project that seeks to expand the income-generating opportunities of vulnerable poor women who are landless and have no active male members in the household. Beneficiaries selected for participation in the 2-year cycle receive cash of which one-eighth is set aside for savings. Each beneficiary receives training in at least two fields of income-generating activities (e.g., trade, tailoring, food catering and processing, livestock production, home gardening, tree nurseries). At the end of the first year, a microcredit is provided to each beneficiary in order to acquire a productive asset. One of the largest and most recent CCT programs in Bangladesh is the Employment Generation Program for the Hardcore Poor. It was developed in 2008 that trains and employs poor persons suing public works during periods of seasonal poverty.

Since the 1990s, Bangladesh has used education conditioned transfers to increase school attendance among children with historically low levels of education. One of the earliest public initiatives began in 1993. The Primary Education Stipend Project (PESP) initially provided food supplements to primary school age children who enrolled in school. In 2002 cash transfers replaced food transfers. Students must attend school at least 85 % of the time and meet minimum grade requirements for school. Another education transfer program is the well-known Female Secondary School Stipend Project (FSSP) in Bangladesh. It was first piloted in 1982 and later established nationwide in 1994 to increase the enrollment and retention of girls in secondary schools to increase female education and delay marriage and childbearing. It pays tuition fees and provides monthly stipends for unmarried rural girls up to class 10 who attend recognized institutions, remain unmarried, maintain at least 75 % attendance, and secure at least 45 % marks in the annual examinations (a pass requires 35 %). FSSP follows previous stipend projects. In 2010, the program was changed to target 30 % of females and 10 % of males in each class based on merit and household status rather than covering all secondary female students, the program targets. Class attendance and minimum examination score criteria have been relaxed to increase inclusion among poor students. The stipend program increased female student enrollment by 2 % above the prevailing trend rate of increase while having no increase in male enrollment. Thus the program closed the gender gap in education by accelerating the trend that had already existed in Bangladesh before the stipend program was introduced in 1994 (Son 2008).

In 2007, the Government of Bangladesh introduced a stipend to increase the enrollment and retention of students with disabilities, particularly those who are from less developed areas in the country known as the Stipend for Students with Disabilities. The stipend is conditional on 50 % school attendance.

India. With a population of more than one billion, about one-third poor (with incomes under $1USD a day) and 80 % with incomes under $2USD a day, income poverty is a major problem. In addition, less than half the female population is literate or two-thirds of the youth population; thus, illiteracy is another major problem. Malnutrition is still another problem, especially in rural areas, as is child labor in urban areas.

In a meeting in New Delhi exploring the relevance of CCTs for India held in December 2009, CCTs were described as part of national development strategies, designed especially to soften the impact of the financial crisis on the urban poor, in addition to its already existing problems. In most Asian countries, there is little in the way of social safety nets – social protection policies – but India does have several social assistance programs. Several of India's social protection schemes such as maternity benefits and the survival and education of the girl child are similar to CCT programs.

The Indian government is currently studying the implications of establishing a CCT to address the countries' nutritional problems. In 2008 India did establish a CCT for girls (Dhanalakshmi or the Conditional Cash Transfer Scheme for the Girl Child) in 11 educationally backward areas across Andhra Pradesh, Uttar Pradesh, Bihar, Orissa, Jharkhand, Chhattisgarh, and Punjab. Cash transfers are provided to families with girls with certain conditions for them to qualify, including birth registration, a full series of immunizations, enrollment, and attendance at school, deferring age of marriage to 18. Several state governments have launched variations of CCT programs, also focused on girls and reducing malnutrition.

A CCT-type approach is also used in the recently revised maternity benefit scheme, Janani Suraksha Yojana, that aims to reduce maternal and neonatal mortality and prevent female infanticide by providing cash rewards for institutional deliveries. The CCT approach was first introduced in 1997 to encourage the development and education of girls. The Balika Samridhi Yojana provides for periodic cash transfers to the girl child at various stages of her life beginning with birth when a postdelivery grant is given to the mother for a surviving girl child. This is followed with annual scholarships at various stages of their education. The scholarship is available to the girl child as long as she is unmarried and attends school regularly.

In 2003, another scheme, the National Programme for Education of Girls at Elementary Level under the Sarva Shiksha Abhiyan (SSA), was introduced for out-of-school girls who are overage but not have completed elementary schooling, working girls, girls from marginalized social groups, and those with low attendance and low achievement levels. The scheme provides direct incentives like free books, uniforms, stationery, and a small cash transfer.

In addition, another scheme, the Kasturba Gandhi Balika Vidyalaya scheme, was merged into the SSA in 2007, to lower the dropout rate of girls in secondary education and ensuring their retention up to age of 18. This builds upon other cash transfer programs by providing a onetime cash transfer deposited in the name of the girl child once the girl child is enrolled in class nine and is not married.

In addition to these national CCT programs, there are numerous state-sponsored programs that go beyond enrollment to include other goals, such as income poverty reduction, increased participation in health checkups, and vaccinations, and all these targeted largely on women and children, especially girl children, and reduction of child labor and increased attendance at school.

The effectiveness of the above described schemes is currently being evaluated. Early results suggest that CCTs are an effective strategy for replacing food aid programs, closing gender gaps in education, and improving child nutrition in India but that targeting and administrative capacity need to be further developed to increase effectiveness (Mehrotra 2010).

Pakistan. Over one-third of all households are classified as poor in Pakistan, and nearly two-thirds are considered vulnerable due to health, illness or disability, or external factors such as natural disasters or the economy (World Bank 2007). Traditionally, Pakistan's social protection system included several social assistance programs (Bait-ul Maal and Zakat) of limited coverage. The poor live mainly in rural areas, are unskilled, and work in the informal sector. Employment opportunities are scarce and real earnings have declined in the last decade. The poor also lack in all of the basic human, physical, and productive assets and have limited or no access to essential social services.

Literacy for girls is a key issue in Pakistan too, and CCTs are viewed as a means of increasing educational levels among girls. Only 57 % of girls and women can read and write. Only 22 % of girls in rural areas have completed primary school as compared with 47 % of boys. CCTs are viewed as a strategy for addressing this literacy and gender equity problem.

In Pakistan's culture, girls can't walk to school or take public transportation, and private transportation is expensive. Families receive a cash benefit if their daughters attend school regularly. The CCT cash benefit offsets these costs and makes attendance at school viable. The CCT program called the Child Support Program is linked to the food support program as well, thus increasing the nutritional intake of children who go to school.

Since 2003, girls' enrollment in secondary school in this area increased by 60 %. The number of 10–14-year-old girls in school increased by 11 percentage points, thus also helping to reduce the gender literacy gap. The impact evaluation of the pilot programs are scheduled to be completed in 2010. Anticipating positive evaluations, there are plans to phase-in the program countrywide and to link it to other existing social protection programs.

Despite its limited resources, Pakistan has increased its spending on social protection. CCTs are an important component of the strategy because CCTs provide incentives for children, especially girls, to stay in school longer even during economic downturns and to forego seeking employment. These human capital investments have long-term consequences but do not address all the obstacles to human development in the country. For example, it is estimated that 35,000 girls drop out of high school in Pakistan each year due to corporal punishment by their teachers. While governments have banned the practice of corporal punishment in schools, implementation is ignored. In 2009, many families in the Swat Valley exhausted their savings fleeing fighting in the area. When they reached Lahore, their children needed to work to help provide income for the survival of their family (Mapp 2011).

Cambodia. Despite significant declines in poverty and deprivation over the last decade, more than one-third of Cambodians live below the poverty line, and poverty is especially pervasive in rural areas and among children, who constitute more than half of the country's population (UNICEF). Cambodia has high infant and under-5 mortality rates and high maternal mortality rates. Malnutrition affects most children and primary school enrollment rates are high, with a declining gender gap. Inequality is growing in the country.

Children are involved in economic activity in Cambodia at very young ages, and economic activity increases sharply with age (Filmer and Schady 2009). About 16 % of children are already economically active at age 6 years, and over half of all children are economically active by the age of 10 years. By the age of 15, the share of children working surpasses that of children attending school. Late school enrollment and early school dropouts are a serious concern in Cambodia.

A food for education program was phased in across 6 provinces between 1999 and 2003 in three different forms: (1) in-school breakfast, (2) in-school breakfast together with take-home ration provided to families of girls in grades 4–6, and (3) the "full package" consisting of in-school breakfast, take-home rations, and deworming medicine to all participating schools. Children were found to stay in school longer where onsite feeding was offered. School enrollment increased generally after the first year of treatment, but the effect waned over several years. This may point to reached supply constraints (such as overcrowding in schools and the resulting deteriorated quality of education).

Another two pilot programs are targeted on girls who have completed sixth grade and are designed to reduce the dropout rate between sixth and seventh grades. They have been successful in achieving their goals, reducing the dropout rate by about 20–30%age points. The average child receiving the cash benefit was 10 percent less likely to work for pay, while adults in recipient households did not reduce their work effort. CCTs reduced the income poverty rate, increased school enrollment, and increased the use of health care. However, it did not necessarily lead to better health and education outcomes, and only a very small proportion of the population was involved. The project's evaluation, which ran over two school years, showed that scholarships worked as a way of getting children to stay in school, but it also found that children who were offered scholarships did not do measurably better on vocabulary or math tests than peers who were not offered scholarships – despite the fact that the former group had higher enrollments and attendance (Filmer and Schady 2009).

Indonesia. Indonesia is an example of how the Asian financial crisis of 1997 triggered political and economic reforms with a new emphasis on social protection programs. To respond quickly to the financial crisis, the Government of Indonesia introduced fuel subsidies, in-kind transfers, and some cash transfers. As the country stabilized economically and politically, the government was interested in implementing programs that would address the root causes of poverty and secure the economic and political future of the country. Indonesia has been phasing out its politically popular fuel subsidies over a number of years and limiting its rice for the poor program, while replacing these programs with community and human investment programs. There is a strong emphasis on community participation and development in Indonesia's antipoverty strategy. Poverty is increasingly understood to be multidimensional and a responsibility of the state, community, and individual.

According to a report issued by the Asian Development Bank (ADB), Indonesia experienced significant human capital barriers to addressing health and education problems including a sharp increase in dropout rates between elementary and junior secondary school, high maternal and infant mortality rates, and high malnutrition rates, particularly in rural areas. Indonesia had established an unconditional cash transfer program earlier, in 2005, with 28 % of the population covered but with further exploration turned to the development of CCTs in 2006. Influenced by the positive CCT evaluation studies in other countries documenting outcomes from the use of CCTs, including improved education and health, Indonesia reshaped its strategy away from using immediate transfers to a more comprehensive strategy that included conditional programs. While reforming its finding for funding for primary education through grade and keeping its scholarships for secondary education, Indonesia introduced a categorical, targeted, conditional cash transfer program known as the Family Hope Program (*Program Keluarga Harapan*, PKH).

Conditions for receipt of the cash benefit include:

- Health-care and nutrition requirements such as a woman obtaining regular pre- and postnatal care, the child receiving a full series of vaccinations by age 6, monthly monitoring of growth, and vitamins for children up to age 8.
- The education conditions included a requirement that all children aged 6–12 be enrolled in primary school and those aged 12–15 be enrolled in junior secondary school, all attending at least 85 % of their school time. Attention was paid to the supply-side (sufficient schools and health-care services) benefit levels.
- Benefits are awarded to mothers, leading to increased spending on children, with better child outcomes. And beneficiaries may participate in the program for a maximum of 6 years.

The outcomes have included reduced poverty, increased enrollment in school, increased use of health care, enhanced nutrition, and reduced child labor. The issues that emerged are very similar to those that have emerged in other countries: implementation problems, the isolation of rural communities thus making access to schools and health-care services challenging, the inability of the poor to afford school costs even with the benefit, mixed parental motivation for sending children to school (rather than work), indexing the benefit, and lowering administrative costs by reducing the frequency with which the benefit is paid from 4 times a year to 3.

The CCT model was extended to community-based antipoverty strategies in 2007. A new community-based program was introduced that combines community empowerment with conditionalities known as *PNPM Generasi*. It has the same health and education objectives for poor households as PKH, but benefits are accrued to the community not an individual. A community council proposes and applies for project funding to develop community infrastructure. In this way, public investment in human capital is created alongside community ownership and development.

Philippines. In the years following the Asian financial crisis, the Philippines's economy experienced boom-and-bust cycles that furthered an unstable and volatile recovery. The ups and downs in the economy were due to increasing poverty and income inequality in the country, high unemployment, and although the Philippines had a foundation of social protection programs in place, there were significant limitations. The 1997 Asian financial crisis exposed weaknesses in coverage, targeting methodologies, and operational constraints. These resulted in significant leakages; resources go unduly to the nonpoor and the near poor amid lack of reliable poverty measures as well as overlaps and redundancies in sectoral or geographical beneficiaries.

In the face of growing concern regarding several problems experienced by children and their families, the government began to explore possible policy strategies. The problems include limited progress in reducing the rate of income poverty, falling education indicators including increased dropout rates and decreased enrollment rates, rising maternal mortality rates, and increased food prices. In an effort at reducing these problems, the Philippine government piloted a CCT program in four provinces and began to implement the program nationally in 2005 (Son 2008).

According to a Philippine government official, CCT programs were viewed as an effective device for strengthening regular attendance among primary school children, obtaining a full set of vaccinations, regular pre- and postnatal checkups, and increased involvement of skilled professionals in childbirth. The pilot called Pantawid Pamilyang Pilipino (CPP) CCTs was established to "enhance the role of parents and help them accomplish their duties and responsibilities to their children" by encouraging them to invest in their future through increasing access to health care, education, nutrition, and food.

Based on the results of the pilot project, Philippines has adopted a CCT in 2010 to provide income support to extremely poor households that encourages increased human capital investment in their children in the 20 poorest provinces in the country. The goal of the *Pantawid Pamilyang Pilipino Program* (the 4Ps) is to break intergenerational poverty improving health outcomes of children and pregnant mothers, improving nutrition in poor households, increasing school attendance and enrollment, and increasing parental participation in their children's lives and the community. The 4Ps address the administrative, grievance, and cultural sensitivity issues identified during the pilot phase such as indigenous groups' use of formal health care, obstacles obtaining benefits from banks due to travel, targeting mechanisms, and increasing accessibility to the grievance process.

Mongolia. Mongolia is one of Asia's poorest countries, with a population of only 2.6 million in 2005. About half the population lives in urban areas. The collapse of the Soviet Union and withdrawal of support led effectively to economic collapse in Mongolia during the early 1990s and the need for radical economic restructuring. One of the most dramatic manifestations of the social and economic breakdown was the sudden increase in numbers of street children, highlighting the need for social and child protection programs in Mongolia. Confronted with the combination of mounting poverty and need, the collapse of universal access to generously funded programs under the Soviet Union regime, the government initiated steps to establish a new system comprising of social welfare services and assistance to protect minimum living standards for the poor and vulnerable, employment services, and social insurance to protect working people from the risk of falling into poverty (Asian Development Bank 2008). The emphasis was on a selective strategy, and targeting was a key factor in developing programmatic responses.

In 2006 the government adopted a new targeted welfare package focused on benefits to newborns, school children, pregnant mothers, or mothers with five or more children – an approach which has been assessed as only modestly performing due to the lack of selectivity and focus on the poorest (Asian Development Bank 2008). Another program implemented was a CCT called the Child Money Program (CMP). The CMP began in 2005 as a targeted, means-tested program but expanded to a universal program in 2006, without a means test but with several conditions (albeit not quite as stringent as the conventional CCT). The conditions included children living with their families, attending school regularly, with their birth registered, and completing a series of vaccinations. However, prohibition of child labor is not a qualifying condition, and street children were not covered, nor are migrants, nor children in institutions.

In July 2006, the Mongolian government made the CMP universal to all families with children under 18 years, and the conditionalities were removed. In 2007, the level of the CMP benefit was increased from 3,000 MNT per month to 136,000 MNT (Sayed 2007). The program is credited with increasing school enrollment particularly among older and poor adolescents and a much smaller effect on reducing poverty among households with children (Sayed 2007). Cash allowances for newlyweds and newborns were also introduced. Persons receiving cash allowances went from 378,700 persons in 2004 to 1.6 million in 2008 (United Nations Country Team in Mongolia 2010). Less than 20 % of the beneficiaries are poor (United Nations Country Team in Mongolia 2010). At the same time, the commodities and economic crises severely impacted government revenues with fiscal consequences for the nation (Walker and Hall 2010). In January 2010, all newly created benefits were abolished and a new universal benefit from the Human Development Fund was introduced, covering all citizens of Mongolia. Recently the Ministry of Social Welfare began discussing the reintroduction of a child benefit adjusted to use existing logistical mechanisms but targeting only families with 3 or more children (United Nations Country Team in Mongolia 2010).

Benefit levels are low but viewed, nonetheless, as making a significant contribution to the incomes of poor families. The program has reduced income poverty. The universal nature of the program is viewed positively by the public, and as a result, the program receives both strong public and strong political support; and despite its being a universal program, it does reach low-income families in large part because low-income families are likely to be large and have more children. The authors note that despite their positive results, CCTs are not a cure-all nor a substitute for services but rather just one component of a social protection system albeit and important one.

Conclusions

In this paper we have described an innovative, increasingly popular, alternative to traditional social assistance, called conditional cash transfers (CCTs), and the experience with its use as a policy tool in several Asian countries. In exploring its use, we sought to identify the major factors leading to successful outcomes, including, in particular, the reduction of income poverty and the increase in human capital. This new means-tested cash benefit was used first and largely in the Latin American countries but now is increasingly used in other regions as well, in this case, in Asia. Qualifying for the benefit is contingent on certain behaviors, in particular, enrolling children in school (and sustaining their participation until a specified age), obtaining regular medical checkups, and improving nutrition and reducing malnutrition. Other desirable outcomes include the reduction of child labor, delay childbearing, and increased literacy, especially among girls. CCTs seek to modify child and parental behavior in ways that will increase the well-being of children and their potential as adults. By complying with the conditionalities imposed, families are rewarded with cash transfers.

There is strong evidence that cash transfers are effective in reducing income poverty in both developed and developing countries; but the evidence appears to be mixed with regard to the value of conditionality in modifying behavior. One scholar (Son 2008), stressing the importance of conditionality, noted that cash benefits alone are not adequate to achieve health and education goals. Other factors leading to successful outcomes include good governance and an adequate social infrastructure, strong political support, effective targeting, and complementary social policies. Changing or modifying individual behaviors requires a social policy strategy that goes beyond CCTs and includes, in addition, an adequate level of child benefits, resources that are sufficient to support more generous cash benefits or other income-generating opportunities, more extensive coverage of social insurance in developing countries, and avoidance of perverse incentives (such as the link, e.g., between poverty reduction and child labor). Despite the factors needed for successful implementation, a World Bank report (2009) points out that the CCT programs were designed primarily to confront long-term poverty, not sudden income shocks or transient poverty, but could reduce poverty by increasing investments in child human capital.

In the Asian countries reviewed here, CCTs tend to be targeted to girls' education to reduce gender disparities in education and are more likely to be linked with food or nutrition than in Latin America. In Asia, as in other parts of the world, CCTs almost always have the dual goals of reducing immediate poverty and a long-term investment in human capital through investments in education, parenting, health services, and nutrition. As CCTs expand throughout countries and within Asian countries, an increasingly relevant challenge will be the effectiveness of imposing conditionalities in more remote regions that have less developed and accessible infrastructure for schooling, health, and even administration.

There are several questions that have emerged with regard to the value of CCTs in general, as well as some questions especially relevant to Asia.

One question is that given the mixed evidence regarding impacts, why has there been such enthusiastic support of such a strategy especially since unconditional cash benefits can be cheaper to provide, support freedom of choice, can also reduce poverty and, appear to achieve desired school and health outcomes as well?

Up to now, the major developments – and successes – have been in middle-income countries of Latin America. Thus a second question is whether CCTs are a viable option for all countries or only for those with an adequate level of resources; and if the latter, what level? Are there certain conditions under which conditional cash transfers work best? For example, it appears that CCTs can expedite the development of social infrastructure, but perhaps in countries in which this is not possible, CCTs may not be the most effective and efficient policy instrument. CCT schemes are complex in design and require administrative skills of a high order to design, implement, and monitor the progress of schemes. The identification of beneficiaries is itself a complex task, and countries with poorly developed data gathering mechanisms are at a disadvantage in this respect. Similarly, the monitoring and evaluation requirements are also very demanding, and unless the country has a sophisticated evaluation system already in place, it would be difficult to adhere to the needs of the scheme.

Both conditional and unconditional transfers can improve the welfare of poor children. Thus third, we need to better understand how conditional and unconditional benefits promote social inclusion and minimize risks of exclusion, an area in which further research is much needed.

Fourth, of special relevance to the Asian countries:

Why has there been so little debate about turning towards a universal policy strategy instead, as attempted in Mongolia, one that stresses social solidarity, equity and efficiency, has a simple administrative structure, and is neither stigmatizing nor paternalistic? (Hanlon et al. 2010; Standing 2007; Hodges et al. 2007).

Of special importance, fifth, many Asian CCTs are targeted on girls' education as in Bangladesh, Cambodia, India, Indonesia, and Pakistan, but it is unclear whether gender makes a difference for all CCTs or significant gender impacts emerge only when it is an explicit goal. Will closing the gender gap in education demonstrate long-term effects as expected and when will these effects become measurable? Or is it targeting on girls that makes the difference, not gender as such? Thus, for example, does gender matter when dealing with the problem of street children, an urban problem associated with boys more than girls?

To conclude, the challenge for both unconditional and conditional cash transfers in developing countries especially is to ensure that in the longer term, these interventions develop into sustainable social policies for children that can be supported by national social protection systems. Only then will child well-being and our futures be enhanced.

References

Adato, M., de la Brière, B., Mindek, D., & Quisumbing, A. (2000). *Final report: The impact of PROGRESA on women's status and intrahousehold relations*. Washington, DC: International Food Policy Research Institute.

Angelucci, M., & De Giorgi, G. (2009). Indirect effects of an aid program: The case of progresa and consumption. *American Economic Review, 99*(1), 486–508.

Asian Development Bank. (2008). *Mongolia: Health and social protection*. Manila: Asian Development Bank.

Attanasio, O., Fitzsimmon, E., & Gomez, A. (2005). *The impact of a conditional cash subsidy on school enrollment in Colombia*. London: Institute for Fiscal Studies.

Barrera-Osario, F., Bertrnd, M., Linden, L., & Perez-Calle, F. (2008). *Conditional cash transfers in education: Design features, peer and sibling effects evidence from a randomized experiment in Colombia, No. 4580*. Wahington, DC: The World Bank, Human Development Network, Education Team.

Barrientos, A., & De Jong, J. (2006). Reducing child poverty with cash transfers: A sure thing? *Development Policy Review, 24*(50), 537–552.

Bastagali, F. (2007, September). *From social safety net to social policy? The role of conditional cash transfers in welfare state development in Latin America*. Paper presented at the International Sociological Association, Research Council 19, Florence.

Chaudhury, N., & Parajuli, D. (2006). *Conditional cash transfers and female schooling: The impact of the female school stipend program on public school enrollments in Punjab, Pakistan* (Policy, Research Working Paper No. WPS 4102, Impact evaluation series, no. IE 9). World Bank. Wahington, DC: The World Bank.

Coady, D. P., Grosh, M., & Hoddinott, J. (2004). Targeting outcomes redux. *World Bank Research Observer, 19*(1), 61–85.

de Britto, T. (2008). The emergence and popularity of conditional cash transfers in Latin America. In A. Barrientos & D. Hulme (Eds.), *Social protection for the poor and poorest* (pp. 181–193). UK: Palgrave MacMillan.

de Janvry, A., & Sadoulet, E. (2006). Making conditional cash transfers more efficient: Designing for maximum effect of the conditionality. *World Bank Economic Review, 20*, 1–29.

Farrington, J., & Slater, R. (2006). Cash transfers: Panacea for poverty reduction or money down the drain? *Development Policy Review, 24*(5), 499–511.

Filmer, D., & Schady, N. (2009). *School enrollment, selection and test scores* (Policy Research Working Paper 4998). Washington, DC: World Bank, Development Research Group, Human Development and Public Services Team.

Fiszbein, A., & Schady, N. (2009). *Conditional cash transfers: Reducing present and future poverty*. Washington, DC: World Bank.

Freeland, N. (2007). Superfluous, pernicious, atrocious and abominable? The case against conditional cash transfers. *IDS Bulletin, 38*(3), 75–78.

Gatenio, G. S., & Kamerman, S. B. (2006). Investing in children: Public commitment in 21 industrialized countries. *Social Services Review, 80*(3), 239–266.

Gatenio, G. S., & Kamerman, S. B. (2009). A global review of new risks and new responses for children and their families. *Asian Social Work and Policy Review, 3*(1), 1–21.

Gertler, P. (2000, November). *Final report: the impact of progresa on health*. Washington, DC: International Food Policy Research Institute. http://www.ifpri.org/themes/progresa/pdf/Gertler_health.pdf

Glewwe, P., & Olinto, P. (2004). *Evaluating of the impact of conditional cash transfers on schooling: An experimental analysis of Honduras' PRAF program*. Washington, DC: USAID.

Gordon, D., Nandy, S., Pantazis, C., Pemberton, S., & Townsend, P. (2003). *Child poverty in the developing world*. Bristol: The Policy Press. http://aa.ecn.cz/img_upload/65636e2e7a707261766f64616a737476/Child_poverty.pdf

Handa, S., & Davis, B. (2006). The experience of conditional cash transfers in Latin America and the Caribbean. *Development Policy Review, 24*(5), 513–536.

Hanlon, J., Barrientos, A., & Hulme, D. (2010). *Just give money to the poor: The development revolution from the global south*. Sterling: Kumarian Press.

Hoddinott, J., & Skoufias, E. (2005). The impact of PROGRESA on food consumption. *Economic Development and Cultural Change, 53*(1), 37–61.

Hodges, A., Dufay, A.-C., Dashdorj, K., Kang, Y. J., Mungun, T., & Budragchaa, U. (2007). *Child benefits and poverty reduction: Evidence from Mongolia's child money program* (Social Science Research Network Working Paper No. 002). New York: UNICEF

Kakawani, N., Soares, F., & Son, H. H. (2006). Cash transfers for school-age children in African countries: Simulation of impacts on poverty and school attendance. *Development Policy Review, 24*(5), 553–569.

Kamerman, S. B., Neuman, M., Waldfogel, J., & Brooks-Gunn, J. (2003). *Social policies, family types, and child outcomes in selected OECD countries: A review of the literature* (OECD Working Paper on Social Policy No. 6). Paris: OECD.

Lagarde, M., Haines, A., & Palmer, N. (2007). Conditional cash transfers for improving uptake of health interventions in low- and middle-income countries: A systematic review. *Journal of the American Medical Association, 298*(16), 1900–1910.

Lund, F., Noble, M., Barnes, H., & Wright, G. (2008). *Is there a rationale for conditional cash transfers for children in South Africa?* (School of Development Studies Working Paper No. 53). Durban: University of KwaZulu-Natal.

Maluccio, J. A., & Flores, R. (2004). *Impact evaluation of a conditional cash transfer program: The Nicaraguan Red de Protección Social* (FCND Discussion Paper No. 184). Washington, DC: International Food Policy Research Institute.

Mapp, S. (2011). *Global child welfare and well-being*. New York: Oxford University Press.

Mead, L. M. (1997). Citizenship and social policy: T. H. Marshall and poverty. *Social Philosophy and Policy, 14*(2), 197–230.

Mehrotra, S. (2010). *Introducing conditional cash transfers in India: A proposal for five CCTs*. Brighton: Institute of Development Studies.

Miller, S. J. (2008, April 29). Schools use cash as an incentive to boost attendance and scores. *The Christian Science Monitor*. Retrieved from http://www.csmonitor.com/USA/Society/2008/0429/p20s01-ussc.html.

Molyneux, M. (2006). Mothers at the service of the new poverty agenda: Progresa/oportunidades, Mexico's conditional transfer programme. *Social Policy and Administration, 40*(4), 425–449.

Patrinos, H. (2007). *The living conditions of children* (Policy Research Working Paper Series 4251). Washington, DC: The World Bank.

Paxson, C., & Schady, N. (2007). *Does money matter? The effects of cash transfers on child health and development in rural Ecuador* (Impact Evaluation Series No. IE 15, Policy, Research working paper No. WPS 4226). Washington, DC: World Bank.

Perry, G. E., Arias, O. S., Lopez, J. H., Maloney, W. F., & Serven, L. (2006). *Poverty reduction and growth: Virtuous and vicious circles. World Bank Latin American and Caribbean Studies*. Washington, DC: World Bank.

Saracostti, M. (2008). The Chile Solidario system: The role of social work. *International Social Work, 51*, 566–572.

Sayed, A. (2007, November). *The social assistance system in Mongolia: An unfinished agenda*. Presentation at the World Bank Cash Knowledge Transfer Workshop. www.sdc-cashprojects.ch/en/Home/document.php?itemID=1770...1. Accessed 15 Nov 2010.

Schady, N., & Araujo, M. C. (2008). Cash transfers, conditions, and school enrollment in Ecuador. *Economia, 8*(2), 43–70.

Skoufias, E. (2005). *PROGRESA and its impacts on the welfare of rural households in Mexico* (Research Report 139). Washington, DC: International Food Policy Research Institute.

Skoufias, E., & Parker, S. (2001). Conditional cash transfers and the impact on child work and schooling: Evidence from the PROGRESA program in Mexico. *Economia: Journal of Latin America and the Caribbean Economic Association, 2*(1.1), 45–96.

Soares, F. V., Soares, S., Medieros, M., & Osorio, R. G. (2006). *Cash transfer programmes in Brazil: Impacts on inequality and poverty* (International Poverty Centre Working Paper No. 21). Brazil: United Nations Development Programme.

Son, H. (2008). *Conditional cash transfer programs: An effective tool for poverty alleviation?* Manila: Asian Development Bank.

Standing, G. (2007, December). *Conditional cash transfers: Why targeting and conditionalities could fail* (International Poverty Centre Working Paper No. 47). Brazil: United Nations Development Programme.

UNICEF Bangladesh. (2010). *Mitigating socio-economic inequalities to accelerate poverty reduction: Investing in vulnerable children*. Dhaka: UNICEF Bangladesh.

UNICEF Innocenti Research Centre. (2007). *Child poverty in perspective: An overview of child well-being in rich countries* (Innocenti Report Card 7). Florence: UNICEF Innocenti Research Centre.

United Nations Country Team in Mongolia. (2010, April 19). *Universal periodic review*. http://www.upr-mongolia.mn/images/xupld/UPRUN.pdf. Accessed 15 Nov 2010.

Vleminckx, K., & Smeeding, T. M. (Eds.). (2001). *Child well-being, child poverty, and child policy in modern nations: What do we know?* Bristol/Toronto: Policy Press/University of Toronto Press (Second printing 2003).

Walker, W., & Hall, D. (2010). *Reforming social protection systems when commodity prices collapse: The experience of Mongolia*. Presentation to the Asian Development Bank. http://www.adb.org/documents/events/2009/poverty-social-development/WG1D-commodity-exports-Mon-Hall-Walker-presentation.pdf

World Bank. (2007). *Pakistan: Promoting rural growth and poverty reduction* (Report No. 39303-PK). Washington, DC: World Bank.

Chapter 13
The Impact of Economic Crises on Health: Past Evidence and Policy Implications for Asia

Phua Kai Hong and Phua Kai Lit

Introduction

Assessment of the social and health effects of the recent global economic crisis is crucial in formulating evidence-based policies to mitigate the impact of the crisis on vulnerable groups. There are lessons from the past, including the Asian financial crisis more than a decade ago, as economic crises are found to have negative impact on employment, poverty, and social services. The long-run impact of the current crisis will not be negligible and should deserve serious considerations and further research. Future research efforts are needed to fully explore the policy implications of short- and longer-term effects (including what they mean to different countries with disparate levels and income classes; vulnerable population groups such as the elderly, mothers, and children; and specific disease categories including mental health and suicides, malnutrition, and infections) and to offer policy options to government services and development agencies on how they can be more responsive towards public policy formulation and implementation.

Analysis of records from the Great Depression reveals serious adverse health effects, including increased morbidity and mortality from heart disease, as well as positive correlations with hypertension and mental health problems, suicides/parasuicides, and alcoholism. Subsequent studies have revealed that vulnerable groups including ethnic minorities, the poor, single mothers, the disabled, and the elderly bear the brunt of cutbacks in public spending on health and social services (Levy and Sidel 2006). Another approach in the study of the

Phua K.H. (✉)
Lee Kuan Yew School of Public Policy, National University of Singapore, Singapore
e-mail: spppkh@nus.edu.s

Phua K.L.
Jeffrey Cheah School of Medicine and Health Sciences, Monash University, Sunway Campus, Selangor, Malaysia
e-mail: phua.kai.lit@monash.edu

W.J.J. Yeung and M.T. Yap (eds.), *Economic Stress, Human Capital, and Families in Asia: Research and Policy Challenges*, Quality of Life in Asia 4,
DOI 10.1007/978-94-007-7386-8_13, © Springer Science+Business Media Dordrecht 2013

impact of economic recession on health is to determine if recession is linked to the incidence of known risk factors for ill health such as poverty, downward social mobility, stress, and substance abuse. There is evidence that economic difficulties such as the debt crisis of the 1980s had resulted in increases in poverty rates, unemployment, and underemployment and decreases in real income in various areas of the world (Abel-Smith 1986; Abrahamson et al. 1986). Similarly, the recent economic crisis which began in December 2007 in the United States and had spread to European nations is expected to impact health through these mechanisms (Horton 2009; Marmot 2009).

What are the lessons from history and what can we learn from the impact of past economic crises? Can policies be taken to prevent, if not mitigate, the negative effects of these shocks? Are the experiences in developed countries similar or different from those of developing countries? How are the effects at the macroeconomic level different from those affecting households and individuals at the microlevel? Are these experiences and lessons applicable to Asia? What are the key policy implications and recommendations to policy makers?

Learning from History: Lessons from Asia

The fiscal crisis of 1998 which engulfed several countries in East Asia, notably Indonesia, Malaysia, Thailand, and South Korea, resulted in a sharp currency depreciation and consequently higher costs of imported drugs and supplies, reduced poor people's access to basic health services, and slashed government health budgets just as demand for public sector healthcare increased. Stringent cost-cutting exposed weaknesses in social safety nets and healthcare financing systems.

A high-profile conference was convened in 2009 by UNICEF in Singapore to warn that economic recession would have far-reaching health effects with the most vulnerable groups bearing a disproportionate burden. Incomes of the unemployed would fall, and they would lose social protection, including occupational health insurance, resulting in a decline in healthcare utilization, especially high-cost catastrophic health expenditure, and reduced consumption of essential medicinal products. A consequent deterioration in health outcomes and long-term increases in morbidity and mortality, in turn, could negatively impact growth and productivity and reverse earlier gains (UNICEF 2009). The vicious cycle of poor health and economic effects is depicted below in Fig. 13.1.

Related research on the East Asian economic crisis investigated the longer-term sequelae including pediatric malnutrition, falling levels of immunization, and the reemergence of infectious diseases. Child mortality in the most severely affected countries spiked in 1997–1998, and undernourishment also became more prevalent, only falling to former levels once the crisis abated (Bhutta et al. 2009). Compared with other countries that were moderately and least affected, child mortality rates were the worst in East Asia during the critical years (see Fig. 13.2).

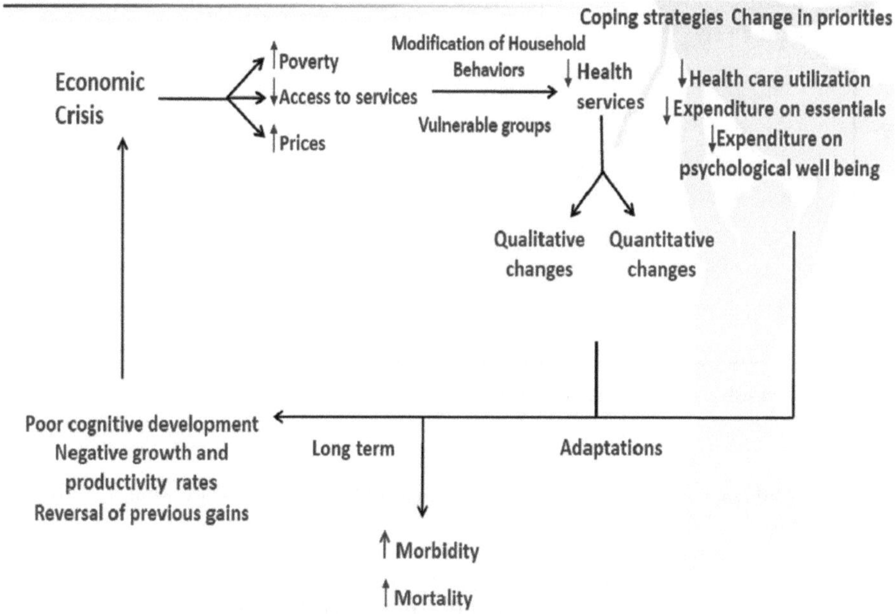

Fig. 13.1 The vicious cycle of economic effects on health (Source: Bhutta et al. 2009)

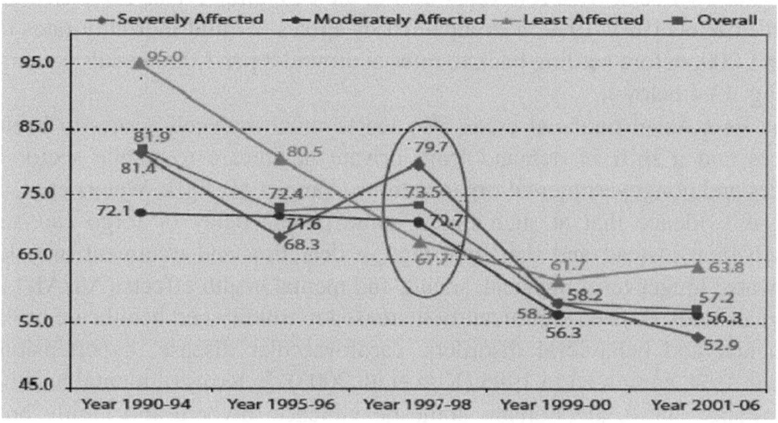

Fig. 13.2 Under-5 mortality rates (per 1,000 live births) during the 1997 crisis (Source: UNICEF 2009)

Even for a rapidly developing country like Thailand that was experiencing progressive improvements in health standards, the declining trends of mortality among children under 5 years of age were suddenly disrupted by a dramatic spike in 1998, before falling back to expected precrisis rates in the following years (see Fig. 13.3 below).

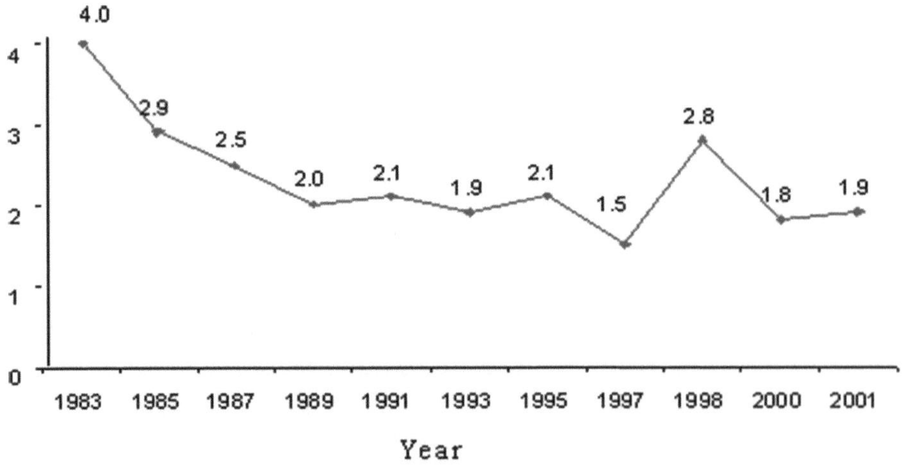

Fig. 13.3 Child mortality in Thailand (Source: Bureau of Policy and Strategy, Ministry of Health, Thailand; cited in Chen L, 2009)

In Malaysia, a middle-income country, there had been steady progress in the reductions in mortality rates for both infants (below 1 year of age) and toddlers (1–5 years of age) along with declining poverty rates. However, these downward trends were set back by a few years during the economic crisis. Poverty rates rose over the period 1997–1999, accompanied by spikes in child mortality rates to over 12 per 1,000, before settling back to rates at around 8 per 1,000 in subsequent years (see Fig. 13.4 below).

The East Asian financial crisis also led to much reduced access to healthcare services and a shift in demand from private healthcare to public sector health services and nongovernmental organizations (Yang et al. 2001; Waters et al. 2003). There is evidence that at such times, some people delay or forgo care-seeking and self-treat instead and that time lags in detection and treatment may lead to even worse longer-term physical, social, and mental health effects (AusAID 2000). A Korean study showed significantly increased morbidity and healthcare utilization for mental and behavioral disorders, cardiovascular disease, hypertension, and injury in 1998 compared to 1995 (Kim et al. 2003). In terms of mental health, rates of substance abuse, alcoholism, domestic violence, divorce and family breakup, depression, and other mental illness, all increased in step with unemployment, poverty, and falling incomes (IMF 2009). There was also a spike in suicides and attempted suicides associated with unemployment at the height of the crisis in Japan, Hong Kong, and Korea (Chang et al. 2009; Kwon et al. 2009).

Based on such bad regional experiences in the past, the Asian Development Bank (ADB) projected early warnings of possible effects of the recent global crisis – an estimated 64 million people in Asia would remain below the poverty line of US$1.25/day (Francisco and Wan 2009). Consequently, progress in reducing

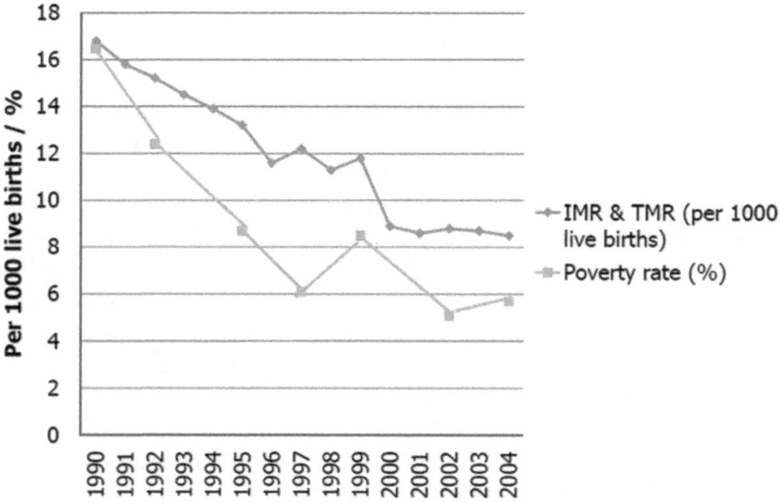

Fig. 13.4 Poverty rate and child mortality for Malaysia, 1990–2004 (Source: Ministry of Health, Malaysia – data on incidence of poverty from the Economic Planning Unit, Malaysia; and under-5 mortality rates from the Demographic Statistics Division, Department of Statistics, Malaysia, various years from 1990 to 2004)

poverty in Asia would be delayed. The social effects of declining affluence in Asia could include increased maternal and infant mortality rates and malnutrition, particularly among the very poor (ESCAP et al. 2008). The ADB thus recommended that policy interventions and donor assistance should prioritize health and that national governments and international agencies should tailor their responses to cater to differing circumstances between countries and sectors.

Studies of Economic Crisis and Health in Developed Countries

Early studies of possible relationships between macroeconomic dynamics and health were carried out in the 1920s and 1930s. Ogburn and Thomas (1923) analyzed the impact of economic recession on mortality in the United Kingdom during the years 1870–1914 and concluded that there was an adverse association between recession and infant mortality rates. Similarly, a later study by Thomas (1925) revealed a relationship between economic cycles and health – although the conclusion arrived at was that mortality rates were positively associated with the early phase of upturns in the business cycle. This indicated the possibility of delayed effects of downturns in the economy on health indicators (time-lagged effects). Studies done by Singer (1937) and by Morris and Titmuss (1944) which utilized longitudinal data revealed adverse effects of unemployment on health at the population level. Morris and Titmuss studied possible relationships between unemployment and the occurrence of heart disease among young people in Britain during the depression years of the 1930s and concluded that there was a 2–4 year lag effect. Emile Durkheim's classic work entitled "Suicide" indicated the existence of possible relationships between periods of socioeconomic disruption and suicide rates, labeled as "anomic suicides" (Durkheim 1951).

Beginning in the late 1960s and 1970s, Brenner conducted a series of studies on the impact of economic instability (as indicated by increased rates of unemployment and slower economic growth followed by periods of rapid recovery) on health in developed nations such as the United States and the United Kingdom and other industrialized Northern countries. He concluded that economic fluctuations did exert negative effects on health. His studies indicated that periods of economic recession were followed by increased morbidity and mortality rates for health problems such as heart disease, alcoholism, and mental illness (Brenner 1967, 1971, 1973a, b, 1975, 1979, 1983, 1984, 1987a, b, c; Brenner and Mooney 1982, 1983). Eyer (1977a, b) also conducted research on possible relationships between the business cycle and health in the United States. However, his view is that the most sustained declines in mortality rates occurred during periods of economic downturn. He attributed this to lowered levels of job stress, longer hours of work, higher migration rates, and greater number of family breakups associated with periods of economic boom.

Another study (Bunn 1979) conducted to investigate the impact of economic recession on health in Australia arrived at the conclusion that ischemic heart disease mortality rates tended to increase a few years after the occurrence of economic recession. Other studies which support the notion that economic fluctuations can adversely affect health include those by Adamchak and Colombino. Adamchak (1979) investigated the relationships between the mortality of infants and community-wide economic and social variables in Toledo, Ohio, from 1959 to 1970 and found that in the 1970s, the marital instability rate, the median income level, and the unemployment rate were the factors most strongly associated with increased risk of postneonatal mortality (which increased in the city between 1960 and 1970). However, he recommended that further research was needed in order to determine if the increase in the postneonatal mortality rate was due to adverse socioeconomic conditions or to medical advances which could have prolonged the lives of weaker infants so that they died in the postneonatal period rather than in the neonatal period. Colombino's (1984) econometric investigation of the impact of economic fluctuations on infant mortality rates in Italy led him to conclude that an adverse impact existed. MacMahon and Yen's (1971) historical study of the United States' experience during the depression years of the 1930s revealed increased rates of some types of birth defects during the period. Bengtsson and Ohlsson's (1985) study of the impact of fluctuations in real wages on age-specific mortality rates in Sweden from 1751 to 1859 using statistical techniques similar to those employed by Brenner led them to conclude that real wage fluctuations were associated with mortality rate fluctuations, i.e., decreases in real wages were positively associated with increases in mortality rates.

Deleterious effects of economic changes on health appear to exist even in countries with highly developed social welfare systems such as Sweden. A group of Swedish researchers (Starrin et al. 1990) found that mortality trends from 1963 to 1983 were associated with economic fluctuations as well as changes in health-related behavior. They carried out synchronic (non-lagged) and asynchronic (lagged) analyses and concluded that the level of employment and overtime work was associated with the suicide rate in the synchronic analysis. In the case of cardiovascular mortality, the synchronic and 2-year time-lagged analyses indicated that alcohol sales and, to a certain extent, the length of periods of unemployment were important factors. The level of unemployment was the only significant factor in an analysis with a 3-year time lag.

Other studies include those by Catalano and Serxner, and Morrell and associates. Catalano and Serxner (1992) attempted to replicate Brenner's earlier finding of an association between economic instability and the neonatal mortality rate while taking into account criticisms of the methodology and potential problems with aggregate time-series research. Their results from ARIMA (autoregressive integrated moving average) models of neonatal mortality among black male birth cohorts in the Los Angeles County and Orange County metropolitan areas led them to conclude that the risks increased due to unexpectedly low levels of employment in the second trimester. They concluded that the " ... implication of the findings ... is that Brenner may have been right, in his contention that economic contraction increases neonatal mortality. The effect, modest as it may be, survives tests that respond to his methodological critics" (p. 284). Morrell and associates' study of suicide and unemployment in Australia from 1907 to 1990 resulted in the following findings: male suicide rates fluctuated sharply, with the peaks coinciding with periods of high unemployment; female suicide rates, in contrast, were generally stable throughout this time period; and from 1966 to 1990, the association was strong for males aged 15–24 (Morrell et al. 1993).

As a result of the US economic turmoil which began in December 2007 and spread to European countries such as Iceland, the United Kingdom, Ireland, Greece, Portugal, and Spain, there has been a recent wave of studies on the relationship between economic instability and health. These include reviews of the literature (Stuckler et al. 2009a; Uutela 2010; Zilko 2010) as well as empirical studies (Stuckler et al. 2009b; Ensor et al. 2010). From their literature review pertaining to three time periods (the Great Depression beginning in 1929, the Post-Communist Depression of the early 1990s, and the East Asian financial crisis of the late 1990s), Stuckler et al. (2009a) found that health was affected during times of rapid economic change, i.e., both during economic booms and during economic busts. Stuckler and his coauthors also concluded that the negative effects could be mitigated by strong social cohesion and social welfare systems.

Uutela (2010) examined the recent literature on whether economic recessions have a negative effect on mental health such as depression and suicides. The conclusion reached was that the consequences of economic recession on mental health are context dependent, with sharp unemployment-related increases in suicide mortality in some East Asian countries (because of the East Asian economic crisis of the late 1990s) and significant short-term increases in deaths from suicides in European Union countries. But in some of the richer countries, active labor market programs appeared to have prevented some of these adverse effects. Zilko's (2010) literature review resulted in skepticism over claims of association between economic contraction and birth weight and neonatal mortality because of inconsistent findings by researchers. As for recent empirical analyses, Stuckler et al. (2009b) studied 26 European Union countries using data from 1970 to 2007 and concluded that increases in unemployment were associated with significant short-term increases in deaths from intentional violence but reductions in traffic fatalities. Ensor et al. (2010) carried out an empirical study of the impact of economic recession on maternal and infant mortality using twentieth-century time-series data from 14 high- and middle-income countries. They concluded that there was a significant association between maternal and infant mortality and economic growth but only for early periods (1936–1965) and not for later periods.

A study on suicides in South Korea (Kwon et al. 2009) revealed that there was indeed an association between economic crisis and suicides in the country. However, another study (Chang et al. 2009) concluded that although there was such an association in South Korea, Japan, and Hong Kong (especially for unemployed males), this was not true for Taiwan and Singapore. The latter two countries were less seriously affected by the East Asian economic crisis and suffered lower rates of unemployment as a result. But are there other mitigating factors present in countries and their social systems to explain these differences?

Studies of Economic Crisis and Health in Developing Countries

What about studies of the impact of economic crisis on health in developing countries and especially in Asia? A study of postwar infant mortality in Sri Lanka (Meegama 1980) noted that an increase in the postneonatal mortality rate (especially among the tea plantation population) during the mid-1970s could be attributed to food shortages (due possibly to halving of the free rice ration in late 1973 and an accompanying sharp increase in bread prices). Wood's study in Brazil (Wood 1982) indicated that infant mortality could even increase during a period of sustained and high rates of national economic growth. In this case, the increase in the infant mortality rate in the Sao Paulo area in the early 1970s was attributed to governmental policies which resulted in downward pressure on real income for some segments of the Brazilian population. When real income began rising again in the late 1970s, the infant mortality rate resumed its downward course. Rosero-Bixby's (1983) study in Costa Rica concluded that downturns in the state of the economy were followed by fluctuations in the rates of health indicators and in the rate of progress in the reduction of infant mortality (deceleration).

A study of infant mortality trends in Mexico (Bronfman 1992) using data derived from their National Fertility and Health Survey (ENFES) found that the steady decline of earlier years continued into the mid-1980s and the years of economic crises. However, an important finding was that the decline occurred at different rates for different social groups. This means that some social classes and groups were more adversely affected by deterioration of economic conditions. The other major finding was that:

> ...certain variables universally accepted as determinants of infant mortality, such as mother's education, seem nonsignificant for some social sectors; and ... certain biodemographic characteristics assumed to have a uniform mortality-related behavior vary among sectors, suggesting that even these constants are determined by social factors." (p. 157)

The literature indicates that the negative effects of economic instability are likely to be stronger for two groups – the poor in urban areas and plantation workers in the rural areas. There is evidence that infectious diseases and malnutrition are major problems for urban slum dwellers. Disease prevalence rates are comparable to or may even exceed those of rural populations. Furthermore, urban life increases the risk of exposure to problems less likely to be found in rural areas such as traffic injuries, occupational ailments, and physical injuries from lax regulation of working conditions in factories. Other problems include those related to the stress, alienation, or disorientation of urban life for rural migrants and from difficult economic conditions. These also include homicide, mental distress, and sexually transmitted diseases (Harpham 1986).

Loewenson (1989) noted that seasonal plantation workers are a subpopulation who are among the most impoverished, unhealthy, and underserved (in terms of access to public social services) in developing countries. As foreign demand for Third World plantation products drops as a result of economic downturn, prices decline and the export earnings of Third World countries follow suit. These are likely to result in increased unemployment for plantation workers or reduced cash incomes for small-scale commercial farmers. Their living standards and welfare are, in turn, likely to deteriorate further. Falagas et al. (2009) carried out a literature review and concluded that economic crises in less affluent nations resulted in increase in all-cause mortality. However, mortality from transport-related injuries actually decreased during economic crises. Jacinto et al. (2010) carried out a study of the effects of macroeconomic conditions on health in Brazil. The unemployment rate was used as a proxy for macroeconomic conditions while mortality rates were used to measure population health. They concluded that Brenner's hypothesis of a negative relationship between macroeconomic conditions and mortality rates was supported in the case of Brazil.

Impact of Economic Crises on Social Expenditure Patterns and Demand for Health Services

The clearest and most easily documented effects of severe economic crises are those pertaining to economic indicators and social expenditure input indicators. In the case of developed nations such as the United States and the United Kingdom, one can safely argue that even if economic problems increase pressure on their respective social welfare systems, owing to the great wealth of these nations, their policy options are not as restricted as those of the much poorer developing nations. Thus, although the governments of nations like the United States and Britain can choose to increase or maintain real levels of expenditure on social welfare, the option taken during the 1980s and more recently under Conservative Prime Minister David Cameron led to the reduction of such expenditure instead (Stuckler et al. 2010). Miller (1985) and Miller et al. (1985a, b) argued that the increased spending on social welfare in the United States during the recession of the mid-1970s had a cushioning effect on the health of children, while the cutbacks of the 1980s were associated with adverse health trends among the most vulnerable population subgroups (such as minorities, the poor, the unemployed, and their children) and resulted in a slowdown in the rate of decline of the infant mortality rate.

In countries like the United States where healthcare costs are high but there is no system of universal coverage through a national health insurance scheme, lack of health insurance is a risk factor for poor health because of financially related delays in care-seeking. Studies on the impact of the recent recession on health insurance coverage reveal that not only have the numbers of uninsured increased because of job loss (Holahan 2011) but there has also been reduced coverage and thus more underinsurance in the case of those who continue to be "covered" by employment-based health insurance (Fronstin 2010).

Abel-Smith (1986) noted the following results of serious economic crises in developing countries – declines in standard of living, serious unemployment and underemployment problems, and substantial social expenditure reductions, leading to disintegration of rural health services in some countries and increases in malnutrition in some countries. As a result of overwhelming dependence on single commodities for earning foreign exchange, countries can be badly hit in terms of trade deterioration and lower demand and reduced prices for commodities. This in turn can result in severe budgetary pressures and input and process indicator erosion for the healthcare system. Severe economic problems may also lead to shortages of essential drugs, transportation problems, and the deterioration of rural health facilities as a result of lack of funds for fuel and vehicle maintenance (Freund 1986).

Jolly and Cornia's (1984) discussion (together with those of Orivel and Lewin) of the impact of the global economic recession and national fiscal difficulties on indicators in the health and education systems of developing nations noted the implementation of cutbacks in spending, declines in real spending, or expenditure per capita as a result of inflation and population growth; although nominal expenditure levels were maintained, subsidies were reduced, user fees and other cost recovery mechanisms were introduced, and there was qualitative deterioration and so on (Jolly and Cornia 1984; Orivel 1986; Lewin 1986). Musgrove documented similar developments in Latin America and the Caribbean. Sharp reductions in domestic investment and imports also occurred. However, some countries were able to maintain the real value of non-investment social expenditure (Musgrove 1987).

Sometimes, cutbacks in expenditure on health and social welfare are carried out in response to pressure from external parties such as the International Monetary

Fund (IMF). Critics such as Stuckler and Basu (2009) pointed out that the conditions tied to IMF loans to economically stricken countries ("IMF conditionality") often necessitate fiscal austerity programs that result in weakened healthcare systems. Currency devaluations can also result in soaring prices for imported medical supplies and equipment. The East Asian Economic Crisis of the late 1990s resulted in reduced access to health services as well as a shift in the demand for medical services from the more expensive private sector to the less expensive public sector (Yang et al. 2001; Waters et al. 2003).

Contrary Findings from Other Research

The literature cited above supports the notion that economic downturns can negatively affect the health and welfare of populations or subpopulations (macrolevel studies). Nevertheless, there also exists a body of literature which states that this relationship may not be so clear-cut (Kasl 1979; Lew 1979; Gravelle et al. 1981; Wagstaff 1985). For example, Stern (1983) argued that the relationship between unemployment and morbidity and mortality rates is not clear because of reasons such as (1) the existence of a multitude of other socioeconomic determinants of mortality and their relationship to the incidence of morbidity and unemployment and (2) the existence of systematic selection factors.

Furthermore, some studies carried out with the aim of replicating and extending Brenner's findings to other places have turned up negative or inconclusive results (John et al. 1983; Forbes and McGregor 1987; Narendranathan et al. 1985). Laporte (2004) argued that the results of Brenner-type analyses could be affected by choice of indicators, the method of analysis, and the time periods examined. Platt and associates' study of possible relationships between unemployment and suicide in Italy from 1977 to 1987 resulted in contradictory and inconsistent findings. They were unable to arrive at any definite conclusions and suggested the importance of individual-level studies utilizing retrospective case-control methodology (Platt et al. 1992). As mentioned earlier, Zilko's (2010) literature review resulted in skepticism over claims of association between economic contraction and birth weight and neonatal mortality because of inconsistency in research findings. Tapia Granados (2005a, b, 2008) and Ruhm (2000, 2007) carried out studies that gave rise to counterintuitive results, i.e., that mortality increased during an economic boom and decreased during a recession. Ruhm estimated that a drop in unemployment by 1 % raised coronary heart deaths by 0.75 % (Ruhm 2007).

Janlert (2009) summarized such contradictory findings well when he wrote that:

> Documentation about the negative health effects of individual unemployment abounds, but many studies of macroeconomic changes point at another result: that mortality increases during a boom and decreases during a recession... (p. 783)
>
> and:
>
> The conflicting results between aggregated macroeconomic studies and the individual unemployment studies, as well as the contradictions between different macroeconomic studies, point at the still very doubtful robustness regarding the studies on aggregate

> data. Obviously an economic downturn has a potential for both negative (loss of income, insecurity) and positive (reduced work hazards, less traffic) effects on the health of different segments of the population. And as the number of unemployed people is in most cases small compared with those still at work .... it is not unreasonable to think that individual unemployment studies and aggregated studies on trade and health could yield different results. (p. 784)

Studies of the Impact of Economic Crises on Individuals

All of the studies cited above can be categorized as macrolevel studies of the impact of macroeconomic dynamics on outcome indicators in the health and demography fields. There also exists a body of literature which may be categorized as microlevel studies, i.e., studies of the impact of unemployment on the mental and physical health of individual unemployed workers and professionals. As Platt et al. (1992) suggested, the controversy over the results of findings of possible relationships between economic instability and health utilizing time-series data is perhaps better investigated by microlevel studies. Such studies often conclude that unemployment does exert a negative effect on the mental health of the unemployed (and even on the mental health of their dependants and on employed people threatened with possible loss of job) but that the negative impact may be cushioned by various factors such as the existence of social support, ethnicity, social class, sex, and age of the people affected. There is also some controversy over the impact of unemployment on the physical health of the unemployed and their family members.

Nevertheless, studies conducted by Moser and associates, Westin, and Grayson indicated that such effects are very likely to exist (Moser et al. 1984, 1986, 1987; Westin et al. 1988; Grayson 1989). Furthermore, studies of unemployed workers showed that unemployment was associated with actual physiological changes, e.g., elevated levels of norepinephrine in the urine of study subjects (Cobb 1974; Baum et al. 1986) and elevated inflammatory status (Hintikka et al. 2009). The studies which were carried out by Liem and associates (Liem and Liem 1978; Liem and Rayman 1982) and Catalano and Dooley are good examples of microlevel studies (Catalano and Dooley 1977, 1979; Dooley et al. 1981; Catalano et al. 1981). Catalano and Dooley believe that a rural geographical location is also a factor in the cushioning of the impact of economic change, possibly because of the existence of more intimate social networks. Other studies by researchers from Sweden (Hammarstrom et al. 1988; Stefansson 1991), the Netherlands (Leeflang et al. 1992a, b), and Australia (Graetz 1993) provide evidence of the negative effects of unemployment on individuals and the importance of cushioning social factors. In the case of developing nations, some studies have proposed that possible negative effects of economic recession on child health may be reduced or neutralized by the response of the state in the form of social policies and programs, e.g., in Cuba and South Korea (Muniz et al. 1984; Suh 1984).

Evidence of the relationship between recession and substance abuse is less clear, although Brenner believes that alcohol consumption is related to trends in the national economy in the case of the United States. His findings indicate that the consumption of distilled spirits tends to increase among some segments of the population under conditions of major economic stress (Brenner 1975). A study of unemployment and consumption of alcohol during the Finish economic crisis of the 1990s concluded that unemployment was weakly but significantly associated with high consumption of alcohol among single people (Luoto et al. 1998).

Studies of the impact of economic instability and unemployment on the mental health of affected individuals continue to be published (Ostamo et al. 2001; Lee et al. 2010; Meltzer et al. 2010; Wang et al. 2010). Ostamo et al. analyzed data pertaining to 2495 persons who attempted suicide in Finland during 1989–1994 and found that unemployment rates were higher among suicide attempters than in the general population, with the rates for males higher than the rates for females during economic recessions. Meltzer and associates (2010) studied the relationship between job insecurity and depression in Britain and found that job insecurity and being in debt were associated with depression after controlling for age and sex. In a study conducted in Alberta province of Canada, deteriorating economic conditions were found to be associated with increased prevalence of major depressive disorder in a cohort of 3579 people (Wang et al. 2010). These two studies echo the findings of the Whitehall II study of Marmot and his research team which revealed that job insecurity had a negative impact on health (Ferrie et al. 2002).

As for research on Asia, Lee et al. (2010) carried out a study of the 2008 East Asian economic crisis and depression in Hong Kong. They found similarly that economic crisis increased the prevalence of depression. They also found that individuals who suffered large investment losses had a significantly higher prevalence of major depressive episodes (20.3 %) than those who experienced little or no investment loss (9.2–13.7 %). Furthermore, the impact was not limited to the unemployed – others such as the employed, homemakers, and high-/middle-income people were also affected. A Finnish study of the impact of economic recession on the mental health of children also showed that "others," including those related and involved with the lives of such children, may be affected. The researchers concluded that the mental health of kids could be affected through increased economic pressure and the resulting negative changes in parental mental health, patterns of marital interaction, and quality of parenting (Solantaus et al. 2004).

Policy Recommendations and Conclusion

The current global recession is the worst since the Great Depression of the 1920s and 1930s and has devastated economies worldwide. Asia appears to have fared better than the western countries, perhaps because of measures taken following the Asian financial crisis of 1997–1998. Nevertheless, projections by the International Monetary Fund indicate that many low-income developing countries will suffer the most severe repercussions of the ongoing crisis, with a significant negative impact of unemployment on health likely to occur after a lag of 1–2 years, depending on factors such as governments' responsiveness and the success of financial stimuli and rescue packages (IMF 2009).

The long-run impacts of the current crisis will not be negligible and should deserve serious considerations and further research. Future research efforts are needed to fully explore the policy implications of short- and longer-term effects (including what they mean to different countries with disparate levels of income classes; vulnerable population groups such as the elderly, mothers, and children; and specific disease categories including mental health and suicides, malnutrition, and infections) and to offer policy options to health-related government services and development agencies on how they can be more responsive in public policy formulation and implementation.

Based on the past lessons of history, and especially from the experience of the last regional financial crisis, the following key public policy priorities during times of crisis have been identified:

- Prevention of negative health consequences by strengthening social welfare and mental health services with protection/expansion of social and healthcare financing
- Early detection and treatment and maintained vigilance in the surveillance and monitoring of risks and symptoms over critical time periods and beyond
- Special attention to high-risk and vulnerable groups and rendering assistance in priority areas of need

Important lessons can be learned from past financial crises and the countries that have managed to avoid the most serious effects of crises. Governments play a critical role in providing social protection but face competing demands for funding (Marmot and Bell 2009). The onus is on health and social policy advocates to lobby strongly for political action to strengthen and maintain safety nets. Access to affordable healthcare is essential, and it may be necessary to re-prioritize resource allocation and find ways to diversify social and healthcare financing. Investment in prevention and early detection and treatment of illness is good public policy in times of economic crisis, and an urgent priority is the strengthening of mental health services in anticipation of the increased demand (Phua and Kua 2009). Economic crises should provide opportunities and the imperative to implement evidence-based health policies, to protect and expand public health budgets in order to avoid longer-term social and economic costs.

References

Abel-Smith, B. (1986). The world economic crisis. Part 1: Repercussions on health. *Health Policy and Planning, 1*(3), 202–213.

Abrahamson, P., Anderson, J., Henriksen, J., Jorgen, E. L., & Andersen, J. (1986). Unemployment and poverty in the contemporary welfare state. *Acta Sociologica, 29*(1), 51–60.

Adamchak, D. J. (1979). Emerging trends in the relationship between infant mortality and socio-economic status. *Social Biology, 26*(1), 16–29.

Australian Agency for International Development (AusAID). (2000). *Impact of the Asian financial crisis on health*. Melbourne: Macfarlane Burnet Centre for Medical Research.

Baum, A., Fleming, R., & Reddy, D. M. (1986). Unemployment stress: Loss of control, reactance and learned helplessness. *Social Science & Medicine, 22*(5), 509–516.

Bengtsson, T., & Ohlsson, R. (1985). Age specific mortality and short-term changes in the standard of living: Sweden, 1751–1859. *European Journal of Population, 1*(4), 309–326.

Bhutta, Z. A., Bawany, F. A., Feroze, A., & Rizvi, A. (2009). *The impact of the food and economic crisis on the nutrition of children*. Report of UNICEF Conference on Impact of the Economic Crisis on Children, 6–7 January 2009, Singapore.

Brenner, M. H. (1967). Economic change and mental hospitalization: New York State, 1910–1960. *Social Psychiatry and Psychiatric Epidemiology, 2*, 180–188.

Brenner, M. H. (1971). Economic changes and heart disease mortality. *American Journal of Public Health, 61*(3), 606–611.

Brenner, M. H. (1973a). Fetal, infant, and maternal mortality during periods of economic instability. *International Journal of Health Services, 3*(2), 145–159.

Brenner, M. H. (1973b). *Mental illness and the economy*. Cambridge, MA: Harvard University Press.

Brenner, M. H. (1975). Trends in alcohol consumption and associated illnesses: Some effects of economic changes. *American Journal of Public Health, 65*(12), 1279–1292.

Brenner, M. H. (1979). Mortality and the national economy. A review, and the experience of England and Wales, 1936–76. *The Lancet, 2*, 568–573.

Brenner, M. H. (1983). Mortality and economic instability: Detailed analysis for Britain and comparative analyses for selected industrialized countries. *International Journal of Health Services, 13*(4), 563–620.

Brenner, M. H. (1984). *Estimating the effects of national economic change on national and social well being*. Joint Economic Committee of the U.S. Congress. Washington, DC: Government Printing Office.

Brenner, M. H. (1987a). Relation of economic change to Swedish health and social well-being, 1950–1980. *Social Science & Medicine, 25*(2), 183–195.

Brenner, M. H. (1987b). Economic change, alcohol consumption and heart disease mortality in nine industrialized countries. *Social Science & Medicine, 25*(2), 119–132.

Brenner, M. H. (1987c). Economic instability, unemployment rates, behavioral risks, and mortality rates in Scotland, 1952–1983. *International Journal of Health Services, 17*(3), 475–487.

Brenner, M. H., & Mooney, A. (1982). Economic change and sex-specific cardiovascular mortality in Britain, 1955–1976. *Social Science & Medicine, 16*(4), 431–442.

Brenner, M. H., & Mooney, A. (1983). Unemployment and health in the context of economic change. *Social Science & Medicine, 17*(16), 1125–1138.

Bronfman, M. (1992). Infant mortality and crisis in Mexico. *International Journal of Health Services, 22*(1), 157–167.

Bunn, A. R. (1979). Ischaemic heart disease mortality and the business cycle in Australia. *American Journal of Public Health, 69*(8), 772–781.

Catalano, R., & Dooley, C. D. (1977). Economic predictors of depressed mood and stressful life events in a metropolitan community. *Journal of Health and Social Behavior, 18*(3), 292–307.

Catalano, R., & Dooley, C. D. (1979). The economy as a stressor: A sectoral analysis. *Review of Social Economy, 37*(2), 175–187.

Catalano, R., & Serxner, S. (1992). Neonatal mortality and the economy revisited. *International Journal of Health Services, 22*(2), 275–286.

Catalano, R., Dooley, D., & Jackson, R. (1981). Economic predictors of admissions to mental health facilities in a non-metropolitan community. *Journal of Health and Social Behavior, 22*(3), 284–297.

Chang, S. S., Gunnell, D., Sterne, J. A., Lu, T. H., & Cheng, A. T. (2009). Was the economic crisis 1997–1998 responsible for rising suicide rates in East/Southeast Asia? A time-trend analysis for

Japan, Hong Kong, South Korea, Taiwan, Singapore and Thailand. *Social Science & Medicine, 68*(7), 1322–1331.

Cobb, S. (1974). Physiological changes in men whose jobs were abolished. *Journal of Psychosomatic Research, 18*, 245–258.

Colombino, U. (1984). An econometric investigation of the condition of children in Italy. *World Development, 12*(3), 365–380.

Dooley, D., Catalano, R., Jackson, R., & Brownell, A. (1981). Economic, life, and symptom changes in a non-metropolitan community. *Journal of Health and Social Behaviour, 22*(2), 144–154.

Durkheim, E. (1951). *Suicide*. New York: Free Press.

Ensor, T., Cooper, S., Davidson, L., Fitzmaurice, A., & Graham, W. J. (2010). The impact of economic recession on maternal and infant mortality: Lessons From history. *BMC Public Health, 10*, 727. doi:10.1186/1471-2458-10-727.

ESCAP, ADB, & UNDP. (2008). *A future within reach*. Bangkok: UN ESCAP.

Eyer, J. (1977a). Prosperity as a cause of death. *International Journal of Health Services, 7*(1), 125–150.

Eyer, J. (1977b). Does unemployment cause the death rate peak in each business cycle? *International Journal of Health Services, 7*(4), 625–662.

Falagas, M. E., Vouloumanou, E. K., Mavros, M. N., & Karageorgopoulos, D. E. (2009). Economic crises and mortality: A review of the literature. *International Journal of Clinical Practice, 63*(8), 1128–1135.

Ferrie, J. E., Shipley, M., Stansfeld, S., & Marmot, M. (2002). Effects of chronic job insecurity and change in job security on self reported health, minor psychiatric morbidity, physiological measures and health related behaviours in British civil servants: The Whitehall II study. *Journal of Epidemiology and Community Health, 56*, 450–454.

Forbes, J. F., & McGregor, A. (1987). Male unemployment and cause-specific mortality in postwar Scotland. *International Journal of Health Services, 17*(2), 233–240.

Francisco, R., & Wan, G. (2009). *How is the global recession impacting on poverty and social spending? An ex ante assessment methodology with applications to developing Asia* (Asian Development Bank (ADB) Sustainable Development Working Paper Series No. 8). The Philippines: Asian Development Bank.

Freund, P. J. (1986). Health care in a declining economy: The case of Zambia. *Social Science & Medicine, 23*(9), 875–888.

Fronstin, P. (2010). The impact of the recession on employment-based health coverage. *EBRI Issue Brief, 342*, 1–22.

Graetz, B. (1993). Health consequences of employment and unemployment: Longitudinal evidence for males and females. *Social Science & Medicine, 36*(6), 715–724.

Gravelle, H. S. E., Hutchinson, G., & Stern, J. (1981). Mortality and unemployment: A critique of Brenner's time series analysis. *The Lancet, 2*, 675–679.

Grayson, J. P. (1989). Reported illness after a CGE closure. *Canadian Journal of Public Health, 80*, 16–19.

Hammarstrom, A., Janlert, U., & Theorell, T. (1988). Youth unemployment and ill health: Results from a 2-year follow-up study. *Social Science & Medicine, 26*(10), 1025–1033.

Harpham, T. (1986). Review article: Health and the urban poor. *Health Policy and Planning, 1*(1), 5–18.

Hintikka, J., Lehto, S. M., Niskanen, L., Huotari, A., Herzig, K.-H., Koivumaa-Honkanen, H., Honkalampi, K., Sinikallio, S., & Viinamaki, H. (2009). Unemployment and ill Health: A connection through inflammation? *BMC Public Health, 9*, 410.

Holahan, J. (2011). The 2007–09 recession and health insurance coverage. *Health Affairs, 30*(1), 145–152.

Horton, R. (2009). The global financial crisis: An acute threat to health. *The Lancet, 373*, 355–356.

International Monetary Fund (IMF). (2009). *The implications of the global financial crisis for low-income countries*. Washington, DC: IMF.

Jacinto, P. A., Tejada, C. A., & Sousa, T. R. (2010). Effects of macroeconomic conditions on health in Brazil. *Revista de Saúde Pública, 44*(2), 310–317.

Janlert, U. (2009). Economic crisis, unemployment and public health. *Scandinavian Journal of Public Health, 37*, 783–784.

John J., Schwefel, D., & Zollner, H. (Eds.) (1983). *Influence of economic instability on health: Proceedings of a symposium*. Munich, Federal Republic of Germany, 9–11 September 1981. Berlin/Heidelberg: Springer.

Jolly, R., & Cornia, G. A. (1984). Editors' introduction. *World Development, 12*(3), 171–176.

Kasl, S. V. (1979). Mortality and the business cycle: Some questions about research strategies using macrosociological and ecological data. *American Journal of Public Health, 69*(89), 784–788.

Kim, H., Chung, W. J., Song, Y. J., Kang, D. R., Yi, J. Y., & Nam, C. M. (2003). Changes in morbidity and medical care utilization after the recent economic crisis in the Republic of Korea. *Bulletin of the World Health Organization, 81*(8), 567–572.

Kwon, J. C., Chun, H., & Cho, S. (2009). A closer look at the increase in suicide rates in South Korea from 1986–2005. *BMC Public Health, 9*, 72. doi:10.1186/1471-2458-9-72.

Laporte, A. (2004). Do economic cycles have a permanent effect on population health? Revisiting the Brenner Hypothesis. *Health Economics, 13*, 767–779.

Lee, S., Guo, W. J., Tsang, A., Mark, A. D., Wu, J., Ng, K. L., & Kwok, K. (2010). Evidence for the 2008 economic crisis exacerbating depression in Hong Kong. *Journal of Affective Disorders, 126*(1–2), 125–133.

Leeflang, R. L., Klein-Hesselink, D. J., & Spruit, I. P. (1992a). Health effects of unemployment – I. Long-term unemployed men in a rural and an urban Setting. *Social Science & Medicine, 34*(4), 341–350.

Leeflang, R. L., Klein-Hesselink, D. J., & Spruit, I. P. (1992b). Health effects of unemployment – II. Men and women. *Social Science & Medicine, 34*(4), 351–363.

Levy, B. S., & Sidel, V. W. (Eds.). (2006). *Social injustice and public health*. New York: OUP.

Lew, E. A. (1979). Mortality and the business cycle: How far can we push an association? *American Journal of Public Health, 69*(8), 782–783.

Lewin, K. (1986). Educational finance in recession. *Prospects, 16*(2), 215–230.

Liem, R., & Liem, J. (1978). Social class and mental illness reconsidered: The role of economic stress and social support. *Journal of Health and Social Behaviour, 19*(2), 139–156.

Liem, R., & Rayman, P. (1982). Health and social costs of unemployment: Research and policy considerations. *The American Psychologist, 37*(10), 1116–1123.

Loewenson, R. (1989). Challenges to health in plantation economies: Recent trends. *Health Policy and Planning, 4*(4), 334–342.

Luoto, R., Poikolainen, K., & Uutela, A. (1998). Unemployment, sociodemographic background and consumption of alcohol before and during the economic recession of the 1990s in Finland. *International Journal of Epidemiology, 27*(4), 623–629.

MacMahon, B., & Yen, S. (1971). Unrecognized epidemic of anencephaly and spinal bifida. *The Lancet, 1*, 31–33.

Marmot, M., & Bell, R. (2009). How will the financial crisis affect health? *BMJ, 338*(858–860), b1314.

Meegama, S. A. (1980, April). *Socio-economic determinants of infant and child mortality in Sri Lanka: An analysis of post-war experience* (World Fertility Survey Sci Reports No. 8). Voorburg, The Netherlands: International Statistical Institute.

Meltzer, H., Bebbington, P., Brugha, T., Jenkins, R., McManus, S., & Stansfeld, S. (2010). Job insecurity, socio-economic circumstances and depression. *Psychological Medicine, 40*(8), 1301–1407.

Miller, C. A. (1985). Infant mortality in the U.S. *Scientific American, 253*(1), 31–37.

Miller, C. A., Coulter, E. J., Schorr, L. B., Fine, A., & Adams-Taylor, S. (1985a). The world economic crisis and the children: United States case study. *International Journal of Health Services, 15*(1), 95–134.

Miller, C. A., Coulter, E. J., Fine, A., Adams-Taylor, S., & Schorr, L. B. (1985b). 1984 update on the world economic crisis and the children: A United States case study. *International Journal of Health Services, 15*(3), 431–450.

Morrell, S., Taylor, R., Quine, S., & Kerr, C. (1993). Suicide and unemployment in Australia 1907–1990. *Social Science & Medicine, 36*(6), 749–756.

Morris, J. N., & Titmuss, R. M. (1944). Health and social change: Recent history of rheumatic heart disease. *The Medical Officer, 72*, 69–87.

Moser, K. A., Fox, A. J., & Jones, D. R. (1984). Unemployment and mortality in the OPCS longitudinal study. *The Lancet, 324*, 1324–1329.

Moser, K. A., Jones, D. R., Fox, A. J., & Goldblatt, P. O. (1986). Unemployment and mortality: Further evidence from the OPCS longitudinal study 1971–81. *The Lancet, 327*, 365–367.

Moser, K. A., Goldblatt, P. O., Fox, A. J., & Jones, D. R. (1987). Unemployment and mortality: Comparison of the 1971 and 1981 longitudinal study census samples. *BMJ, 294*, 86–90.

Muniz, J. G., Fabian, J. S., Manriquez, J. C., & Hertenberg, R. (1984). The recent worldwide economic crisis and the welfare of children: The case of Cuba. *World Development, 12*(3), 247–260.

Musgrove, P. (1987). The impact of the economic crisis on health and health care in Latin America and the Caribbean. *International Journal of Health Services, 17*(3), 411–441.

Narendranathan, W., Nickell, S., & Metcalf, D. (1985). An investigation into the incidence and dynamic structure of sickness and unemployment in Britain, 1965–1975. *Journal of the Royal Statistical Society Series A (General), 148*(P3), 254–267.

Ogburn, W., & Thomas, D. (1923). The influence of the business cycle on certain social conditions. *American Statistical Association Bulletin, 38*, 137–144.

Orivel, F. (1986). Economic crisis and educational crisis: Looking ahead. *Prospects, 16*(2), 197–204.

Ostamo, A., Lahelma, E., & Lonnqvist, J. (2001). Transitions of employment status among suicide attempters during a severe economic recession. *Social Science & Medicine, 52*(11), 1741–1750.

Phua, K. H., & Kua, E. H. (2009). Economic crisis and mental health services in Asia. *Asia Pacific Psychiatry, 1*(2), 55–57.

Platt, S., Micciolo, R., & Tansella, M. (1992). Suicide and unemployment in Italy: Description, analysis and interpretation of recent trends. *Social Science & Medicine, 34*(11), 1191–1201.

Rosero-Bixby, L. (1983, February 28–March 4). *Social and economic policies and their effects on mortality: The case of Costa Rica*. Paris: IUSSP-INED.

Ruhm, C. J. (2000). Are recessions good for your health? *The Quarterly Journal of Economics, 115*, 617–650.

Ruhm, C. J. (2007). A healthy economy can break your heart. *Demography, 44*, 829–848.

Singer, H. W. (1937). *Unemployment and health* (Pilgrim Trust Enquiry, Interim Paper No. 4). Transcipt by The National Archives of the UK is available online at http://www.nationalarchives.gov.uk/education/topics/going-short.htm

Solantaus, T., Leinonen, J., & Punamaki, R. L. (2004). Children's mental health in times of economic recession: Replication and extension of the family economic stress model in Finland. *Developmental Psychology, 40*(3), 412–429.

Starrin, B., Larsson, G., Brenner, S. O., Levi, L., & Petterson, I. L. (1990). Structural changes, ill health, and mortality in Sweden, 1963–1983: A macroaggregated study. *International Journal of Health Services, 20*(1), 27–42.

Stefansson, C. (1991). Long-term unemployment and mortality in Sweden, 1980–1986. *Social Science & Medicine, 32*(4), 419–423.

Stern, J. (1983). The relationship between unemployment, morbidity and mortality in Britain. *Population Studies, 37*(1), 61–74.

Stuckler, D., & Basu, S. (2009). The International Monetary Fund's effects on global health: Before and after the 2008 financial crisis. *International Journal of Health Services, 39*(4), 771–781.

Stuckler, D., Basu, S., Suhrcke, M., & McKee, M. (2009a). The health implications of financial crisis: A review of the evidence. *The Ulster Medical Journal, 78*(3), 142–145.

Stuckler, D., Basu, S., Suhrcke, M., Coutts, A., & Mckee, M. (2009b). The public health effect of economic crises and alternative policy responses in Europe: An empirical analysis. *The Lancet, 374*(9686), 315–323.

Stuckler, D., Basu, S., & McKee, M. (2010). Budget crises, health, and social welfare programmes. *BMJ, 340*, c3311. doi:10.1136/bmj.c3311.

Suh, S. M. (1984). Effects of the current world recession on the welfare of children: The case of Korea. *World Development, 12*(3), 329–338.

Tapia Granados, J. A. (2005a). Increasing mortality during the expansion of the US economy, 1900–1996. *International Journal of Epidemiology, 34*, 1194–1202.

Tapia Granados, J. A. (2005b). Recessions and mortality in Spain, 1980–1997. *European Journal of Population, 21*, 393–422.

Tapia Granados, J. A. (2008). Macroeconomic fluctuations and mortality in postwar Japan. *Demography, 45*, 323–343.

Thomas, D. S. (1925). *Social aspects of the business cycle*. London: Routledge.

UNICEF. (2009). *Report of UNICEF conference on Impact of the Economic Crisis on Children*, 6–7 January 2009, Singapore.

Uutela, A. (2010). Economic crisis and mental health. *Current Opinion in Psychiatry, 23*(2), 127–130.

Wagstaff, A. (1985). Time series analysis of the relationship between unemployment and mortality: A survey of economic critiques and replications of Brenner's studies. *Social Science & Medicine, 21*(9), 985–996.

Wang, J., Smailes, E., Sareen, J., Fick, G. H., Schmitz, N., & Patten, S. B. (2010). The prevalence of mental disorders in the working population over the period of global economic crisis. *Canadian Journal of Psychiatry, 55*(9), 598–605.

Waters, H., Saadah, F., & Pradhan, M. (2003). The impact of the 1997–98 East Asian economic crisis on health and health care in Indonesia. *Health Policy and Planning, 18*(2), 172–181.

Westin, S., Norum, D., & Schlesselman, J. J. (1988). Medical consequences of a factory closure: Illness and disability in a four year follow-up study. *International Journal of Epidemiology, 17*, 153–160.

Wood, C. H. (1982). The political economy of infant mortality in Sao Paulo, Brazil. *International Journal of Health Services, 12*(2), 215–229.

Yang, B. M., Prescott, N., & Bae, E. Y. (2001). The impact of economic crisis on health-care consumption in Korea. *Health Policy and Planning, 16*(4), 372–385.

Zilko, C. E. (2010). Economic contraction and birth outcomes: An integrative review. *Human Reproduction Update, 16*(4), 445–458.

Chapter 14
Policy Responses in an Unstable Globalized Economy: Multi-stressed Low-Earning Families in Singapore

Irene Y.H. Ng and Kong Weng Ho

Introduction

Since the 1980s, the income divide in Singapore has been on an upward trend (Ng 2010), and more recently, low-skilled wages have been stagnating (Yeoh 2007: 7–12). The 2008 income trends reported by the Department of Statistics showed that a family in the bottom 10 % earned less than S$1,310 per month or less than S$340 per capita per month (Department of Statistics Singapore 2009). Compared to the year 2000 and in real terms, this was a decrease for household earnings and an increase of only 2 % for per capita earnings.

Traditionally, Singapore has relied on a social protection model based on economic growth and its trickle down benefits. It provided welfare only to the aged or disabled, who are unable to work. Heavy investments were and still are being made in human capital development to meet the economic objectives of growth and competitiveness, through building quality yet affordable housing, education, and healthcare. In recent years, as it became more evident that low-wage earners are finding it harder and harder to eke out a living despite their best efforts, the social safety net in Singapore was expanded to include workfare.

Workfare, which I define as financial aid conditional on work, began in Singapore in 2006, when a workfare bonus and the Work Support Program (WSP) were introduced. The workfare bonus, which in 2007 became a permanent scheme called the Workfare Income Supplement (WIS), is a cash and savings payout to low-wage workers (Central Provident Fund Board 2009). WSP offers job placement and other assistance to remove barriers to work, besides a monthly cash assistance (Ministry of

I.Y.H. Ng (✉)
Department of Social Work, National University of Singapore, Singapore
e-mail: swknyhi@nus.edu.sg

K.W. Ho
Department of Economics, National University of Singapore, Singapore
e-mail: ecshkw@nus.edu.sg

W.J.J. Yeung and M.T. Yap (eds.), *Economic Stress, Human Capital, and Families in Asia: Research and Policy Challenges*, Quality of Life in Asia 4,
DOI 10.1007/978-94-007-7386-8_14, © Springer Science+Business Media Dordrecht 2013

Community Development, Youth and Sports 2010b). WIS is available to individuals whose monthly earnings are $1,500 or less and WSP to those whose household earnings are $1,500 or less.[1] Clearly, workfare is only for earners in the very bottom.

The 2008 global recession put many families in financial difficulties. Real economic growth slowed from 8.9 % in 2007 to 1.7 % in 2008 and turned negative to −1.0 % in 2009. The resident unemployment rate increased from 3.2 % in 2008 to 4.3 % in 2009. Although still low relative to other countries, the 34 % increase from a low base was significant (Department of Statistics Singapore 2011). What might the plight of bottom earners be during the recession and in the future? What about low-wage earners whose earnings are not low enough to qualify for workfare? This paper analyzes the impact of the recession and subsequent policies on low-wage earners. It is not interested in those in the middle or upper classes. Nor is it about the poor who cannot work. The focus is on those who are considered to be work-capable, yet struggle to make ends meet on their stagnating and low wages. This group is particularly vulnerable in several ways. First, compared to the poor who cannot work, the social safety net for the working poor is less clear. Some may argue that the safety net for the nonworking poor is insufficient, but public assistance for them has at least been permanently in place for decades, with periodic review. Second, the economic well-being of low-wage earners is increasingly uncertain. The current skill-biased globalized economic development will continue to erode jobs and wages of those with low education and skills. Third, economic stress of low earnings is often interrelated with social factors in the family that compound or are compounded by low earnings. Hence, the effects being analyzed are socioeconomic effects; the social and economic effects are interdependent.

The rest of the paper proceeds as follows. First, the socioeconomic conditions of low-earning families are explicated through a model of the multiple stressors experienced by low-wage earners. Next, policies and programs introduced in the aftermath of the 2008 recession are described. The multi-stressed low-earning family model is then illustrated with statistics and case examples from a pilot study of recipients of WSP, followed by a presentation of administrative data showing the duration of WSP assistance, and changes in economic conditions of recipients before and after WSP. Finally, the policies and programs are discussed in light of the data showing that recipients of a short-term program are experiencing multiple disadvantages.

A Model of Multi-stressed Low-Earning Families

Adapting from the family stress model outlined by Conger and Dogan (2007: 433–460), Fig. 14.1 depicts the multiple stressors on a family in economic hardship. In Conger and Dogan, economic pressures from financial hardship create familial

[1]This criterion has been revised in April 2012 to household income not exceeding $1,700 or per capita income not exceeding $550.

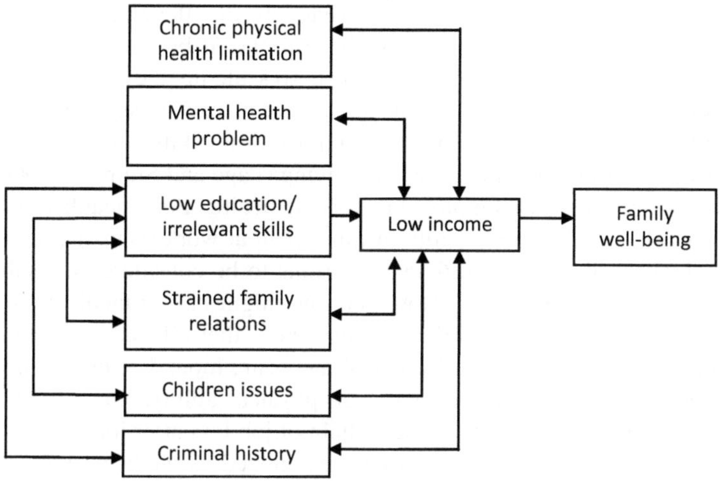

Fig. 14.1 A model of multi-stressed low-earning families (*Note*: A simplified version of the model is also published in Ng 2013)

conflict or withdrawal (leading to separation or divorce) and cause emotional distress. Such conflict and distress in turn result in child maladjustment. The model in this paper extends on the family stress model by specifying the kinds of stressors interrelated with low earnings (indicated by double-headed arrows). The stressors in the modified model, which I shall name a model of multi-stressed families, were identified by their repeated attribution in government reports, media articles, the author's participant observations at meetings with practitioners, as well as results from a pilot study with recipients of WSP. The relationships between the stressors and earnings were also informed by theories and findings in current scholarly research.

While the stressors identified in the model might affect families independently of earnings, anchoring family functioning and well-being on earnings is generally reflective of stressed families in the current economic order. The current world order is based on the economic market. In an urban society like Singapore in particular, livelihood depends on employment-based income – either you hire somebody, somebody hires you, or you hire yourself. Without a job, one has limited means of sustenance.

There was a time when globalization brought more jobs for everyone in Singapore. Being an open economy meant increasing trade and foreign direct investments, bringing with them employment opportunities as well as the opportunities to better education. Today, however, globalization means that low-skilled wages are kept down by relocation of standardized processes to cheaper destinations and the importing of foreign workers (Yeoh 2007). This globalized economic order is a threat to those with low education and irrelevant skills. I use the term "irrelevant skills" because the skills that are valued in today's technology-intensive economy are very different from the skills of yesteryears. To me, the clog maker or hawker has skills, but theirs are skills that have been replaced by machines and that are difficult to scale up to the global mass market. To scale up, they will need the skills of professionals such as logistics engineers, marketing executives, or web designers. So at first base, those with low education and irrelevant skills will have greater and greater difficulty improving their means of living (Page and Simmons 2000).

Another reason for low employability is ill health. Poor health affects one's quality of work and also the quantity of time spent at work (Danziger et al. 2002). If the medical condition was sufficiently serious to be considered a disability, the individual could receive welfare. However, one might have a medically minor but chronic condition – such as arthritis or migraine – that affects work but does not qualify one for government aid. Physical ailments are more deleterious in unskilled jobs because manual jobs depend more on physical ability. Worse still, a work-related injury might be the start of one's chain of job loss after job loss.

Mental health conditions are even less recognized as medical or valid reasons for missing work or decreased effectiveness at work (Danziger et al. 2002). Again, such health problems might have resulted from work, as anxiety and depression over financial difficulties from a low-paying job exacerbates one's inability to work.

Individuals with low earnings might also struggle with family problems (Voydanoff 1990: 1099–1115). Long hours at work translate into less family time, and stress over financial problems put a strain on relationships. In the other direction, problems at home affect productivity at work (Forthofer et al. 1996: 597–605). Marital conflict might worsen to the point of marital breakup. Yeung and Hofferth (1998) found that families that experienced substantial income loss were more likely to divorce or separate. When that happens, pooled resources are split, putting in particular women with low education and irrelevant skills in a vulnerable financial situation. Similarly, single parents have much fewer resources for bringing up children (Lerman 2002).

As economic distress takes its toll on parents' mental health and marital relationships, parenting is affected too. The result is problems in children's cognitive-socio-emotional development as well. Conger and Dogan (2007) related low earnings to children's outcomes only through parenting, but since the model here aims to show the relationship between low earnings and other stressors and not between the stressors, I simplify the model by a direct bidirectional line between low earnings and children's problems. The line is bidirectional because while work problems affect children's development, children's problems such as intensive caregiving for a sickly child or emergency response to a wayward adolescent take parents' time and attention from work.

Difficulty finding gainful employment creates another set of very specific problems when one turns to unlawful means of living. Criminology studies have shown the strong correlation between low earnings and crime (Freeman 1999: 3529–3571; Messner et al. 2001: 591–614). Economics of crime literature have also shown that criminals often flow in and out of crime and employment (Freeman 1999: 3529–3571). Afterall, compared to someone with a high-paying job, they have less to lose if they are caught and imprisoned. Thereafter, the stigma of a criminal record becomes a barrier to employment.

A final set of interrelations are between low education and the other stressors. Low education has been shown by research to relate with marital relationships, children's upbringing (Lareau 2003), and crime (Lochner 2004: 811–843; Lochner and Moretti 2004: 155–189). Given the importance of education and skills in the current economy, Fig. 14.1 therefore also shows bidirectional arrows between low education and family relationships, children, and crime.

While richer families might also face similar social stressors, their financial resources enable them to purchase services to cope. Health, for example, can be greatly improved and maintained with preventive care and medication. For the poor, a minor health condition might be left alone until it needs emergency attention. The need for caregiving can also be resolved with paid services. When a marriage breaks up, a woman with low education will have much more difficulties finding a sustainable livelihood than a more educated woman. In terms of adapting to income loss, Yeung and Hofferth (1998) found that families with more preexisting resources, such as income and assets, and living in an area with low unemployment were more able to adapt by cutting expenses, moving, or increasing work hours of another family member.

This model of multi-stressed low-earning families leads to two policy implications. First, temporary assistance focused on financial aid will have limited effectiveness in uplifting low-earning families. Second, the challenges faced by low-income families in the current globalized economy transcend economic booms and recessions and require more structural interventions. This article does not have the data to evaluate a particular policy or program. Instead it provides an analysis of the policy responses in Singapore during the 2008 financial crisis in terms of their possible effects on multi-stressed low-earning families.

Policy Response

The Singapore government responded swiftly to the 2008 recession. The government budget for 2009 was announced a month earlier, so that new countermeasures could be quickly rolled out. The initiatives were bold. For the first time in Singapore's history, the budget was so large that the government was to incur a deficit of 6 % of GDP and had to dip into its reserves. The key initiatives were aimed at saving companies in order to save jobs. The government shared up to 80 % of the risk of business loans, gave per employee jobs credits to employers, and lowered the corporate tax rate. Other interventions to safeguard jobs included a temporary top-up to WIS and expansion of the Skills Program for Upgrading and Resilience (SPUR). While the former clearly supports low-wage earners, SPUR was expanded to "step up training across all levels of the workforce, including our PMETs (professionals, managers, executives, and technicians)." Additional help for PMETs was introduced, for example, through on-the-job training for fresh graduates and co-sharing with companies for training of engineering and technical jobs (Ministry of Finance 2009).

The initiatives from the then Ministry of Community Development, Youth and Sports (MCYS) (MCYS has been renamed Ministry of Social and Family Development with effect from 1 November 2012) during that time recognized the economic as well social hardships of families. In a press release by MCYS on 21 May 2009, the Ministry listed the target populations of its commitment to "provide hope and assurance for the needy" as "(a) those who are permanently unable to work and have no family support; (b) those who are usually able to cope in good times, but are thrown into distress by the economic downturn; and (c) dysfunctional families plagued by multiple and chronic problems." For group (a), public assistance quanta were increased (Ministry of Community Development, Youth and Sports 2009a). For group (b), besides the employment and skills upgrading initiatives previously highlighted, MCYS made the eligibility and duration of WSP more flexible in order to extend help to those who were retrenched. ComCare Transitions had also been introduced the year before, providing "medium-term" help for those who are unable to work (Ministry of Community Development, Youth and Sports 2010a).

It was, however, the third group that the Minister for Community Development, Youth and Sports focused his 2009 budget speech on. Defining dysfunctional families as "those who experience multiple or severe problems that adversely affect the well-being of the family," MCYS would set aside $25 million a year over the next 5 years to identify at-risk families early, intervene to strengthen their resilience, and resource the community to better help such families (Ministry of Community Development, Youth and Sports 2009b). The newest initiative was a pilot Intensive Case Management program with 150 high-risk families. Social workers would work with at most 10 families at any one time, a sharply reduced load from regular case work of 40–50 families (Ministry of Community Development, Youth and Sports 2009b, c).

Multiple Stressors Experienced by Work Support Program Recipients

Anchored on the model of multi-stressed low-earning families, how responsive low-wage earners would have been to the policy initiatives will depend on how prevalent the multiple stressors are among low-income families in Singapore. An indication that the model does hold is provided by a pilot research study of recipients of the Work Support Program. As introduced earlier, WSP provides financial and other assistance to recipients who are work-able. For families with children below 18 years of age, case management is provided. A case officer draws up an action plan of steps to take in consultation with the family to enable them to become financially independent and monitors the progress of the family in achieving action steps. The action items in the case management framework cover seven areas that might act as barriers to financial independence, including employment, finance, health, children, shelter, food, and social support. Case managers refer clients to relevant

Table 14.1 Pilot WSP respondents by Community Development Council and sex

CDC/sex	Male	Female	Total
Northeast	3	5	8
Northwest	2	10	12
Southeast	5	6	11
Southwest	2	3	5
Central	3	11	14
Total	15	35	50

agencies when a particular area of need is identified. WSP is a voluntary program, where recipients have to apply for assistance. It is disbursed by five Community Development Councils (CDCs) which are distributed across Singapore to represent different geographical areas.

The pilot was conducted to test the survey questionnaire and the interview guide for a longitudinal study that would follow WSP recipients from program entry until 3 years after they leave the program. The pilot also served as a starting point to understand the backgrounds of WSP recipients. The study focused on recipients who were being case managed and who therefore had children younger than 18 years old. The pilot surveyed 50 recipients who had been placed on WSP for less than a month. It also conducted more in-depth interviews with five of the recipients.

Beginning in September 2009, names of approved applicants were given by the CDCs. Applicants were contacted to participate in the research until January 2010, when 50 respondents was reached. Respondents were selected to have a representation by CDC, sex of recipient, and ethnicity of respondent. Table 14.1 provides the distribution of the 50 respondents by the CDCs and sex.[2] The numbers reflect roughly the relative sizes of the CDCs and sex profile of the applicants.

Table 14.2 reveals high prevalence rates in each of the stressors among respondents. While providing a helpful appreciation for the life struggles of WSP recipients, it must be noted that due to the small sample size, the results cannot be taken as representative of WSP recipients in general.

Consistent with the criteria for receiving assistance through WSP, the top reasons given for what prompted respondents of the pilot study to apply for assistance included utilities (54 %), mortgage/rental (44 %), and other arrears (44 %), followed by job loss (26 %). Mean household income was $1,061 per month, with a minimum reported of $20 and maximum $2,300. Income from other sources besides work amounted to an average of $238.58. Dividing by household size gives a per capita income of only $304.48. These numbers suggest that WS families are among the bottom tenth percentile of the income distribution, with a few exceptions whose earnings were higher. According to the Income Trends Report by the Department of Statistics (2009), the tenth percentile monthly income from work in 2008 was $1,310 for the whole household and $340 per household member. In contrast, the mean income levels of the pilot sample were lower, and it included nonwork income such as financial aid and informal support.

[2]Statistics on ethnicity will not be published.

Table 14.2 Socioeconomic statistics of 50 Work Support recipients

	No.	%	Mean	Min	Max	*N*
Reasons for approaching CDC						
Owed too much utility bills	27	54				50
Owed HDB too much mortgage/rent arrears	22	44				50
Owed too much of other bills	22	44				50
Lost his/her job	13	26				50
Income per month						
Household income			$1,060.72	$20	$2,300	44
Income from nonwork sources			$238.58	$0	$850	37
Per capita household income			$304.48	$6.67	$2,300	44
Past year employment status						
Males less than full time	14	36				39
Females less than full time	29	67				43
Main reasons for males less than full-time work						
Ill health or disability	4	29				14
Criminal record	4	29				14
Need more education	2	14				14
No jobs available	2	14				14
Main reasons for females less than full-time work						
Prefer/need to stay at home with children	13	45				29
Need to care for ill/disabled child/children	6	21				29
Cost of child care	4	14				29
Ill health or disability	4	14				29
Highest educational level attained						
PSLE and below	26	52				50
"N" level/ITE	19	38				50
"O" level	2	4				50
"A" level/diploma	3	6				50
Degree and above	0	0				50
Physical health						
Has chronic health condition that limits work	21	44				48
Mental health						
Generally depressed	18	37				49
Generalized anxiety disorder	23	47				49
Marital status						
Divorced	9	18				50
Child's health						
Has a child with a physical, learning, or mental health condition that limits regular activities	16	33				48
Asthma	8	16				50
Learning/behavioral problem	4	8				50
Mental retardation	3	6				50

(continued)

Table 14.2 (continued)

	No.	%	Mean	Min	Max	*N*
Mental/emotional illness	3	6				50
Child's physical, learning, or mental health Interfered work or regular activities	11	24				46
Parenting						
Completely agree that being a parent is harder than I thought	26	52				50
Completely agree with feeling trapped by responsibility as a parent	18	37				49
Completely agree that taking care of child (children) is much more work than pleasure	13	26				50
Completely agree with often feeling tired, worn out, or exhausted from raising a family	13	26				50
Completely agree with all four statements	6	12				50
Criminal record						
Criminal record	11	22				50
Spouse with a criminal record or is in prison	6	12				50

In the past year, combining responses on self and spouse, 36 % of male respondents worked less than full time. Their reasons for working less than full time included needing more education, unavailability of jobs, ill health or disability, criminal record, transportation problems, and needing to stay at home with children. For females, 67 % worked less than full time. The most common reason given was the need to stay at home with children (45 %). Another two common reasons included ill health or disability and the need to care for a sick or disabled child. These reasons echo the stressors in the model.

Other questions in the survey reveal that the stressors in the model applied to many respondents. Respondents had very low education: about half had only PSLE as their highest qualification and none had a degree. Many respondents were in poor physical health, with 44 % reporting a chronic health or medical condition that prevents them from attending work, affecting their work performance, or preventing them from regular exercise. Common conditions cited included arthritis, asthma, back problems, headaches, and high blood pressure. Divorce rate among the respondents (18 %) was higher than the national average of 0.8 % (Ministry of Community Development, Youth and Sports 2009d). Mental health of respondents was also poor. Applying the Kessler-6 psychological distress scale, 37 % of the pilot respondents could be considered emotionally depressed (Kessler et al. 2002: 959–976; $\alpha = 0.89$). Further, 47 % met the conditions for generalized anxiety disorder – being worried more than half the time, finding it difficult to control worry, and at least having three of six symptoms of anxiety (Liebowitz 1996: 432–436; $\alpha = 0.72$). A substantial number also had challenges bringing up children. In a set of four statements indicating difficulties in parenting, six out of 50 respondents completely agreed with all four statements. 33 % had a child with a physical, learning, or mental health condition that limited regular activities. The most commonly cited conditions included asthma (8), learning/behavioral problems (4), mental retardation (3), and mental or emotional illness (3). Finally, a high percentage of respondents had criminal records, with 11 % self-reporting a criminal record and 12 % reporting that spouse had a criminal record or were in prison.

While the statistics from the pilot study show high rates among WSP respondents of individual stresses in life, how many of them face multiple stressors? All the respondents had low earnings. This is one source of stress. Six other sources of stress were aggregated. They included low education (highest education level at PSLE), poor physical health (health limited work), poor mental health (depressed and generalized anxiety disorder), single parenthood, children problems, and self or spouse with criminal record. Including low earnings, the mean, median, and mode number of stressors experienced by respondents was three. Sixteen (32 %) faced four or more types of stressors. More strikingly, the majority of the respondents experienced three or more stressors, that is, two other stressors besides low earnings.

Two out of the five cases where in-depth interviews were conducted provide a richer picture of the multiple stresses these vulnerable families were experiencing. The two cases illustrate two kinds of multi-stressed families. For family B, they were just getting by, but one trigger event unraveled into a series of events including imprisonment, job loss, and piling arrears. For family C, several series of events led to one episode of financial hardship after another.

Mr B (29 years old) and Mrs B (26 years old) have five young children, aged 7, 5, 4, 3, and 2. They got into financial difficulties just as things were looking up:

> Based on the husband's work as a delivery man, they had just saved up enough money to purchase a HDB flat. However, the new mailing address from the flat purchase triggered the authorities to dispatch notices of unpaid compounded parking summons incurred several years ago with a former company. The former boss was supposed to pay the fines but did not. Unable to pay the fines, Mr B was sentenced to jail and had his driving license, his primary source of livelihood, suspended. They then had to sell their flat because they could not make regular housing loan payments. Life began to sink rapidly as Mr B was in jail for a period and could not find a job after his release. (Ng et al. 2010)

With education only up to primary 6, a criminal record, and driving his only skill, Mr B felt frustrated idling at home instead of working. Mrs B had an 'N' level qualification. However, as she had to fetch her young children to and from school and look after them, she could only take on part-time jobs. Both, however, aspired to move out of their rental apartment into a bigger apartment of their own. They also tried not to skimp too much in spending on their children.

Ms C (28 years old) was in her second marriage and had three young children, aged 9, 5, and 4. Her husband (40 years old) had a criminal record. Both had studied only up to primary 6. Ms C had also experienced financial hardship in her first marriage, when she was married to her first husband who was a drug addict and was in and out of prison. Ms C is under treatment for diabetes and depression. However, she had stopped working not because of her ill health, but because her husband had found a full-time job and one of them needed to stay at home to take care of the children. One of the children had bronchitis. However, her husband lost his job due to a heart problem, and this triggered them to apply for government assistance.

From Administrative Data: Program Information of WSP Recipients Who Exited in 2009

That WSP adopts a case management approach suggests that the program has the potential for working with recipients on their different stressors that prevent work. However, MCYS is also clear in its publicity that WSP is meant to be a temporary program. The maximum duration of assistance is 24 months. With administrative data from MCYS on WSP recipients who completed WSP in 2009 (and therefore a different group from the pilot sample who started WSP at the end of 2009), this section shows the temporary nature of WSP and the lack of change in recipients' economic situation before and after the program.

Table 14.3 reports the mean duration of WSP assistance for recipients exiting the program in 2009. On average, WS participants received 6.72 months of assistance in 2009. A very low percentage of the WS participants, with an average of 1.20 % in 2009, reached the maximum of 24 months of assistance. Table 14.4 provides supporting evidence that WS had been an interim program aimed to deal with short-term economic stress, as the average duration of assistance was slightly more than half a year.

Table 14.4 gives the mean change in gross[3] monthly household income, gross monthly individual income, total household expenditure, and total debt[4] between the time of entry into and exit from the program of WSP recipients who completed the program within the year 2009. Overall, the changes are in the desired directions, with increases in income and decreases in expenses and debt. However, with large standard deviations, no indicator is statistically different from zero. In other words,

Table 14.3 Mean duration in program of recipients who exited WSP in 2009

Months of exit	Months in program	Percent with duration 24 months and above (%)
Jan–Mar	8.10	1.32
$N = 228$	(6.56)	
Apr–Jun	6.08	1.58
$N = 252$	(5.32)	
Jul–Sep	6.06	0.92
$N = 434$	(4.45)	
Oct–Dec	7.05	1.20
$N = 415$	(4.93)	

Note: N refers to the sample size for each quarter. The sample sizes reported in Table 14.3 are different from those reported in Table 14.4 because of missing observations in some variables. Figures in parentheses refer to the standard deviations

[3]Gross income refers to income before deduction of contribution to one's Central Provident Fund (CPF), a compulsory savings scheme.

[4]Total debt includes mortgage, rent, utilities, and conservancy charges.

Table 14.4 Mean change in income, expenditure, and debt between program entry and exit of recipients who exited WSP in 2009

Exit months	Change in gross monthly household income (S$)	Change in gross monthly individual income (S$)	Change in monthly household expenditure (S$)	Change in total debt (S$)
Jan–Mar	191	114	−93	85
$N = 199$	(739)	(445)	(497)	(12,359)
Apr–Jun	369	180	−49	−1,924
$N = 223$	(1,140)	(587)	(474)	(13,422)
Jul–Sept	335	239	−195	−633
$N = 394$	(932)	(651)	(1,050)	(13,680)
Oct–Dec	412	183	−73	−572
$N = 364$	(841)	(982)	(512)	(7,391)

Note: N refers to the sample size for each quarter. The changes are expressed in Singapore dollars S$. Figures in parentheses refer to the standard deviations

there was no improvement in their household income or individual income and no reduction in household expenditure or total debt. It could be that their economic performance might have worsened without participation in WSP. However, noting that late 2008 was when the global financial crisis hit and that recovery began in late 2009, the lack of change in WSP recipients' economic performance might also suggest that the struggles of many in this group and the assistance to them transcend economic trends.

Discussion

How much did the postrecession policy responses help multi-stressed families? I would like to offer three observations. First, the recession was both a bane and a boon to multi-stressed families. At the same time that it increased their risk of financial hardship through retrenchment or pay cut, the recession also increased government and societal aid to them. Where assistance used to be restrictive and stringently guarded, they became more generous in criteria and amounts during the recession. Figure 14.2 gives the numbers of WSP (self-reliance) applications from quarter four of 2008, around when the financial crisis hit, to the third quarter of 2009. It shows the high numbers of applications at the end of 2008 and beginning of 2009 and the tapering off in the second half of 2009. While WSP increased its intake such that approval rates were slightly higher than usual, the much larger number of applications during the peak of recession also implies that a larger number of people who requested assistance did not receive help through WSP. They might have received help through other programs and agencies, but the programs in the recession package were well targeted for those at the bottom as well as for professionals. Low-wage earners who did not clearly meet the criteria for

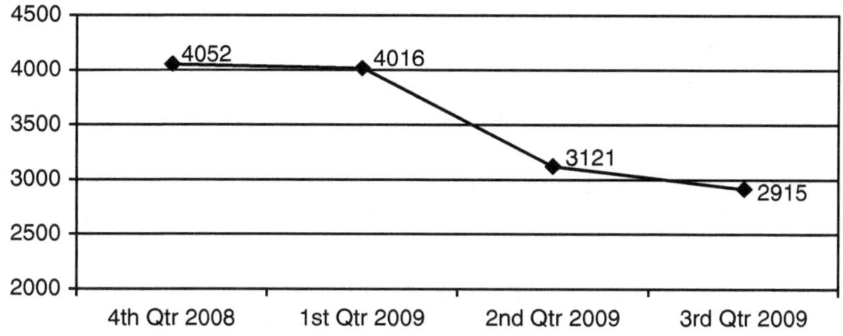

Fig. 14.2 Applications to Work Support self-reliance, 2008 Quarter 4–2009 Quarter 3 (*Source*: Data provided by MCYS)

assistance through programs such as WIS, ComCare Transitions, or WSP might have received inadequate assistance. These might include workers who had their wages cut suddenly, but not to levels below the eligibility criteria of the programs.

My second observation is that policies and programs introduced during the recession were probably effective to help many families tide through the recession, but not (1) some families with multiple challenges and not (2) families through longer-term hardships. For one, the programs introduced in response to the recession would be slowly withdrawn. However, for the low-wage multi-stressed household, the problems of stagnating wages and employability are permanent problems and not problems during the recession only. Further, multi-stressed families face not just economic problems, but other social challenges that nevertheless affect their economic functioning. The results of the pilot survey of WS recipients reflect this. The pilot was conducted in the last quarter of 2009, when the worst of the recession ended. However, the WSP pilot findings clearly show that respondents were experiencing multiple challenges that go beyond recession woes, challenges such as own and children's health, and criminal history. Although Intensive Case Management was introduced to help families facing multiple problems, currently it is targeted only for families facing the most challenging issues, while WSP provides only interim help. The results from the WSP administrative data in 2009 bears this out. Duration of assistance is short, and economic conditions of recipients did not significantly improve.

My third observation is that low-earning multi-stressed families need help beyond recession measures and economic assistance. Commentators such as Tan (2009) have cautioned that to be forward-looking, the plight of low-skilled workers would be a continuing challenge requiring government intervention. The Singapore government is well aware of this challenge. On 1 February 2010, the Economic Strategies Committee (ESC) released its recommendations for Singapore's economic development. With the aim "to sustain Singapore's development as well as ensure that growth is inclusive" (Economic Strategies Committee 2010), its prescription for inclusive growth included the following two noteworthy proposals for low-wage workers: (a) increasing productivity through innovation, continued education and training (CET), and reducing reliance on foreign workers and (b) reviewing the WIS (Chia 2010). Through these efforts, low-wage workers would be supported for working, and their earnings could be improved by higher productivity. The Singapore government is also well aware of the social struggles of low-income families, besides economic distress. Social programs such as Intensive Case Management and WSP were introduced exactly in recognition that families need to be helped holistically in various manners.

These initiatives are promising. They target the socioeconomic factors that have been identified as key to social and economic functioning. However, the current policies to support multi-stressed low-income families might be insufficient for two reasons. First, while the policy as stated looks adequate, how recipients are helped ultimately depends on the implementation of the policies. As a first example, many programs in Singapore continue to emphasize self-reliance with temporary help from the government although low wage and employability are structural problems that will likely worsen. On the WSP website, the words "if your household needs assistance to tide over a difficult period" clearly spell out that help is only for a temporary duration (Ministry of Community Development, Youth and Sports 2010b). While such a position has well-founded wisdom in preventing dependency, evaluation results in the USA have shown unsustainable self-sufficiency in welfare-to-work programs, especially from those that gave lower amounts of assistance (Hamilton et al. 2001; Swartz and Corbett 2001; Department of Workforce Development 2001; Nightingale and Mikelson 2000; Piliavin et al. 2003). Well-known poverty experts in the USA such as Sheldon Danziger, William Julius Wilson, and Peter Gottschalk have begun proposing the need for a "guaranteed work" policy (Page and Simmons 2000: 224). Due to the eroding of jobs and earnings of low-wage workers, workfare programs will have limited effectiveness, especially for workers who face multiple barriers to work, because they predicate on jobs being available. Therefore, government assistance might need to go beyond mandating work to providing work.

As a second example of implementation making a difference, the case management aspect of WSP is important in addressing the various barriers to employment that recipients might have. However, how the case management is conducted could make a crucial difference. A collection of articles on welfare-to-work programs in different countries in Hoefer and Midgley (2006) found that the USA (generally) emphasizes mandates and sanctions, whereas the UK apparently takes a more support-oriented approach. From the perspective of the multi-stressed model, the UK way should be more effective, since it is more empathic towards the stressful experiences of recipients. The Singapore Work Support Program seems more similar to the US model. After all, we started workfare-type schemes not from a welfare model, but from a work-based model. Welfare in the form of public assistance in Singapore had been stringently guarded. We had no safety net for those who were working but poor. So in introducing WIS and other workfare schemes such as WSP, we came with a philosophy of mandating work. In the case management in WSP, recipients sign an action plan with their case officer, which case officers monitor.

The third example of implementation affecting effectiveness of policies highlights some limitations that might arise from how the government will roll out the ESC recommendations. The ESC recommendations rightly target the macro-level structural issues of earnings and employment cautioned by evaluation studies and poverty experts. The implementation question is how to improve employment, productivity, and wage of the low skilled. At first base, as pointed out by Law Professor Tan (2010), there are "severe constraints in significantly raising the productivity of low-skilled workers." Indeed, a recommendation to enhance WIS is recognition of this fact. One of the ways mooted to improve productivity is to increase the foreign workers' levy. To this, Economist Lim (2010) cautioned that raising the foreign workers' levy might have similar effects to the high labor costs in the 1980s that were said to have contributed to the subsequent recession. For some low-wage earners, the upward push in wages in this scenario might mean unemployment. This brings us back to the conundrum of workfare: no job, no workfare. The current recommendations to improve productivity, in particular for those with low skills, are largely employment based, through MNCs and SMEs. Economist Choy's (2010) suggestion to promote "home-grown businesses catering to domestic demand" could be given further thought as an alternative to supporting a means of living for those with low skills. One shift away from employment-based assistance for low-income earners might be to provide more support to starting and sustaining small local businesses such as hawker stalls and retail stores. All in all, it remains to be seen how the policies will be adopted and, later on, how they will be implemented.

The second reason for the inadequacy of current social policies to help low-wage earners is that the focus might be too narrow, in terms of eligibility by income as well as by "dysfunction." For the former, stagnating of median wages puts many who do not meet the $1,500 earnings cutoff in economic hardship. For the latter, MCYS classifies families who need interim help such as WSP differently from dysfunctional families who need intensive help. However, the pilot survey results of WSP recipients indicate that individuals who have been placed in WSP also face multiple challenges that require assistance from multiple sources. As highlighted above, while WSP does provide case management for families with children, the case management might be focused more on mandating compliance than dealing with the social issues. As a program with the aim to support work, the emphasis on job placement might also insufficiently deal with the social issues that the multi-stressed model indicates that directly affect work effort.

Figuring out how effective the social policies and programs really are would require rigorous research. One would need a longitudinal study of the families before, during, and after the recession to answer this question. A longitudinal study of Work Support recipients is currently underway. Evaluation research of other policies and programs would provide a knowledge pool to tease out the effects of various programs individually or in accumulation and in response to different socioeconomic trends.

Conclusion

In conclusion, the policies in Singapore have probably helped to stave off poverty for many low-income households. However, as the economy picks up and government assistance shrinks back, the problems faced by multi-stressed low-earning families will be insufficiently addressed by the current slate of social policies. The problems faced by this population are structural and would only worsen as skill-biased globalized development continues its course. The challenges that this population struggle with are also social and interconnected in nature, calling for social and multisystemic solutions. The current economic-centric and growth-oriented policies will not only inadequately address the needs of this population but even contribute to exacerbating their condition. Lim (2009), for example, argues the case for "growth for people" instead of "people for growth" that lower growth might be necessary in order that growth is distributed among beneficiaries.

The Singapore government is keenly aware of the tensions in growth and social protection, and the recent ESC recommendations have acknowledged the need for inclusive growth. Without a doubt, there will be more investments to improve the social safety net and support for families in distress. The question would be how much more relative to investments in pursuing high growth. It remains to be seen how willing the Singapore government would be to forego the venerable aim of maintaining competitiveness and growth. With new questions like these coming up, good and rigorous research becomes key to understanding the social and economic impacts of socioeconomic trends and policies.

Acknowledgements We gratefully acknowledge the Ministry of Social and Family Development (previously the Ministry of Community Development, Youth and Sports) for their permission to report findings from the collaborative research of the Work Support Program and for their comments on the paper. We thank Helen Sim for research assistance and the Work Support Program research team (Alex Lee, Ngiam Tee Liang, and Nesam Tharmalingam) for their inputs. The opinions expressed in this paper are, however, our own and do not reflect the positions of the ministry or our research collaborators.

References

Central Provident Fund Board. (2009). *FAQs on Workfare Income Supplement Scheme (WIS).* http://mycpf.cpf.gov.sg/CPF/Templates/SubPage_Template.aspx?NRMODE=Published&NRORIGINALURL=%2fMembers%2fGen-Info%2fWIS%2fFAQs_WIS%2ehtm&NRNODEGUID=%7b0AFCD966-2976-44BA-ABB8-FF6084F17A72%7d&NRCACHEHINT=Guest#2. Accessed 19 Jan 2009.

Chia, S. A. (2010, February 8). More help on the way for low-wage workers. *The Straits Times.*

Choy, K. M. (2010, February 3). A blueprint for fundamental change. *Today.*

Conger, R. D., & Dogan, S. J. (2007). Social class and socialization in families. In J. E. Grusec & P. D. Hastings (Eds.), *Handbook of socialization: Theory and research* (pp. 433–460). New York: The Guilford Press.

Danziger, S. K., Corcoran, M., Danziger, S., Heflin, C., Kalil, A., Levine, J., Rosen, D., Seefeldt, K., Siefert, K., & Tolman, R. (2002). *Barriers to the employment of welfare recipients*. Ann Arbor: Population Studies Center, University of Michigan, http://www.psc.isr.umich.edu/pubs/pdf/rr02-508.pdf. Accessed 20 Jan 2011.

Department of Statistics Singapore. (2009). *Key household income trends, 2008*. http://www.singstat.gov.sg/pubn/papers/people/op-s15.pdf. Accessed 21 July 2009.

Department of Statistics Singapore. (2011). *Statistics: Time series on GDP at 2005 market prices and real economic growth*. http://www.singstat.gov.sg/stats/themes/economy/hist/gdp1.html. Accessed 20 Jan 2011.

Department of Workforce Development. (2001). *An evaluation: Wisconsin Works (W-2) Program*. Madison: Wisconsin Legislative Audit Bureau.

Economics Strategies Committee. (2010). *ESC recommendations*. http://www.esc.gov.sg/recommendation.html#esc1. Accessed 12 Feb 2010.

Forthofer, M. S., Markman, H. J., Cox, M., Stanley, S., & Kessler, R. C. (1996). Associations between marital distress and work loss in a national sample. *Journal of Marriage and Family, 58*(3), 597–605.

Freeman, R. B. (1999). The economics of crime. In O. C. Ashenfelter & D. Card (Eds.), *Handbook of labor economics* (pp. 3529–3571). Amsterdam: North Holland Publishers.

Hamilton, G., Freedman, S., Gennetian, L., Michalopoulos, C., Walter, J., Ciardullo-Adams, D., & Gassman-Pines, A. (2001). *National evaluation of welfare-to-work strategies*. US Department of Health and Human Services. http://aspe.hhs.gov/HSP/NEWWS/

Hoefer, R., & Midgley, J. (Eds.). (2006). *International perspectives on welfare to work policy*. New York: The Haworth Press.

Kessler, R. C., Andrews, G., Colpe, L. J., Hirippi, E., Mroczek, D. K., Normand, S.-L. T., Walters, E. E., & Zaslavsky, A. M. (2002). Short screening scales to monitor population prevalences and trends in non-specific psychological distress. *Psychological Medicine, 32*(6), 959–976.

Lareau, A. (2003). *Unequal childhoods: Class, race and family life*. Berkeley: University of California Press.

Lerman, R. I. (2002). *How do marriage, cohabitation and single parenthood affect the material hardships of families with children?* Washington, DC: Urban Institute and American University. http://www.urban.org/publications/410539.html. Accessed 20 Jan 2010.

Liebowitz, M. R. (1996). Generalized Anxiety Disorder (includes Overanxious Disorder of Childhood). In T. A. Widiger (Ed.), *DSM-IV Sourcebook* (2nd ed., Vol. 2, pp. 432–436). Washington, DC: American Psychiatric Association.

Lim, L. (2009). Singapore's economic growth model: Too much or too little? *Ethos* (6), 36–42. http://www.cscollege.gov.sg/cgl/pdf/ETHOS_IS06.pdf. Accessed 29 Jan 2010.

Lim, L. (2010, February 6). Opening a window to the future. *The Straits Times*.

Lochner, L. (2004). Education, work, and crime: A human capital approach. *International Economic Review, 45*(3), 811–843.

Lochner, L., & Moretti, E. (2004). The effects of education on crime: Evidence from prison inmates, arrests, and self-reports. *American Economic Review, 94*(1), 155–189.

Messner, S. F., Raffalovich, L. E., & McMillan, R. (2001). Economic deprivation and changes in homicide arrest rates for white and black youths, 1967–1998: A national time-series analysis. *Criminology, 39*(3), 591–614.

Ministry of Community Development, Youth and Sports. (2009a). *Addendum to President's Address*. http://app.mcys.gov.sg/web/corp_press_story.asp?szMod=corp&szSubMod=press&qid=4774. Accessed 29 Jan 2010.

Ministry of Community Development, Youth and Sports. (2009b). *Assurance and hope for needy: New measures to help dysfunctional families*. http://www.mcys.gov.sg/MCDSFiles/Press/Articles/05-2009.pdf. Accessed 29 Jan 2010.

Ministry of Community Development, Youth and Sports. (2009c, February 11). *Speech by Dr Vivian Balakrishnan, Minister, Ministry of Community Development, Youth and Sports at the FY 2009 Committee for Supply Debate*. http://www.mcys.gov.sg/MCDSFiles/Speeches/Articles/13-2009.pdf. Accessed 29 Jan 2010.

Ministry of Community Development, Youth and Sports. (2009d). *Singapore social statistics in brief 2008*. Singapore: Ministry of Community Development, Youth and Sports.
Ministry of Community Development, Youth and Sports. (2010a). *CCT: Comcare transitions*. http://www.mcys.gov.sg/web/serv_E_CCT.html. Accessed 3 Feb 2010.
Ministry of Community Development, Youth and Sports. (2010b). *Help and assistance: Work Support (WS) Scheme*. http://www.mcys.gov.sg/web/serv_E_WS.html. Accessed 29 Jan 2010.
Ministry of Finance. (2009). *Budget speech 2009*. http://www.mof.gov.sg/budget_2009/speech_toc/index.html. Accessed 29 Jan 2010.
Ng, I. Y. H. (2010). Globalized intentions in tension: The case of Singapore [Globalisation and indigenisation]. *International Social Work, 53*(5), 671–685. doi:10.1177/0020872810371202.
Ng, I. Y. H. (2013). Multistressed low-earning families in contemporary policy context: Lessons from Work Support recipients in Singapore. *Journal of Poverty, 17*(1), 86–109
Ng, I., Lee, A., Ngiam, T. L., Ho, K. W., & Nesamani, T. (2010). *Longitudinal study of families placed on longer term assistance under the Work Support Programme: Phase One Report*. Singapore: National University of Singapore.
Nightingale, D. S., & Mikelson, K. S. (2000). *An overview of research related to Wisconsin Works (W-2)*. Washington, DC: The Urban Institute. http://www.urban.org/UploadedPDF/wisc_works.pdf. Accessed date?
Page, B. I., & Simmons, J. R. (2000). *What government can do: Dealing with poverty and inequality*. London: University of Chicago Press.
Piliavin, I., Dworsky, A., & Courtney. M. E. (2003). *What happens to families under W-2 in Milwaukee County, Wisconsin? Report from Wave 2 of the Milwaukee TANF Applicant Study*. Chicago: Chapin Hall Center for Children, University of Chicago; Institute for research on poverty, University of Wisconsin. http://www.irp.wisc.edu/research/welreform/pdfs/w2milw-wav2.pdf. Accessed 9 Sept 2009.
Swartz, R. J., & Corbett, T. (2001). *W-2 achievements and challenges: An overview and interpretation of the white papers commissioned by the Department of Workforce Development*. Hudson Institute and the Institute for Research on Poverty. http://dcf.wi.gov/w2/pdf/whitepaper_overview.pdf. Accessed 9 Sept 2009.
Tan, K. G. (2009, January 25). Sticking to sound principles. *The Straits Times*.
Tan, E. K. B. (2010, February 6). For the prescription to work . . . mindset change and inclusive growth must be abiding commitments. *Today*, p. 6.
Voydanoff, P. (1990). Economic distress and family relations: A review of the eighties. *Journal of Marriage and Family, 52*(4), 1099–1115.
Yeoh, K. L. (2007). Rethinking a new social compact for Singapore. *ETHOS* (3), 7–12. http://www.cscollege.gov.sg/cgl/pdf/ETHOS_IS03.pdf. Accessed 29 January 2010.
Yeung, W. J., & Hofferth, S. L. (1998). Family adaptations to income and job loss in the U.S. *Journal of Family and Economic Issues, 19*(3), 255–283.

Chapter 15
Conclusion and Policy Implications

Mui Teng Yap

While the twenty-first century has been hailed by some as the Asian century, the region has, since the turn of the century, also seen its share of man-made and natural disasters, including financial crises, earthquakes, and tsunamis, and the consequent rise in commodity prices. While Asia, unlike the USA, recovered quickly from the most recent crisis of 2008 sparked off by the US housing crisis and the collapse of Lehman Brothers, it is now watching closely the unfolding of the Euro-zone crisis and its potential fallout on the region. The slow recovery in the USA and the slowdown of China are also potential triggers for further economic distress in the region. It does not help that natural disasters also appear to be occurring with increasing frequency in the region, impacting the lives and livelihoods of many.

The various contributors in this volume have pointed out the vital role of social safety nets for the protection of the vulnerable. At the macro level, while governments may be tempted or, indeed, forced to cut their budgets for welfare programs in times of economic stress, they should heed the suggestion of UNESCAP Executive Secretary Noeleen Heyzer that such expenditure be viewed as investment for the future. This is because of the long-term negative consequences that economic stress can have, particularly on children (see contributions by Thapa and Patel of UNICEF and by Duncan and Magnuson). This is particularly important as parents tend to disinvest in their children's education (see contribution by Wong) and even pull them out of school totally in times of economic crisis. Food and healthcare expenditure may also be cut, affecting child development. These have long-term implications for human capital development. Moreover, as Phua and Phua point out, the effects of economic stress on some aspects of population health may take time to emerge.

M.T. Yap (✉)
Institute of Policy Studies, Lee Kuan Yew School of Public Policy,
National University of Singapore, Singapore
e-mail: yap.muiteng@nus.edu.sg

W.J.J. Yeung and M.T. Yap (eds.), *Economic Stress, Human Capital, and Families in Asia: Research and Policy Challenges*, Quality of Life in Asia 4,
DOI 10.1007/978-94-007-7386-8_15,

Several contributors call for social protection not only for children but also for their parents (see contributions by Duncan and Magnuson and by Gatenio Gabel and Kamerman). Support should also be extended to the young adults at the age of family formation as it has been shown that, under conditions of economic stress and greater labor market competition, they are unable to achieve their desired family sizes (see contribution by Kim). In an ultra-low fertility society like Korea, this in turn has implications for their old-age care and security. Such situations are likely to apply to the other East Asian countries like China, Japan, Singapore, Taiwan, and Thailand which have undergone rapid fertility decline and ageing of the population and where there is strong emphasis on family care for the elderly. Apart from policies to improve labor market conditions, Kim also suggests that more pro-natalist assistance be given to the less well educated, given that they are the most affected in terms of their family size achievement.

In countries such as China which has a considerable proportion of elderly in spite of its developing country status (because of its sharp fertility decline over the last three decades), Yeung and Xu call for more safety nets for the elderly, which, they point out, would be very much needed as family sizes decline and more of the young migrate for job opportunities. In this regard, this contribution again calls into question the sustainability of the family care model which is highly popular among Asian governments.

Very often too, women become the victims of family violence and abuse at the hands of their husbands under conditions of unemployment and economic stress. While some may be able to escape such fate temporarily or permanently through migration (see contribution by Arnado), they often suffer in their destination countries and have no support when they return home. Support for these migrant women in both the destination and source countries are called for.

In an important contribution, Ng and Ho remind us that families are often stressed by multiple factors, of which economic crisis may only be one aspect. Thus, they call for safety nets that also look after the long-term needs of such families and not just needs due to financial crisis.

Should the task of social protection be left to governments and policy makers alone? The contribution on the Wenchuan earthquake shows the importance of social networks in delivering support, especially in emergencies. A "many helping hands" approach, involving self-help as well as help by the community, the government, and even international agencies, seems to be suggested as most effective. Local communities may be able to respond to emergencies more rapidly because they are closer to the ground and, for this reason, are also more knowledgeable about the needs. Likewise, Heyzer also calls for the use of traditional knowledge available in rural communities.

Wong's contribution on migrant mainland Chinese families and their children in Hong Kong also shows that the social support and human capital investment for children can be adversely affected during economic hard times. In this regard, he welcomes the Hong Kong government's Community Investment and Inclusion Fund set up in 2002 to promote the development of mutually supportive communities, including migrants. This is an example where governments, which are usually better-resourced, complement the efforts of the community.

Finally, in a highly interconnected world where economic distress in one nation or region can spread rapidly to another, it behooves the better off in the international community to come together to support the less well-off, developing economies in caring for the vulnerable in their midst.

Contributors in this volume also point out the importance of research, particularly longitudinal research (see, e.g., contributions by Duncan and Magnuson, Thanakwang, and Yeung and Xu). In this regard, academia could play its part by providing the evidence base for appropriate policies and programs to be introduced and implemented. As Tang and Midgley (2010) point out, while East Asian governments have been critical of "Western 'welfare statism'," they are now more open to expanding welfare spending given the global economic situation since 2008. In this regard, they would be "receptive to research that shows which policy interventions are the most effective" (p. 14).

Be that as it may, it would not be possible to recommend a single welfare model that would be universally applicable or transferable across the region. Each system has its strengths and weaknesses, and each country will have to decide how to deal with its vulnerable population, which will also depend on its culture and resources. To quote White and Goodman (1998: 14), writing on whether there is a distinctive East Asian welfare model, despite common elements, "the evolution of each country's welfare system has its own distinctive trajectory and they differ today in consequences."

References

Tang, K.-l., & Midgley, J. (2010). Introduction: Poverty and social policy responses in East Asia. In J. Midgley & K.-l. Tang (Eds.), *Social policy and poverty in East Asia; the role of social security* (pp. 3–15). London: Routledge.

White, G., & Goodman, R. (1998). Welfare orientalism and the search for an East Asian welfare model. In R. Goodman, G. White, & H.-j. Kwon (Eds.), *Welfare orientalism and the search for an East Asian welfare model* (pp. 3–24). London: Routledge.

References

Index

W.J.J. Yeung and M.T. Yap (eds.), *Economic Stress, Human Capital, and Families in Asia: Research and Policy Challenges*, Quality of Life in Asia 4, DOI 10.1007/978-94-007-7386-8, © Springer Science+Business Media Dordrecht 2013

N

O

P

MIX
Papier aus verantwortungsvollen Quellen
Paper from responsible sources
FSC® C105338

If you have any concerns about our products,
you can contact us on
ProductSafety@springernature.com

In case Publisher is established outside the EU,
the EU authorized representative is:
Springer Nature Customer Service Center GmbH
Europaplatz 3, 69115 Heidelberg, Germany

Printed by Libri Plureos GmbH
in Hamburg, Germany